Advances in Hepatology
http://dx.doi.org/10.5772/intechopen.91512
Edited by Luis Rodrigo, Ian Martins, Xiaozhong Guo and Xingshun Qi

Contributors
Syed Manzoor Kadri, Marija Petković, Anja Geerts, Sander Lefere, Simona Claudia Cambrea, Elena Dumea, Bouchra Kitab, Michinori Kohara, Kyoko Tsukiyama-Kohara, Waleed Al-Hamoudi, Saad Alghamdi, Laura Iliescu, Alberto Frosi, Eira Cerda, Saraid Cerda-Reyes, Graciela Elia Castro-Narro, Perla Flores-Rangel, Alicia Sarahi Ojeda-Yuren, Julian Torres-Vázquez, Maria Del Rosario Herrero-Maceda, Martín Uriel Vázquez-Medina, Yailin Fabiola Velásquez-Palacios, Arshpal Gill, Ruby Sangha, Rachelle Hamadi, Dhineshreddy Gurala, Zeeshan Zia, Ra'ed Nassar, Suzanne El-Sayegh, Abureesh Mohammed, Rebeca Pérez-Cabeza De Vaca, Tomás Cortés Espinoza, Balasubramaniyan Vairappan, Juan Antonio Suárez Cuenca, Paul Mondragón Terán, Diana Selene Morgan Penagos, Chrisitan Navarro Gerrard, Brenda Maldonado Arriaga, Victoria Chagoya De Sanchez, Cuauhtemoc Licona Cassani, Anıl Delik, Yakup Ülger, Hassan M. Heshmati, Halyna Kuznietsova, Olexandr Ogloblya, Talari Praveen

First published in London, United Kingdom, 2021 by IntechOpen
IntechOpen is the global imprint of INTECHOPEN LIMITED, registered in England and Wales, registration number: 11086078, 5 Princes Gate Court, London, SW7 2QJ, United Kingdom
Printed in Croatia

British Library Cataloguing-in-Publication Data
A catalogue record for this book is available from the British Library

Additional hard and PDF copies can be obtained from orders@intechopen.com

Advances in Hepatology
Edited by Luis Rodrigo, Ian Martins, Xiaozhong Guo and Xingshun Qi
p. cm.
Print ISBN 978-1-83968-623-8
Online ISBN 978-1-83968-624-5
eBook (PDF) ISBN 978-1-83968-625-2

For EU product safety concerns:
IN TECH d.o.o., Prolaz Marije Krucifikse Kozulić 3, 51000 Rijeka, Croatia, info@intechopen.com or visit our website at intechopen.com.

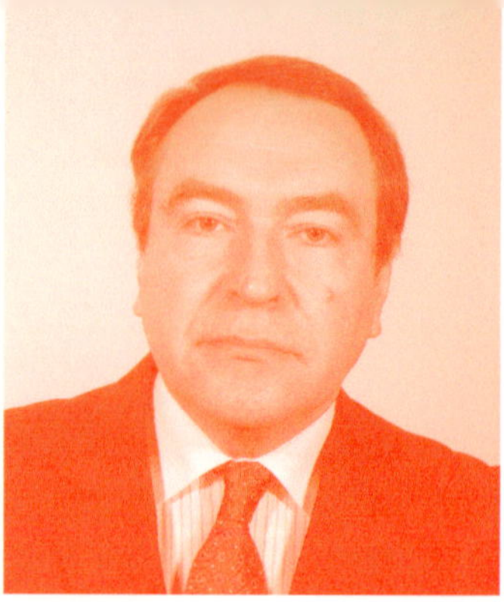
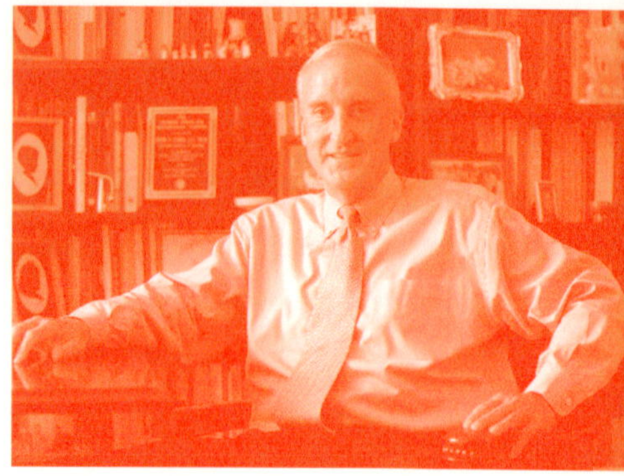
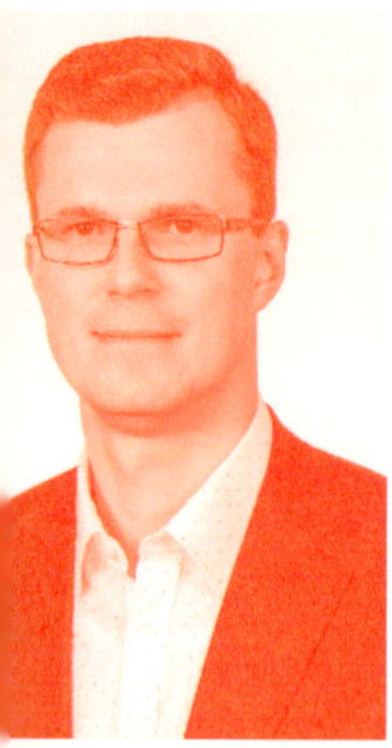
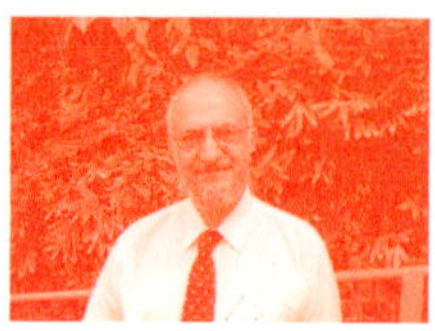
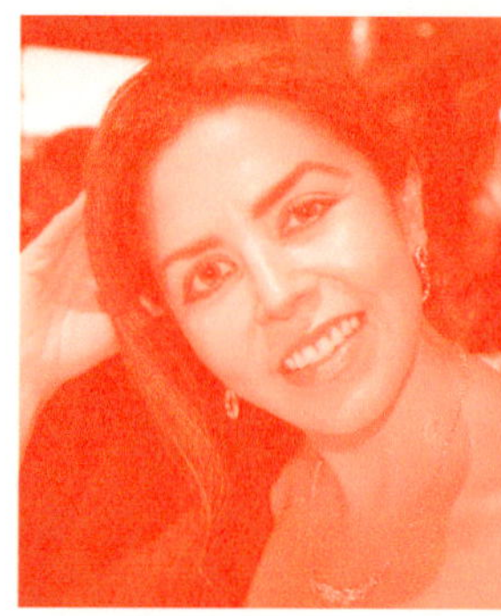

Supporting open minds since 2005

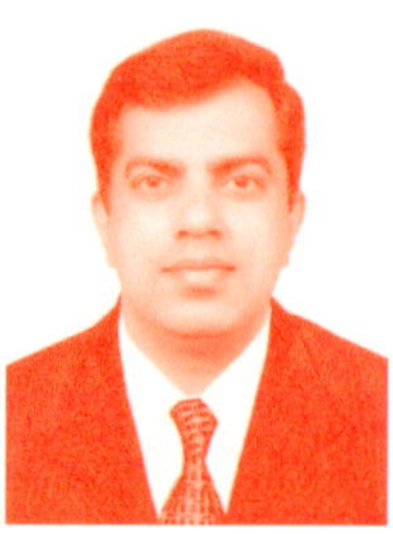
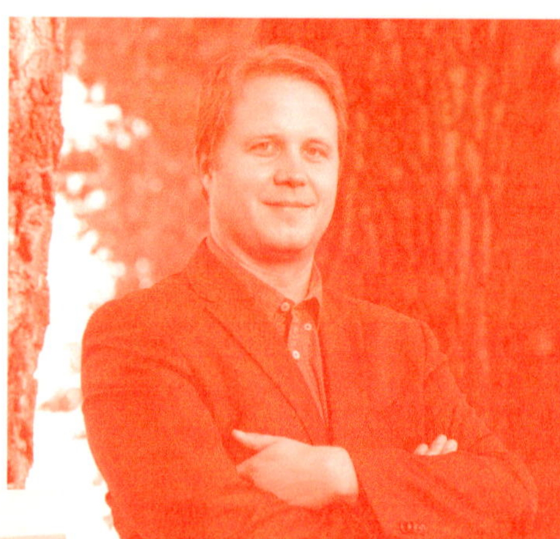
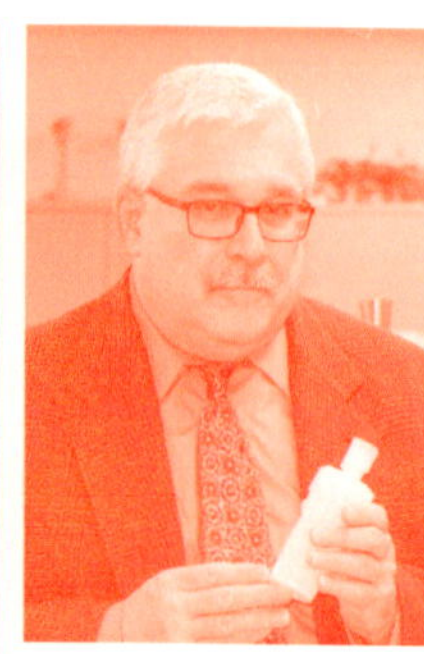
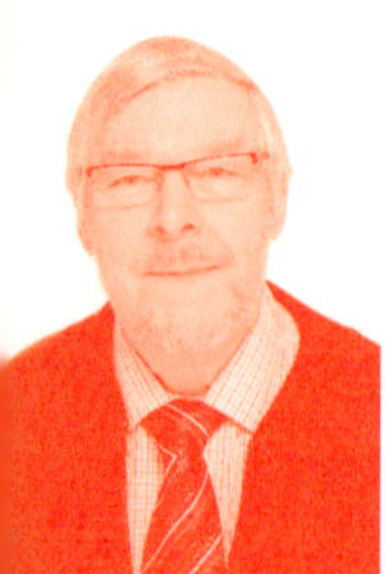
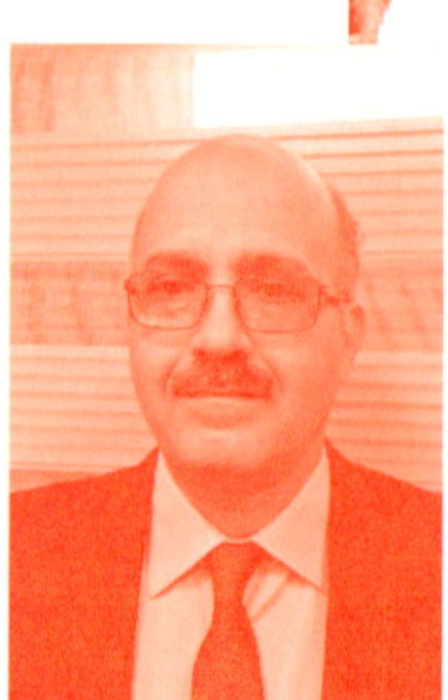
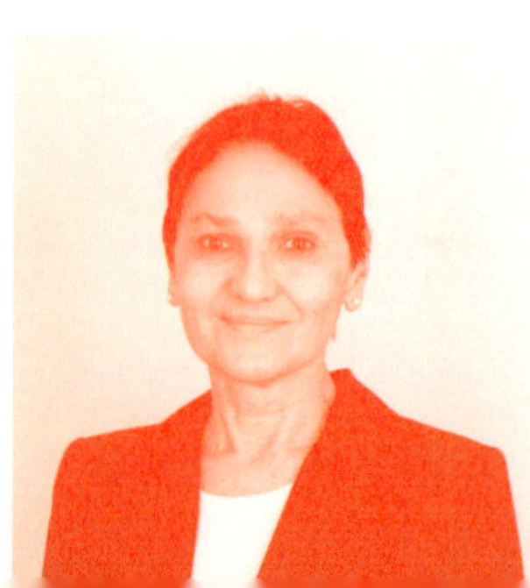
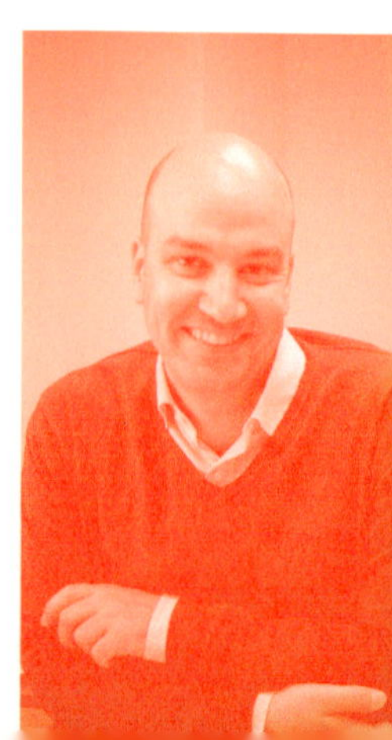

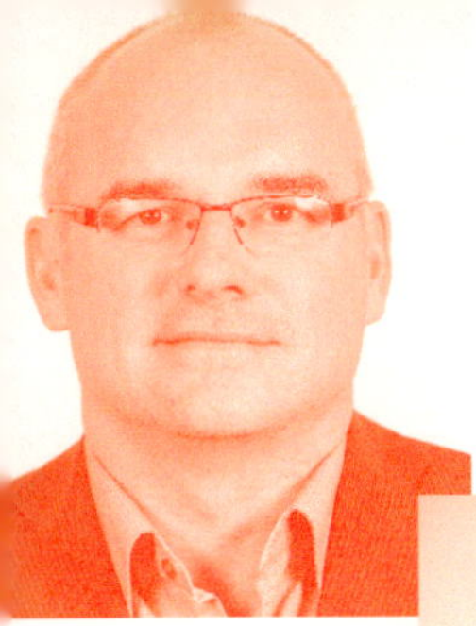
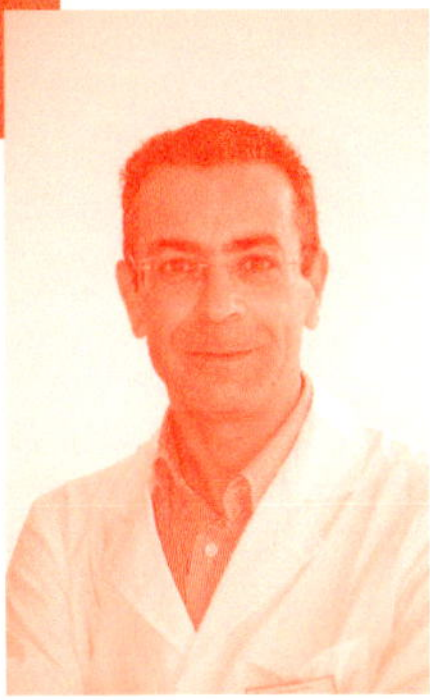
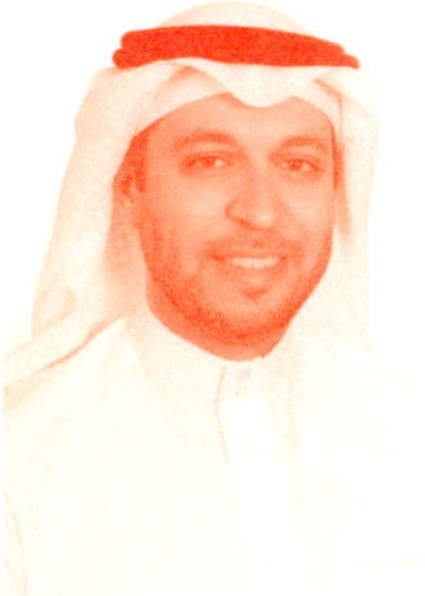
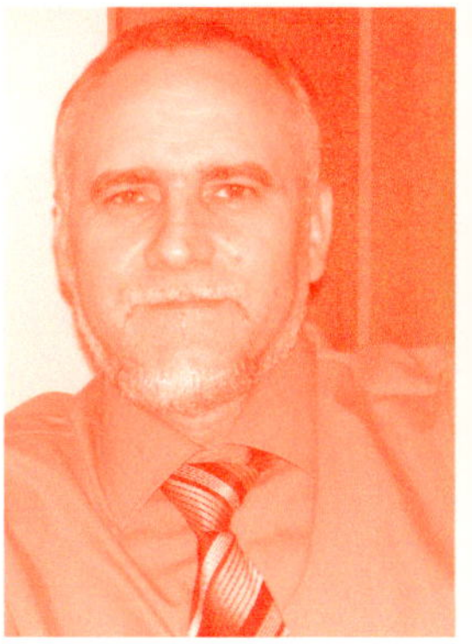
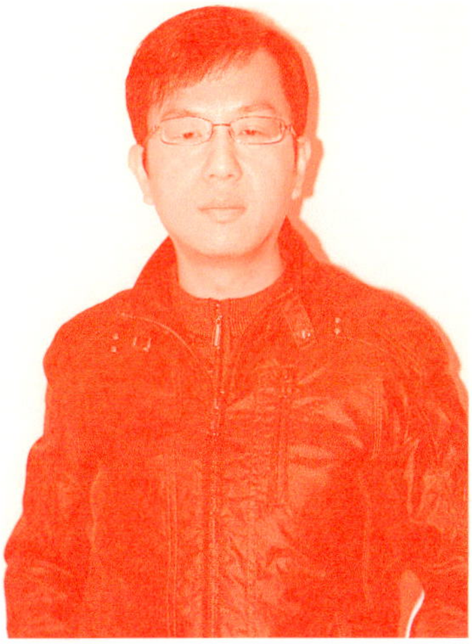
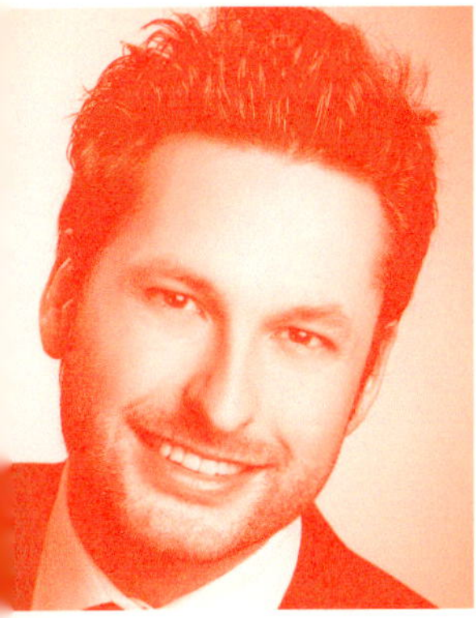
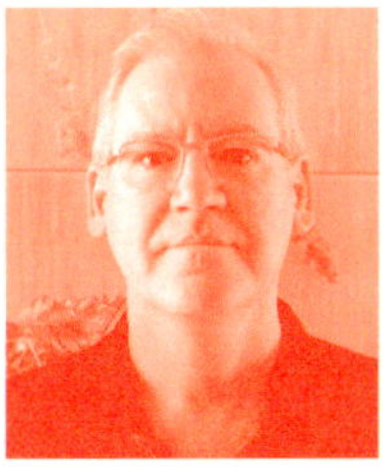

IntechOpen

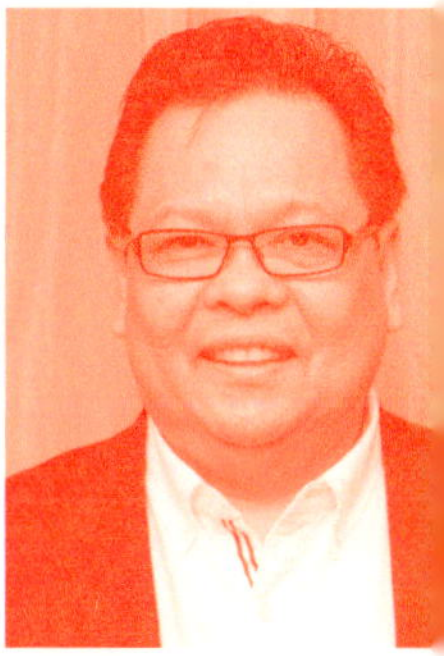
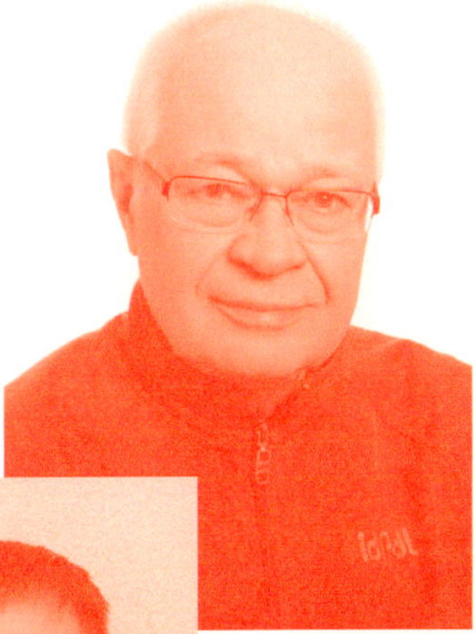
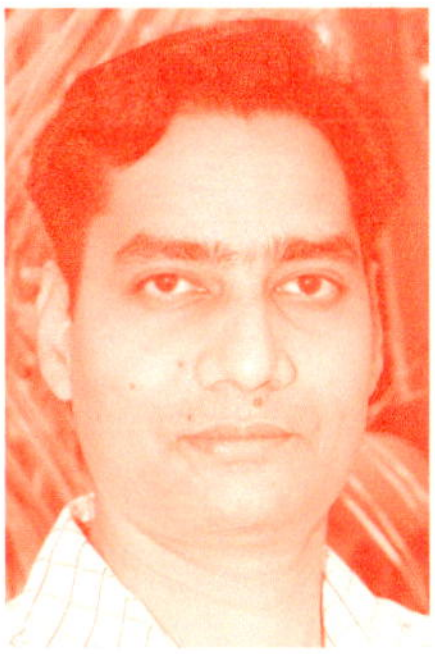
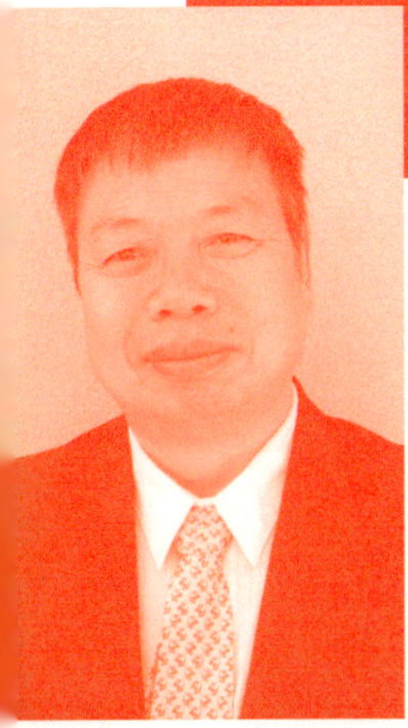
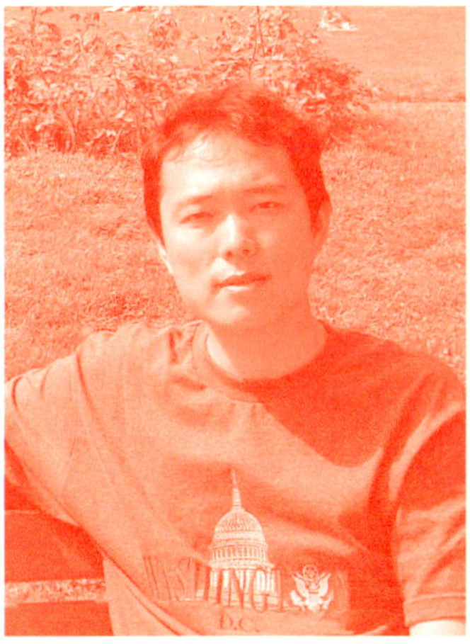
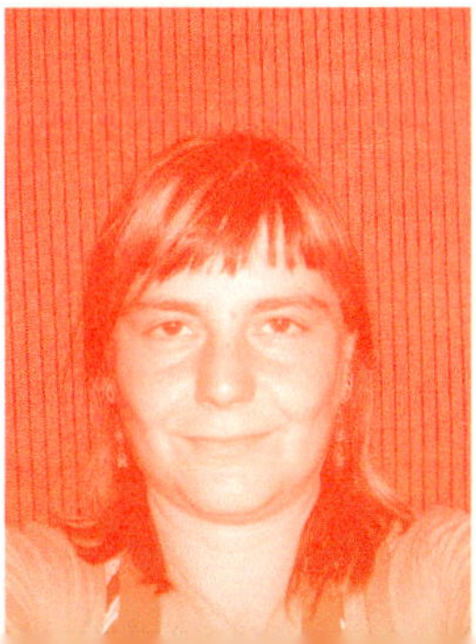

Advances in Hepatology

*Edited by Luis Rodrigo, Ian Martins,
Xiaozhong Guo and Xingshun Qi*

Published in London, United Kingdom

Meet the editors

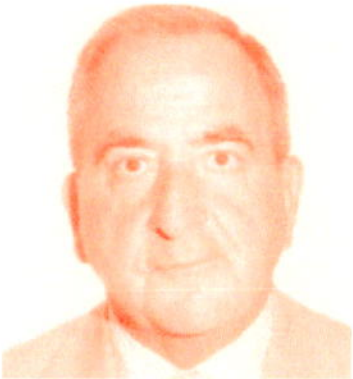

Dr. Luis Rodrigo, MD, is an Emeritus Professor of Medicine at the University of Oviedo, Spain. He has been the chief of Gastroenterology Service at the HUCA Hospital in Oviedo for more than forty years. He obtained a Ph.D. in 1975 and since then has developed a long career in teaching and research. He has published 707 scientific papers, 425 written in English and 282 in Spanish. He has participated as the main investigator in forty-five clinical trials and has directed forty doctoral theses. He has contributed actively to the formation of about 100 specialists in gastroenterology working in his hospital and other centers in Spain and abroad. He has written around thirty-five chapters in books and edited twenty-four books in gastroenterology and hepatology. His areas of interest are celiac disease and autoimmune-associated diseases.

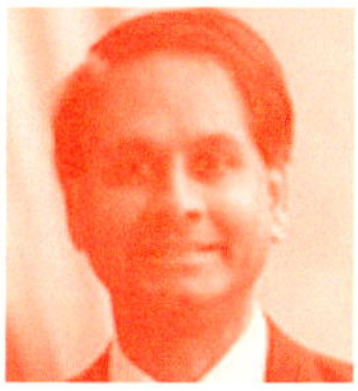

Dr. Ian James Martins is an editor and reviewer for Open Acess Pub/MDPI journals, *Frontiers* and *Scientific Reports* (Nature) and various other international journals. He is also an advisory board member for *Photon Journal* and a member of the BIT Congress. Dr. Martins is a 2021 Distinguished Scientist (International Scientist Awards on Engineering, Science and Medicine, Pondicherry Awards). He was also recognized as a top peer reviewer by the Global Peer Review Awards in 2019,.PUBLONS, RANKING TOP 1% in the field, 22 Essential Science Indicators research fields. BIT Member (BIT Congress. Inc) with an *h-index* of 132, citations have accumulated to >15,474 in the past 27 years. INTERNATIONAL CERTIFICATES from journals, conferences, congresses and summits. RESEARCH GATE ANALYSIS: RG score (> 97.5%) of international SCIENTISTS. ORCID CONNECTING RESEARCHER: Editorial Team www.macrothink.org/journal/index.php/jfs/about/editorialTeamBio/13511. Editorial Team. Ian James Martins. · http://orcid.org/0000-0002-2390-1501.

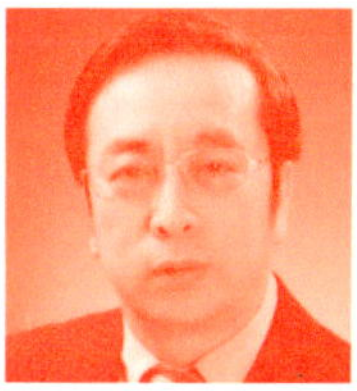

Prof. Xiaozhong Guo is the director of the Department of Gastroenterology, General Hospital of Northern Theater Command (formerly General Hospital of Shenyang Military Area). He has practiced in the field of digestive diseases and digestive endoscopy for more than thirty years. His major achievements include experimental and clinical research on the management of pancreatic diseases, especially pancreatic cancer, and stem cells for digestive diseases, such as liver cirrhosis and ulcerative colitis. He has published more than 500 papers and edited more than ten books. He has received six funds from the National Natural Science Foundation of China. He received first prizes from the Natural Science and Science and Technology Progress Awards of Liaoning Province.

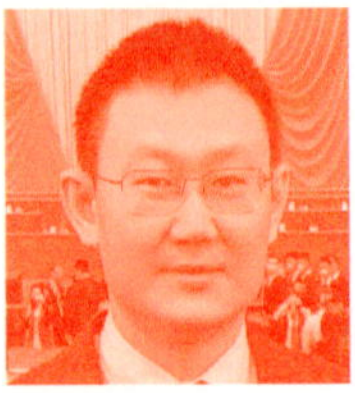

Dr. Xingshun Qi obtained his medical doctoral degree at the Fourth Military Medical University, China, and completed his post-doctoral fellowship at the General Hospital of Shenyang Military Region. Currently, he is a deputy director at the Department of Gastroenterology, General Hospital of Northern Theater Command (formerly General Hospital of Shenyang Military Region). His research interests include the etiology, diagnosis, and management of liver cirrhosis, portal hypertension (especially portal vein thrombosis and Budd-Chiari syndrome), and hepatocellular carcinoma. He serves as an associate editor of *BMC Gastroenterology*, an academic editor of the *Canadian Journal of Gastroenterology and Hepatology*, and an academic editor of *Frontiers in Medicine*. His H-index is 37 with 4546 citations.

Contents

Preface

Advances in Hepatology presents new achievements in the clinical management of chronic liver disease patients, including effective treatments for chronic infection mainly related to the hepatitis C virus (HCV). It examines the relationship between obesity and liver diseases such as nonalcoholic fatty liver disease (NAFLD) and nonalcoholic steatohepatitis (NASH). To prevent and treat deleterious liver effects, bariatric surgery may be indicated in selected patients, which the book also discusses.

The development of direct-acting antiviral (DAA) agents for the treatment of HCV infection has completely transformed the management of this disease in the last decade. The advantages of using DAA therapies include high efficacy (sustained virological response (SVR) rate > 95%) with minimal side effects, good tolerability, easy drug administration (once-daily oral dosing), and short duration of treatment (8–12 weeks).

Hepatitis C is a high-prevalence disease, representing a global impact health problem. Lately, many changes have been made in treatment guidelines because of the commercialization of second-generation DAAs due to their high effectiveness, few side effects, and pangenotypic action.

In one recently published study (Liver Int. 2021;41: 456-73) using a mathematical program, the authors evaluated the possibilities of the complete elimination of HCV from the world by the end of 2030, as defined by the World Health Organization (WHO), considering that is attainable with the availability of highly efficacious therapies. This study reports progress made in the timing of HCV elimination in forty-five high-income countries between 2017 and 2019.

Disease progression models of HCV infection for each country were updated with the latest data on chronic HCV prevalence and annual diagnosis and treatment levels, assumed to remain constant in the future. Modeled outcomes were analyzed to determine the year in which each country would meet the WHO 2030 elimination targets.

Of the forty-five countries studied, eleven (Australia, Canada, France, Germany, Iceland, Italy, Japan, Spain, Sweden, Switzerland, and United Kingdom) are on track to meet the WHO's elimination targets by 2030; five countries (Austria, Malta, Netherlands, New Zealand, and South Korea) by 2040; and two (Saudi Arabia and Taiwan) by 2050. The remaining twenty-seven countries are not expected to achieve this elimination before 2050. Compared to progress in 2017, South Korea is no longer on track to eliminate HCV by 2030, three countries (Canada, Germany, and Sweden) are now on track, and most countries (thirty in total) saw no change.

The authors conclude that assuming high-income countries will maintain current levels of diagnosis and treatment, only 24% are on track to eliminate HCV by 2030, and 60% are off track by at least twenty years. If current levels of diagnosis and treatment continue falling, achieving the WHO's 2030 targets will be more challenging. With less than ten years remaining, screening and treatment expansion is crucial.

In relation to benefits obtained in the treatment of hepatocellular carcinoma (HCC) patients with DAA agents, the current opinion is that the risk may persist up to ten years after obtaining an effective sustained viral response (SVR) with complete disappearance of this virus from the human body because HCV infection appears to leave behind an epigenetic scar, inducing carcinogenesis.

The discrepancy between the number of potentially available kidneys and the number of patients listed for kidney transplant continues to widen all over the world. Transplantation of kidneys from HCV-infected donors into HCV-naïve recipients has increased recently because of persistent kidney shortage and the availability of DAA agents. This strategy has the potential to reduce waiting times for transplants as well as the risk of mortality in dialysis.

The many possibilities of eliminating HCV infection with different types of treatment and the expectation of new vaccines in the near future have the potential to cure this chronic viral infection in different settings and circumstances with possible eradication in the future.

Luis Rodrigo MD
Professor,
School of Medicine,
University of Oviedo,
Oviedo, Asturias, Spain

Ian Martins
Independent Scientist,
Australia

Xiaozhong Guo and Xingshun Qi
General Hospital of Northern Theater Command,
China

Section 1

Discovery of Hepatitis C Virus

Chapter 1

Discovery of Hepatitis C Virus: Nobel Prize in Physiology and Medicine 2020

Talari Praveen

Abstract

Scientists were successful in discovering Hepatitis A and B, but there is another virus which has a long incubation period, many people are asymptomatic and cause adverse effects. Three scientists Harvey J Alter, Michael Houghton and Charles M Rice who have contributed their work in discovering a non-A, non-B hepatitis virus called Hepatitis C. Hepatitis is a disorder associated with the functioning hepatic cells in the liver. The person infected with Hepatitis C will have poor functioning of liver, vomiting, fatigue, jaundice and appetite. In this paper, I am going to explain about the Hepatitis C virus, and the work was done by three scientists and various research around it.

Keywords: Hepatitis C, Post-transfusion, non-A non-B hepatitis, Gene expression, Antigen antibody reaction

1. Introduction

Hepatitis C virus is a blood-borne pathogen. The person infected with this virus has defects in the functioning of the liver and blood. The progress of the virus in the human body is slow acting. The incubation period varies from person to person, it is about 2–3 months [1]. Hepatitis C is associated with chronic hepatitis which means inflammation of the liver and may also lead to liver failure sometimes cancer called Hepatocellular carcinoma [2]. According to the World Health Organization, it was estimated that there are about 70 million of the total world population infected with the Hepatitis C virus [3, 4]. If the treatment is delayed, the disease will progress and cause liver cirrhosis and hepatocellular carcinoma [5]. Hepatitis C is causing 400 000 deaths annually [4].

2. Discovery of hepatitis A and B

In 400 B.C., Hippocrates called hepatitis infection as 'Epidemic Jaundice' and told that "The bile contained in the liver is full of phlegm and blood, and erupts.. Such an eruption, the patient soon raves, becomes angry, talks nonsense and barks like a dog" [6]. During the second world war, the infection to the liver was thought of infection by several viruses and called it 'Viral Hepatitis'. After that, in 1947,

British hepatologist F.O. MacCallum has classified viral hepatitis into Hepatitis A which is Epidemic hepatitis and Hepatitis B which is serum hepatitis [7].

Baruch Blumberg (1925–2011) was a geneticist at National Institute of Health in Bethesda who is working on human disease susceptibility. He collected blood samples of people from many places in the world to study inherited diseases and susceptibility [7]. He found an unfamiliar reaction taking place in the serum of a hemophilic patient who needs blood and an Australian aborigine who is a donor. He initially thought that he discovered a new lipoprotein. After that, in the serum of a hemophilic patient, he could find detection of a new antigen, he called that as 'Australian-antigen' [7, 8]. In 1967, Blumberg linked the Australian-antigen with viral hepatitis, and in 1968, Alfred Price used Immuno-electrophoretic technique to explain that serum antigen that Blumberg discovered was related to hepatitis and called it as Serum hepatitis antigen. Later, both Australian-antigen and Serum hepatitis antigen were confirmed that these are viral particles. Blumberg performed several serological tests using chimpanzees to confirm the antigens are of Hepatitis B virus. In 1976, Blumberg got Nobel Prize Physiology and Medicine [9]. At that time, it was impossible to identify who are carriers of diseases and who are healthy donors, the effect of disease on a person is silent and progressive [4].

3. Discovery of hepatitis C

3.1 Harvey J Alter

Along with Blumberg, there is another person who also contributed his work in discovering Hepatitis B is Harvey J Alter. Alter also worked at National Institute of Health in Bethesda [10]. In the 1970s, people started studying the relationship between blood donors infected with Hepatitis B and post-transfusion hepatitis [8]. While they were studying about this, Alter found out that, though Hepatitis B positive donors prevented from donating blood, he found that blood transfused people were still infected with other 'Hepatitis related infections' [11]. Alter came across a patient who had a mild form of the disease and later that patient had Hepatitis associated diseases after a long incubation period. Based on this, he proposed that there may be two different viruses causing 'post-transfusion hepatitis' [11]. In 1975, Feinstone, Purcell and other scientists tested patients who are non-B hepatitis and found that Hepatitis A is not causing the disorders [12, 13].

The blood transfusion of non-B hepatitis was spreading to more numbers of people. They were sure the infection was not because of Hepatitis A or B, then came up with a term called 'non-A, non-B hepatitis' (NANBH) [12, 13]. Alter and his colleagues were clear that NANBH is responsible for post-transfusion hepatitis, but they were unable to show what NANBH is? Since there is no tool to diagnose NANBH, many people got affected by blood transfusion. The only animal model which is susceptible to NANBH is chimpanzees, Tabor et al. [14] have infected chimpanzees to study the hepatocyte infection and agents causing the disease. They have taken plasma from NANBH people and infected chimpanzees, and they found cirrhosis and hepatocellular carcinoma disorders in animal [4]. After several experiments, Alter and his colleagues found that NANBH has essential lipids which are enveloped around the virus which are different from Hepatitis B [15, 16]. Alter did not give conclusive results to state the causative agent is causing post-transfusion hepatitis.

3.2 Michael Houghton

In 1982, Houghton worked at Chiron Corporation and came up with molecular methods called cDNA library. Houghton and his colleagues infected chimpanzees with NANDH virus and have taken plasma from them, that plasma they have centrifuged to get a pellet of virus and they have extracted the nucleic acid from it. They have denatured the nucleic acid because they do not know whether it is DNA or RNA. After denature, they synthesized the cDNA [17]. They transduced the cDNA to a bacterial vector using a bacteriophage λ gt11 strain, the method is called transduction [18]. The bacterial vector undergoes translation to display cDNA-encoded polypeptides. They also looked for whether similar antigen that is expressed in the serum of NANBH patients by using screening techniques. If an antigen is found in the body, the immune system will generate antibodies against it. They have considered those patients as sources of viral antibodies, they have taken plasma by centrifuging blood of NANBH patients [18]. The bacterial vector has expressed the cDNA proteins, and by introducing plasma of the patient to the bacterial colony, the antibodies in the plasma will bind to polypeptides of bacteria [4]. Based on this idea of Molecular Biology and Immunology, they performed several screenings of the above experiment about 10^6 and found there is one colony that did not match human or chimpanzee DNA sequence, it matched with the sequence of a virus family called Flaviviridae [4]. They named it as cDNA clone 5–1-1 and named it as Hepatitis C virus (**Figure 1**) [17–20].

Houghton and his colleagues have immediately taken this knowledge further. They have collected suspected blood samples from Alter and performed the above experiment on those samples. They found all the blood samples they have tested are positive Hepatitis C. Using this diagnostic technique, donors were tested blood samples before transfusion which decreased the number of hepatitis cases [4]. But, Houghton has not evidently proved that Hepatitis C is only the causative agent or a mix of viruses causing disorder?

3.3 Charles M Rice

To find out what is actually causing chronic liver cirrhosis, two scientists Kunitada Shimontohno and Charles Rice came up with a new experiment. Blight and Rice [21], they have sequenced the viral genome and found that it is positive RNA strand about 96000 nucleotides, the RNA undergoes direct translation to form proteins, the primary transcription process is eliminated. The viral genome is a long

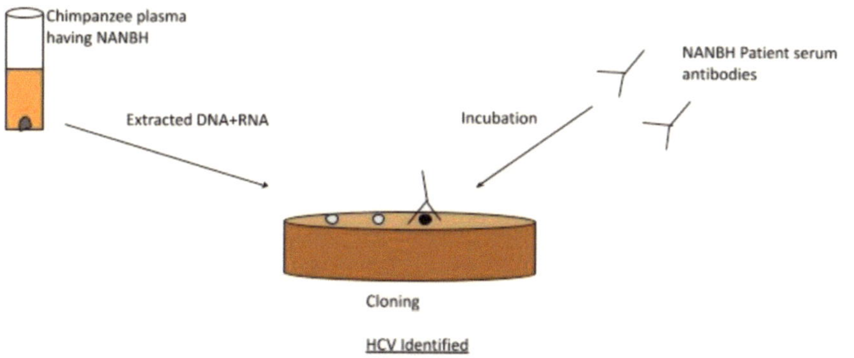

Figure 1.
Summary of Houghton work.

open reading frame (ORF), different types of proteins are translated from one ORF which has several translation initiation and termination codons [21].

They have found that there is a non-coding region at the 3'and 5′ ends of the viral RNA genome which is responsible for replication of the virus [21, 22]. Kolykhalov et al. [23] have constructed a viral genome which has conserved 3′ region at 5′ nontranslated region (5' NTR) and rest in long ORF (**Figure 2**). That genome gene they have injected to the chimpanzee liver to check the viral replication, but unfortunately the experiment failed, they did not find new viruses in the blood. While finding reasons for failure of experiment, they came across that during replication, mutations are common in the viral genome. To eliminate the mutations, they have engineered a few new sequences with silent markers. With all new sequences, they have created a new repaired conserved 3′ region (**Figure 3**) [4, 23, 24]. They repeated the above experiment with a newly engineered genome and the experiment worked resulting in chimpanzees having liver cirrhosis and hepatocellular carcinoma. Based on this, Rice gave the conclusion that only Hepatitis C virus alone causes hepatitis, there no other causative agent involved.

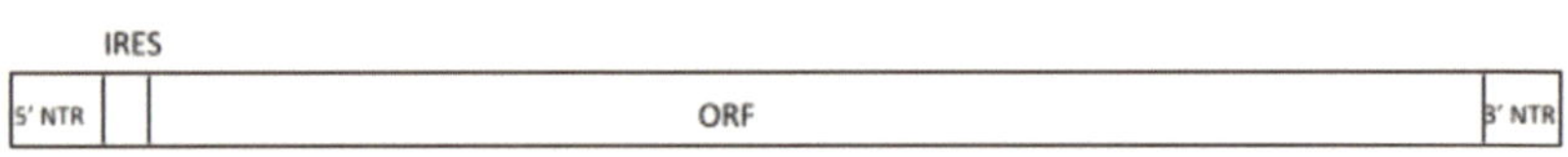

Figure 2.
Viral genome with conserved 3' region.

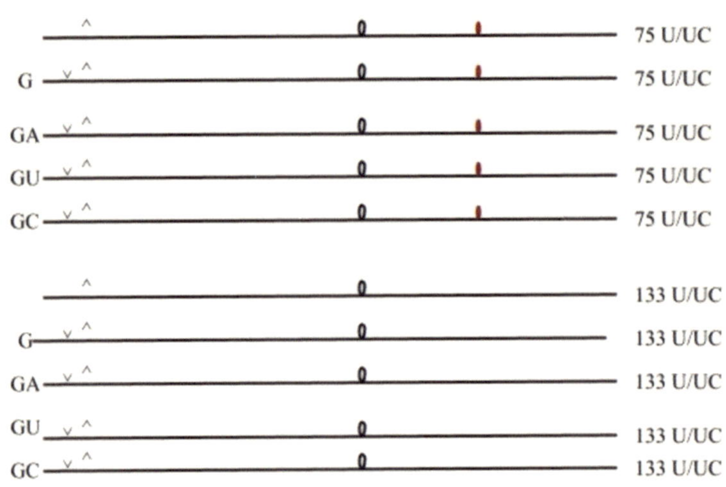

Figure 3.
Repaired conserved 3' region Genomes [23].

4. Mode of infection and diseases

Virus Type	Family	Genetic material	Disorders	Disorders
Hepatitis A	Picornaviridae	RNA	Contaminated food and water	Abdominal pain, nausea, fatigue
Hepatitis B	Hepadna	DNA	Blood transfusion	Liver failure, jaundice
Hepatitis C	Flaviviridae	RNA	Blood transfusion	Inflammation of liver and hepatocellular carcinoma

5. Molecular mechanisms of replication

Structure of Virus: Hepatitis C is a single-stranded RNA virus belonging to the family of Flaviviridae and there are seven genotypes (gt 1–7) and 67 subtypes which states genetic diversity is high [5]. The size of the virus is about 56–65 nm in diameter and the viral core about 45 nm. In the viral envelope, there are viral spikes which are formed by E1 and E2 glycoprotein heterodimers. Viral membranes consist of several lipoproteins those are low-density lipoprotein (LDL), very-low-density lipoprotein (VLDL) and apolipoproteins (Apo) which are A1, B, C (**Figure 4**) [5].

Viral Genome: As described above, viral genomes contain 96000 nucleotides and one ORF with the coding region of 3010 to 3033 nucleotides and 5′ and 3′ ends have non-translational (NTR) regions. The translation of viral RNA takes place in the endoplasmic reticulum of hepatic cells in the liver which is initiated by the IRES region which is adjacent to 5’NTR (**Figure 3**). The translation results in the formation of three structural proteins which are core, E1 and E2 and seven non-structural proteins which are p7, NS2, NS3, NS4A, NS4B, NS5A, NS5B. The structural proteins form viral components and non-structural proteins regulate viral growth and replication (**Figure 5**) [5].

Viral Cycle: When a person has blood transfusion from the Hepatitis C infected person, the virus reaches to the liver cell and binds to the lipoviral receptor proteins and the whole virus is engulfed into the cell by a process called clathrin-mediated endocytosis. The virus reaches the endoplasmic reticulum and releases its RNA. The ORF of RNA is translated to form structural and non-structural proteins.

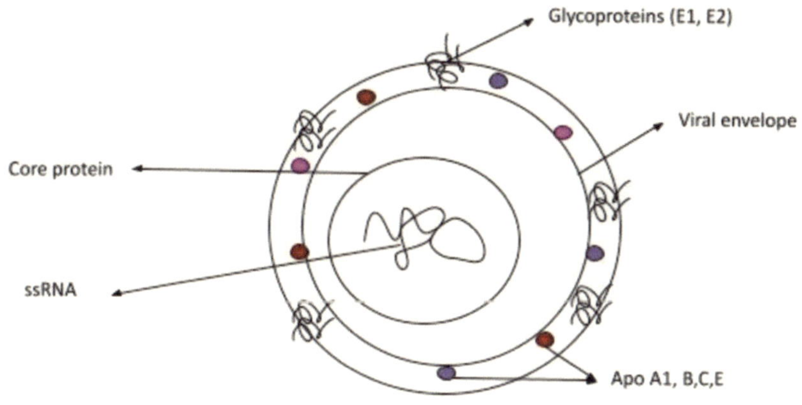

Figure 4.
Structure of hepatitis C .

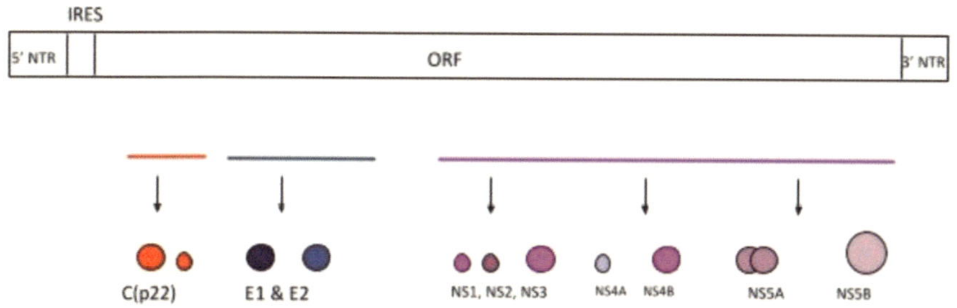

Figure 5.
Viral genome expression [5].

As I mentioned, the structural proteins form viral components and non-structural proteins regulate viral growth and replication using cellular components. The viral components and replicated RNA fragments reach the Golgi apparatus and unite to form mature viruses. The formed viruses enter the blood by bursting the liver cell. One single entry produces millions of viruses that cause liver dysfunction by bursting hepatic cells [5].

6. Research: a way to discovery of vaccine

Phosphatidylinositol 4-kinase III α (PI4KA) is a hepatic cellular protein which converts phosphatidylinositol to phosphatidylinositol 4-phosphate (PI4P) [25]. This protein has several roles in the viral replication and growth in an infected cell. PI4KA interacts with structural proteins in shaping the virus and also interaction with the non-structural protein of NS5B will accumulate the essential cellular material for viral growth [26]. When the Phosphatidylinositol 4-kinase III?? is knocked down, the replication and production of viral components are affected. Harak et al. [26] have done an in-vitro gene knockdown method to inhibit viral growth. Sarhan et al. [27] have also done similar experiments. They found other proteins called GSK3 α and β interacting with viral NS5A. The GSK3 α and β phosphorylates the NS5A. The phosphorylation of NS5A results in multiple functions such as viral maturation and release. If the GSK3 α and β genes are knocked down, the viral maturation and release is inhibited [27].

When any foreign particles enter the body, our immune system will identify that antigen. The human immune system has B cells, T cells and Natural killer cells play essential roles in detecting antigens. Hepatitis C virus has E2 glycoprotein in the core. CD81 markers which are present on B-cells will interact with E2 glycoprotein [28]. The binding of E2 and CD81, B-cells release serum antibodies to neutralize the viral activity. Research around Molecular Biology and Immunology will increase the chances of discovering the vaccine. Research is the stepping stone to discovering new things in science.

7. Diagnosis and treatment

When Hepatitis C is infected, the majority of the people are asymptomatic. The incubation period varies from person to person. In order to detect the virus, there are diagnostic tests to be performed. There are two ways to direct the virus, one is an indirect method based on antibodies production and direct method based on viral detection. In the indirect method, a person's blood sample will be taken which consist of serum, blood and plasma. To that blood, recombinant viral proteins core, NS3 and NS4 antigen are added. Along with recombinant proteins, colloidal gold labeled protein A is added. If the antibodies bind to antigens, the recombinant protein generates reddish-purple lines. This screening test will reveal that antibodies are present. To confirm the person infected with Hepatitis C, Recombinant Immunoblot Assay (RIBA) is antibody specific test which will direct anti-hepatitis C antibodies [29]. In the direct method diagnosis, Reverse-transcriptase polymerase chain reaction (RT-PCR) is performed which directly gives confirmatory results whether the virus is present or not [29].

The current work going on Hepatitis C is discovering a vaccine. To cure Hepatitis C, there is no vaccine. If the disorder is in advanced stages, the person needs liver transplantation. If Hepatitis C is directed at early stages like at chronic hepatitis stage, there are antiviral drug treatments which cure disorder to some extent. These antiviral drugs interfere with viral replication and maturation [3]. There are several classes of drugs which interfere with viral growth. The nonstructural 3/4A inhibitor drugs Boceprevir and telaprevir interfere with NS3/4 A proteins to inhibit the viral protein formation. Nonstructural 5A inhibitors like Ledipasvir, ombitasvir, daclatasvir etc., will interfere with NS5A protein which plays an important role in viral replication and assembly of viral particles. Nonstructural 5B inhibitors like sofosbuvir interfere with NS5B which synthesizes viral RNA [3]. Treating patients with antiviral drugs will inhibit viral progress in the body. These drug targets cure the disease if the disease is at an early stage.

8. Conclusion

Alter, Houghton, Rice and their colleagues have contributed their work to the world of science. They have come up with new molecular and immunological techniques to detect the presence of viruses. Alter and his colleagues discovered an Australian antigen and it was non-A, non-B hepatitis (NANBH). He introduced a model organism chimpanzees to study the disease post-transfusion hepatitis. Houghton and his colleagues have brought Molecular Biology and Immunology together and diagnosed NANBH and named it as Hepatitis C virus. Rice and his colleagues sequenced the viral genome and explained its properties of replication and gene expression. He discovered that alone Hepatitis C is causing Liver cirrhosis and Hepatocellular carcinoma.

Author details

Talari Praveen
Centre for Human Genetics, Bangalore, Karnataka, India

*Address all correspondence to: talaripraveen2000@gmail.com

References

[1] D'Souza, Raymond., & Foster, Graham R. (2004). "Diagnosis and treatment of hepatitis C." Journal of the Royal Society of Medicine, 97(5), 223-225. https://www.ncbi.nlm.nih.gov/pmc/articles/PMC1079461/.

[2] Bukh, Jens. (2016). "The history of hepatitis C virus (HCV): Basic research reveals unique features in phylogeny, evolution and the viral life cycle with new perspectives for epidemic control." Journal of Hepatology, 65(1), S2-S21. https://doi.org/10.1016/j.jhep.2016.07.035.

[3] Horsley-Silva, Jennifer L., and Vargas, Hugo E. "New Therapies for Hepatitis C Virus Infection." *Gastroenterology & Hepatology*, 13(1), 22-31. https://pubmed.ncbi.nlm.nih.gov/28420944/.

[4] Nobel Prize. (2020, October 6). "Announcement of the 2020 Nobel Prize in Physiology or Medicine."[Video]. *You Tube*. https://youtu.be/BTu6uOWLKR4.

[5] Morozov, Vladimir Alexei., and Lagaye, Sylvie. (2018). "Hepatitis C virus: Morphogenesis, infection and therapy." World Journal of Hepatology, 10(2), 186-212. https://pubmed.ncbi.nlm.nih.gov/29527256/.

[6] Ginsau, M A., and Ahmed, U A. (2019) "Examination of Blood for Hepatitis B Virus (HBV) and possible Transmission by Mosquito (Aedesaegypti)." *IOSR Journal of Environmental Science, Toxicology and Food Technology (IOSR-JESTFT)*, 13(2), DOI: 10.9790/2402-1302014851.

[7] Thomas et al. (2015). "Viral Hepatitis: Past and Future of HBV and HDV." *Cold Spring Harbor Perspectives in Medicine*, 5(2), 1-11. https://pubmed.ncbi.nlm.nih.gov/25646383/.

[8] Gerlich, Wolfram H. (2013). "Medical Virology of Hepatitis B: how it began and where we are now." Virology Journal, 10(1), 239. http://www.virologyj.com/content/10/1/23.

[9] Pilcher, Carl B. (2015). "Explorer, Nobel Laureate, Astrobiologist: Things You Never Knew about Barry Blumberg." Astrobiology, 15(1), 1-14. https://doi.org/10.1089/ast.2013.1401.

[10] Palese, Peter. (2016). "Profile of Charles M. Rice, Ralf F. W. Bartenschlager, and Michael J. Sofia, 2016 Lasker-DeBakey Clinical Medical Research Awardees." *Proceedings of the National Academy of Sciences*, 113(49), 13934-13937. https://doi.org/10.1073/pnas.1616592113.

[11] Alter et al. (1972). "Posttransfusion Hepatitis After Exclusion of Commercial and Hepatitis-B Antigen-Positive Donors". *Annals of Internal Medicine*, 77(5), 691-699. https://pubmed.ncbi.nlm.nih.gov/4628213/.

[12] Alter et al. (1975a). "CLINICAL AND SEROLOGICAL ANALYSIS OF TRANSFUSION-ASSOCIATED HEPATITIS." *The Lancet*, 306(7940), 838-841. https://doi.org/10.1016/S0140-6736(75)90234-2.

[13] Alter et al. (1975b). "The emerging pattern of post-transfusion hepatitis." *The American Journal of the Medical Sciences*, 270(2), 329-334. https://pubmed.ncbi.nlm.nih.gov/1235474/.

[14] Tabor et al. (1978). "TRANSMISSION OF NON-A, NON-B HEPATITIS FROM MAN TO CHIMPANZEE." *The Lancet*, 311(8062), 463-466. https://doi.org/10.1016/S0140-6736(78)90132-0.

[15] Feinstone et al. (1983). "Inactivation of Hepatitis B Virus and Non-A, Non-B Hepatitis by Chloroform." *Infection and Immunity*, 41(2), 816-821. https://iai.asm.org/content/41/2/816.

[16] He et al. (1987). "Determining the Size of Non-A, Non-B Hepatitis Virus by Filtration." *Journal of Infectious Diseases*, 156(4), 636-640. https://pubmed.ncbi.nlm.nih.gov/3114389/.

[17] Houghton, Michael. (2019) "Hepatitis C Virus: 30 Years after Its Discovery." *Cold Spring Harb Perspect Med*, 9(12):a037069, 1-9. https://pubmed.ncbi.nlm.nih.gov/31501269/

[18] Choo et al. (1989). "Isolation of a cDNA clone derived from a blood-borne non-A, non-B viral hepatitis genome." *Science*, 244(4902), 359-362. https://pubmed.ncbi.nlm.nih.gov/2523562/.

[19] Alter, Harvey J., Houghton, Michael.,and Rice, Charles M. "Press release: The Nobel Prize in Physiology or Medicine 2020." *The Nobel Prize*. https://www.nobelprize.org/prizes/medicine/2020/press-release/.

[20] Houghton, Michael. (2009). "Discovery of the hepatitis C virus." Liver International, 29(s1), 82-88. https://doi.org/10.1111/j.1478-3231.2008.01925.x.

[21] Blight, Keril J., and Rice, Charles M. (1997). "Secondary Structure Determination of the Conserved 98-Base Sequence at the 39 Terminus of Hepatitis C Virus Genome RNA." Journal of Virology. 71(10), 7345-7352. https://jvi.asm.org/content/71/10/7345.

[22] Tanka et al. (1996). "Structure of the 39 Terminus of the Hepatitis C Virus Genome." *Journal of Virology*. 70(5), 3307-3312. https://jvi.asm.org/content/70/5/3307.

[23] Kolykhalov et al. (1997). "Transmission of Hepatitis C by Intrahepatic Inoculation with Transcribed RNA." *Science*, 277(5325), 570-574. https://science.sciencemag.org/content/277/5325/570.

[24] Wakita et al. (2005). "Production of infectious hepatitis C virus in tissue culture from a cloned viral genome." *Nature Medicine*, 11(7), 791-796. https://doi.org/10.1038/nm1268.

[25] Ilboudo et al. (2014). "Over-expression of phosphatidylinositol 4-kinase type III?? is associated with undifferentiated status and poor prognosis of human hepatocellular carcinoma." *BMC Cancer*, 14(7), 1-8. https://doi.org/10.1186/1471-2407-14-7.

[26] Harak et al. (2016). "Tuning a cellular lipid kinase activity adapts hepatitis C virus to replication in cell culture." *Nature Microbiology*, 2, 1-13. https://doi.org/10.1038/nmicrobiol.2016.247.

[27] Sarhan et al. (2017). "Glycogen synthase kinase 3?? inhibitors prevent hepatitis C virus release/assembly through perturbation of lipid metabolism." *Scientific Reports*, 7(1), 1-12. https://doi.org/10.1038/s41598-017-02648-6.

[28] Rosa et al. (2005). "Activation of naive B lymphocytes via CD81, a pathogenetic mechanism for hepatitis C virus-associated B lymphocyte disorders." *PANS*, 102(5), 18544-18549. https://doi.org/10.1073/pnas.0509402102.

[29] Li, Hui-Chun., and Lo, Shih-Yen. (2015). "Hepatitis C virus: Virology, diagnosis and treatment." World Journal of Hepatology, 7(10), 1377. https://www.ncbi.nlm.nih.gov/pmc/articles/PMC4450201/.

Section 2

Hepatitis C Virus Characteristics and Evolution

Chapter 2

Hepatitis C: An Overview

Syed Manzoor Kadri and Marija Petkovic

Abstract

Hepatitis C virus (HCV) has infected approximatelly 130–170 milion individuals in the form of chronic liver infection and hepatocellular carcinoma. In the majority of patients with the increased risk for hepatocellular carcinoma the initial rearrangement is fibrosis. HCV is a bloodborne virus. The most common route of the infection are drug use, injections, unsafe health care performance, transfusion and sexual transmission. The incubation period ranges from 2 to 6 weeks in case of HCV. HCV infection is diagnosed in the process of detecting of anti-HCV antibodies and if positive, a nucleic acid test for HCV ribonucleic acid (RNA) is done. Currently, the most promising treatment agents are direct-acting antivirals (DAAs). They have shown limited viral resistance, long treatment duration and higher cost with no proven benefits in the prevention of graft reinfections in HCV individuals. In the light of the aforementioned, there is a need to a more dubious research in the quest for the effective therapeutic modalities.

Keywords: HCV, diagnosis, management, vaccine

1. Introduction

The word "hepatitis" is defined as the liver inflammation. In the majority of individuals it is due to genetic diseases, iatrogenic effect (certain medications), sexual intercourse, being born to a mother who has hepatitis C, transfusion, tattooing, illegal drug use or high alcohol intake. Prior to 1992, while the screening of the blood supplies started in the US, hepatitis C was most commonly spread through blood transfusions, organ transplants and haemodialysis treatment. Hepatitis C virus (HCV) has infected approximately 130–170 million individuals in the form of chronic liver infection and hepatocellular carcinoma [1].

In the majority of patients with an increased risk for hepatocellular carcinoma, the initial rearrangement is fibrosis. HCV is a bloodborne virus (**Figure 1**) [2].

Chronic hepatitis C (CHC) patients are at high risk to develop life-threatening complications, including cirrhosis in 20% of cases and hepatocellular carcinoma (HCC) at an incidence of 4–5% per year in cirrhotic patients [3].

Recommended HCV routine testing is based on the high-risk individuals such as risk the use of illegal drugs, clotting factors prior 1987, received blood/organs before 1992, chronic haemodialysis, liver disease, healthcare, emergency, healthcare workers after needlestick injuries in case of to HCV-positive blood, children born to HCV-positive women [4].

The routine HCV testing is not recommended in the healthcare setting, especially in the emergency and public safety professionals, pregnant individuals, in-home contacts of HCV-positive individuals etc.

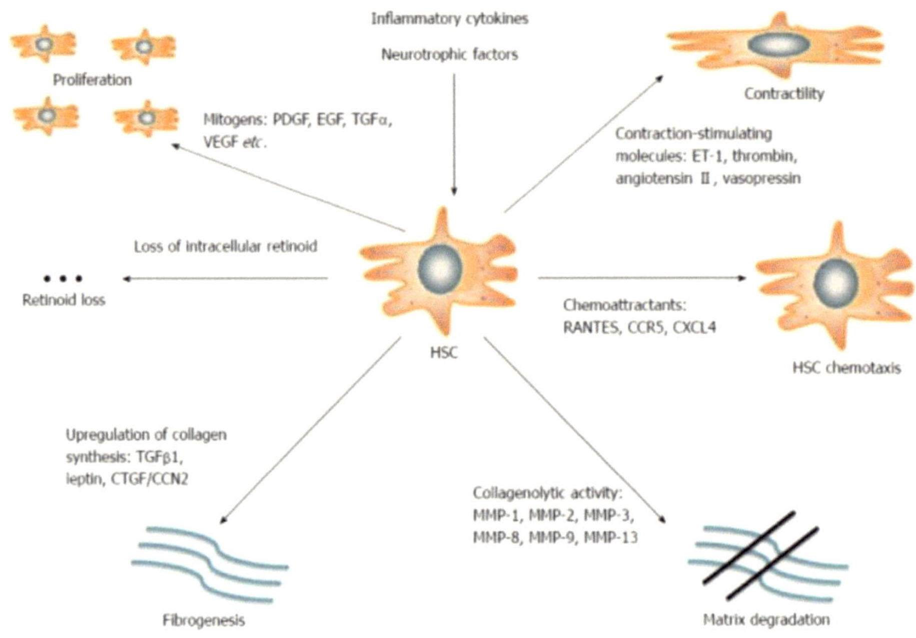

Figure 1.
Fibrogenesis. World J Gastroenterol. 2014. Doi: 10.3748/wjg.v20.i32.11033.

2. Epidemiology of hepatitis C virus

Hepatitis C is a disease with a worldwide burden, with the variable prevalence among major geographic areas. WHO estimates that about 170 million people or 3% of the world's population are infected with HCV [5].

The regions with high incidence are Eastern Mediterranean and European, with a prevalence of 2.3% and 1.5% respectively (**Figure 2**).

The estimated global prevalence of HCV infection is 3% which translates to over 180 million people worldwide [6].

High seroprevalence is noted in Asian and African countries. Egypt reported a seroprevalence of about 22% [7] and is highest in the world. A substantial regional difference exists in the distribution of HCV genotypes in the world. In Mexico, the estimated prevalence of HCV (2001–2002) was 1.2%. In the UK region, it has been estimated that nearly 200,000 adult individuals are HCV carriers. In Australia, the prevalence is estimated to be 2.3%. In Pakistan, HCV prevalence studies detected

WHO Region	Total Population (Millions)	Hepatitis C prevalence Rate %	Infected Population (Millions)	Number-of countries by WHO Region where data are not available
Africa	602	5.3	31.9	12
Americas	785	1.7	13.1	7
Eastern Mediterranean	466	4.6	21.3	7
Europe	858	1.03	8.9	19
South-East Asia	1 500	2.15	32.3	3
Western Pacific	1 600	3.9	62.2	11
Total	5 811	3.1	169.7	57

Figure 2.
HCV prevalence.

that 751 out of 16,400 (4.57%) patients are +HCV Ab, while the rated are lower in Saudi Arabia and Yemen.

In Asia, the HCV prevalence among blood donors has been estimated lower than 0.49% (1995–2000.), with higher rates in Thailand (3.2–5.6%).

3. HCV characteristics

3.1 HCV genotype

Hepatitis C virus is an RNA viral microorganism. This virus belongs to the Flaviviridae family, genus Hepacivirus. It has one serotype, but minimum 6 major genotypes and over 80 subtypes [8].

The HCV virion is 55–65 nm in diameter. It consists of a 9.6 kbp positive-sense single-stranded RNA genome composed of a long open reading frame (ORF) flanked by untranslated regions (UTR's) at both the ends (**Figure 3**).

The genome of HCV is thought to encode at least 10 proteins, of which 3 are structural (core, envelope glycoproteins E1, E2) and 6 nonstructural proteins (NS2, NS3, NS4A, NS4B, NS5A, NS5B).

HCV also expresses p7, a membrane-associated ion channel that may function during assembly or infection (**Figure 4**).

Two viral proteases are involved in the processing of HCV nonstructural proteins: NS2, a zinc-dependent metalloproteinase that cleaves between proteins NS2 and NS3, and NS3/4A, a serine protease that cleaves between the NS3-NS4A, NS4A-NS4B, NS4B-NS4B, NS4B-NS5A and NS5A-NS5B junctions [9].

3.2 Genetic variations of HCV

The HCV RNA sequences are highly heterogeneous. HCV is classified into 11 genotypes [1–11]. The several genotypes form further subtypes such as a, b, c etc.

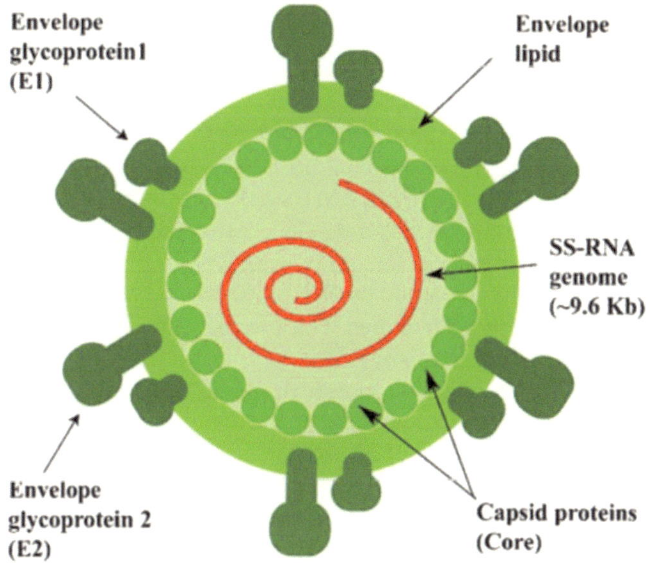

Figure 3.
Hepatitis C virus- an overview. 2018. Sagar Aryal

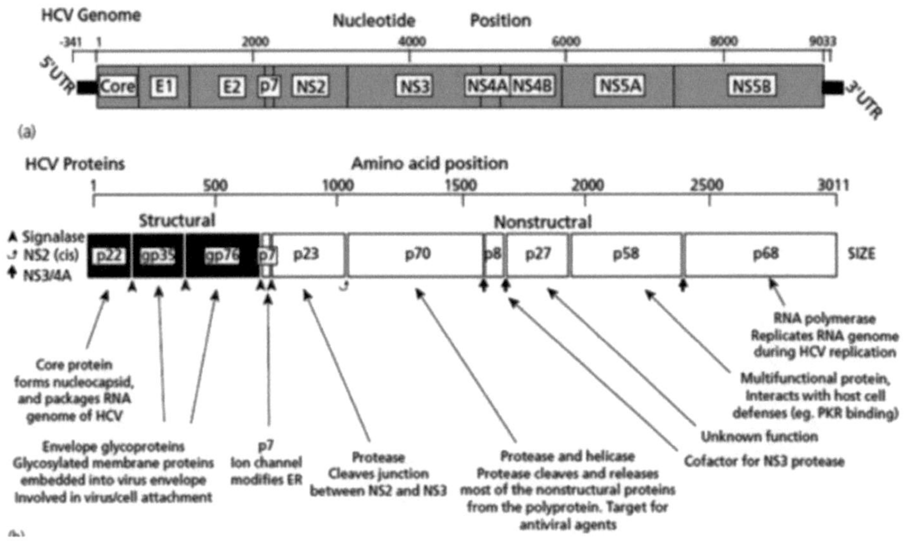

Figure 4.
HCV genome.

The classification is made according to the nucleotide sequence, variable infectivity and pathogenicity determining the progression rate of cirrhosis and hepatocellular carcinoma [11].

At this point, genotype 1 is the most prevalent (46%), then genotype 3,2 and 4 [12].

Core, a 191-amino acid polypeptide, may be involved in hepatocarcinogenesis and steatosis [13].

The importance of HCV genotype is highlighted in the case of the treatment response and the therapy duration.

The HCV genotype is characterised by the detection of antibodies against HCV genotype-specific epitopes with the application of competitive EIA.

HCV subtyping is of paramount importance in case of epidemics/pandemics, especially in case of epidemiological studies.

4. Pathogenesis of hepatitis C virus

The most common route of the infection is drug abuse, injections, unsafe health care performance, transfusion and sexual transmission.

The incubation period ranges from 2 to 6 weeks in case of HCV. HCV infection is diagnosed in the process of detecting anti-HCV antibodies and if possible, a nucleic acid test for HCV ribonucleic acid (RNA) is done [14].

The pathogenesis is characterised by HCV infected hepatocytes that may be destructed by HCV-specific CTL clones. The apoptotic mechanism is Fas ligand, TNF-α or perforin-based mechanism [15].

In the majority of cases, there is a slowly progressive asymptomatic hepatitis, with persistent viremia. The chronic form of the disease has a higher rate of progression to cirrhosis over a period of 20 years.

The exacerbation of the disease is characterised by elevated alanine aminotransferase activity. HCV –specific antibodies are detectable 7 to 31 weeks after the initial infection. Thus, the humoral immunity is highly variable and aimed towards the HCV core, envelope, NS3 and NS4 proteins [16].

The characteristic parenchyma impairments are the triad of steatosis, bile duct damage and the portal tracts [17].

Hepatic steatosis presents with large droplets of fat vacuoles in the cytoplasm of hepatocytes. In 20% of chronic hepatitis C cases, there is an eosinophilic deposit in the cytoplasm of periportal hepatocytes. Furthermore, the level of necroinflammation, fibrosis and cirrhosis depends on the serum alanine aminotransferase activity.

Predisposing factors such as viral co-infection (HBV etc.) and high alcohol consumption increase the risk of hepatic disease progression.

Chronic active hepatitis frequently leads to the onset of hepatocellular carcinoma (HCC) [18].

It has been postulated that in the case of HCV infection, the HCV-immune specific reaction is not adequate to control the viral replication due to high level of T-cell response.

The variety of polymorphism is associated with HCV prognostic diversity. The major cytokine involved in the molecular HCV infection pathway is the interleukin 28B [19].

5. Clinical manifestations of hepatitis C virus

5.1 Acute hepatitis

The incubation period for HCV is 7 weeks (2–26 weeks) after the initial exposure. The acute HCV infection presents with fever, fatigue, decreased appetite, nausea, vomiting, abdominal cramps, dark coloured faeces, grey facial skin, joint pain and jaundice [20].

5.2 Chronic hepatitis

In the patient with chronic hepatitis, the hepatic function is impaired. Additional symptoms are anorexia, nausea, right upper quadrant pain, dark coloured urine and pruritus. The serum level of ALT is either normal or elevated [21].

5.3 Hepatocellular carcinoma

The oncogenesis in the patients with chronic virus inflammation leads to the onset of necrosis, regeneration and cirrhosis [22].

6. Diagnostic assessment

In the majority of individuals, HCV viremia may be present in spite of normal serum ALT levels. Thus, the virological confirmation of HCV infection is more significant [23].

There is an HCV testing protocol such as to test the asymptomatic individuals: EIA for anti-HCV if negative (non-reactive) test no further if positive repeat testing or RIBA for anti-HCV. Recombinant immunoblot assays (RIBA) can be used to confirm the presence of anti-HCV antibodies.

The other possible testing pathway is to perform RT-PCR for HCV RNA if negative or if the positive result, proceed with medical evaluation [24].

In case RIBA test for anti-HCV is negative, [25] do not perform the further evaluation. In case the test is indeterminate (PCR negative, ALT normal or positive PCR, abnormal ALP continue with medial evaluation. In case both tests are positive, continue with the medical evaluation.

A serologic screening test is recommended to perform on individuals in the high-risk groups and nucleic acid tests are recommended to confirm the active HCV infections.

6.1 Laboratory diagnosis of HCV

Nowadays, HCV infection is detected by the use of serologic tests to detect HCV antibodies. Enzyme immunoassay (EIA) shows false negative in patients on haemodialysis. Immunodeficiency, and false-positive in an autoimmune disorder.

Recombinant immunoblot assay (RIBA) is a molecular assay that targets the amplification technique to detect HCV RNA.

A positive polymerase chain reaction (PCR) confirms HCV infection.

At present, the second-generation enzyme immunoassay (EIA-2) for antibodies to HCV (anti-HCV) is the most recommended diagnostic modality. If positive, the diagnosis may be confirmed by RIBA to detect antibodies to individual HCV antigens.

Anti-HCV is detected by the enzyme-linked immunosorbent assay (ELISA). In EIA, conserved antigens from the HCV core, NS3,NS4 and NS5 are used in the diagnostic laboratory.

EIAs to detect anti-HCV antibody are recommended for screening the HCV infections. It is not recommended in infants younger than 18 months due to the possible reactivity with the maternal antibody [26].

The serological window period is 40 days.

A screening test is the rapid, point-of-care test (POCTs) developed to detect anti-HCV antibodies with high sensitivity and specificity (OraQuick, OraSure Technologies). This test detects anti-HCV antibodies in different specimens (fingerstick, venipuncture whole blood, serum, plasma, oral fluid [27].

Confirmatory test such as recombinant immunoblot assay (RIBA) is used to confirm the presence of antibodies against each of the several HCV proteins is assessed as individual bands on a membrane strip [28].

HCV RNA level in the serum is probably the first detectable marker of acute HCV infection – a few weeks prior to the appearance of anti-HCV antibody by several weeks [29].

In the period prior and after the treatment, detection of HCV RNA is used to monitor the disease status. The level of HCV RNA is not in correlation with the hepatic disease stadium.

6.2 Molecular diagnosis of HCV

Qualitative reverse transcription-polymerase chain reaction (RT-PCR) assays for HCV RNA are simpler than quantitative tests and adequate for confirmation of the diagnosis of HCV [30].

Serum alanine aminotransferase level (ALT) is inexpensive, routine and noninvasive. It is great value for monitoring the disease activity.

6.3 Detection of viral RNA

Detection of HCV RNA by PCR and nucleic acid amplification tests (NAT) is performed, such as Transcript-Mediated Amplification (TMA).

Qualitative HCV RNA detection is defined as the use of conventional RT-PCR or transcription-mediated amplification (TMA) [31].

Quantitative NAT test is available in the form of quantitative RT-PCR (qRT-PCR) and branched deoxyribonucleic acid (bDNA) technology.

The indirect tests detect antibody induced by virus replication, IgM for recent infection, IgG for recent or past infection. The direct tests are virus isolation, detection of viral antigens and viral nucleic acids.

6.4 Detection of HCV core antigen

NATs test has higher specificity and sensitivity, but it is more time-consuming and in need of more sophisticated techniques. Currently, there are several generations of ELISA developed such as the one that uses the recombinant c100–3 epitope from the NS4 region, c22–3 and c33c from the HCV core and NS3 regions. The 4th generation of the anti-HCV assay is designed from the core, NS3, NS4A, NS4B and NS5A region.

6.5 Liver biopsy

The liver biopsy provides use of full information about the degree of fibrosis in HCV infected individuals [32].

The main benefit is to further manage the treatment protocol. The liver biopsy can assess the degree of inflammation, fibrosis, co-morbidities and therapeutic modalities [33].

Activity (necro-inflammation) severity and progress. May fluctuate with disease activity or therapeutic intervention [34].

Fibrosis implies possible progression to cirrhosis or in advanced disease defined as 'bridging fibrosis.'. To assess the degree of fibrosis, non-invasive tests (APRI or FIB4) are recommended.

7. Treatment

The initial HCV treatment was based on the application of interferon alfa, peginterferon and ribavirin [35].

The antiviral activity of interferon and peginterferon is based upon their ability to stimulate interferon-stimulated genes (ISGs) that have endogenous antiviral activities. Ribavirin is a nucleoside analogue that potentiates the effects of interferon against hepatitis by as yet undefined mechanisms [36].

Until 2020, the standard chronic HCV therapy was the combination of peginterferon and ribavirin given for 24 or 48 weeks. This combination led to sustained clearance of HCV and remission disease in 40–50% of patients. The response rate is higher in genotypes 2 and 3 [37].

In 2010, several HCV-specific protease inhibitors were approved for use: boceprevir, telaprevir and simeprevir specific to genotype 1 HCV. In 2013, sofosbuvir (HCV specific RNA polymerase inhibitor) was approved for the clinical treatment [38].

Other oral regimens become available in 2015, 2016 and 2017. They represented a combination of several HCV RNA polymerase regimens – nucleoside and non-nucleoside, HCV NS5A antagonists and the HCV protease inhibitors.

In individuals with cirrhosis, there is a higher risk of developing HCC and end-stage liver disease [39].

The combination of pegylated interferon plus ribavirin (PR) was the gold treatment standard (2000.). anti-HCV therapy requires weekly injections and is associated with numerous systemic side effects (flu-like symptoms, fatigue, etc.) [40].

The first approved in the USA according to FDA – boceprevir (Victrelis) and telaprevir (Incivek) for the treatment of chronic HCV genotype I infection [41].

Both drugs are classified as NS3/4A protease inhibitors, 24-28wk duration therapy, administered in combination with PR. FDA approved the different NS3/4A protease inhibitor named simeprevir (2013).

The HCV NS5B protein is an essential enzyme (RNA-dependant RNA polymerase) in HCV viral replication and has been a prime target in the search for antiviral therapies [42].

Adverse effects with interferon treatment: anaemia, neutropenia, rash, skin reactions, anorectal signs, elevated uric acid, bilirubin levels etc [43].

In the early 2000s, pegylated interferon plus ribavirin became the standard anti-HCV treatment. In 2014, boceprevir, telaprevir, simeprevir, sofosbuvir and Harvoni were approved by the FDA.

The highly significant antiviral treatment regimens are PEG-IFN + Ribavirin, – Telaprevir or boceprevir in genotype 1, -Sofosbuvir + Ribavirin ± PEG-IFN in genotypes 1,2,3 and 4, Simeprevir +PEG-IFN + Ribavirin in genotype 1 [44].

HCV has several genotypes detected. Therefore, an effective vaccine must be multivalent to have a beneficial treatment outcome.

There is no vaccine for Hepatitis C. The only way to prevent Hepatitis C is by avoiding behaviour that can spread the disease, especially injection drug use.

8. Prevention and control of hepatitis C

Screening of blood donors and screening for the presence of HCV prior to any transfusion of blood.

The use of sterile needles in case of medical and dental procedures, tattooing, or other percutaneous exposures [45].

Alcohol-intake decreased consumption or reduction will improve the overall health of an individual.

9. Conclusion

Currently, the most promising treatment agents are direct-acting antiviral (DAAs). They have shown limited viral resistance, long treatment duration and higher cost with no proven benefits in the prevention of graft reinfections in HCV individuals.

In light of the aforementioned, there is a need for more dubious research in the quest for the effective therapeutic modalities.

In summary, the diagnostic algorithm of Hepatitis C depends on the clinical context. In asymptomatic, low-risk subjects, who are found to be anti-HCV positive by EIA-2, the diagnosis of HCV infection needs to be confirmed, especially if the initial biochemical tests reveal normal ALT levels.

Author details

Syed Manzoor Kadri[1*] and Marija Petkovic[2]

1 Disease Control, Directorate of Health Services, Kashmir, India

2 University of Medicine, Belgrade, Serbia

*Address all correspondence to: kadrism@gmail.com

References

[1] Takafumi Saito, Yoshiyuki Ueno. Transmission of hepatitis C virus: self-limiting hepatitis or chronic hepatitis? 2013 Nov 7;19(41):6957-61. World J Gastroenterol

[2] Dakhil N, Junaidi O, Befeler AS. Chronic viral hepatitis. Mo Med. 2009 Sep-Oct;106(5):361-5.

[3] *Chen SL, Morgan TR.* The natural history of hepatitis C virus (HCV) infection.*Int J Med Sci. 2006; 3(2):47-52.*

[4] Catelyn Coyle, MPH, MEd, Helena Kwakwa, MD, MPH, Kendra Viner, PhD, MPH.. Integrating Routine HCV Testing in Primary Care: Lessons Learned from Five Federally Qualified Health Centers in Philadelphia, Pennsylvania, 2012-2014. Public Health Rep. 2016 May-Jun; 131(Suppl 2): 65-73.

[5] Meryem Jefferies, Bisma Rauff, Harunor Rashid, Thao Lam, and Shafquat Rafiq. Update on global epidemiology of viral hepatitis and preventive strategies. World J Clin Cases. 2018 Nov 6; 6(13): 589-599.

[6] Ekta Gupta, Meenu Bajpai, and Aashish Choudhary. Hepatitis C virus: Screening, diagnosis, and interpretation of laboratory assays. Asian J Transfus Sci. 2014 Jan-Jun; 8(1): 19-25.

[7] Asmaa GomaaNaglaa Allam, Aisha Elsharkway,[2] Mohamed El Kassas, Imam Waked. Hepatitis C infection in Egypt: prevalence, impact and management strategies. Hepat Med. 2017; 9: 17-25.

[8] *Catanese MT, Uryu K, Kopp M, Edwards TJ, Andrus L, Rice WJ, Silvestry M, Kuhn RJ, Rice CM.* Ultrastructural analysis of hepatitis C virus particles. Proc Natl Acad Sci U S A. 2013 Jun 4; 110(23):9505-10.

[9] Peter Simmonds. Proposed update to the taxonomy of the genera *Hepacivirus* and *Pegivirus* within the *Flaviviridae* family. J Gen Virol. 2016 Nov; 97(11): 2894-2907.

[10] Donald B. Smith, Paul Becher, Jens Bukh, Ernest A. Gould, Gregor Meyers, Thomas Monath, A. Scott Muerhoff, Alexander Pletnev, Rebecca Rico-Hesse, Jack T. Stapleton,

[11] *Gower E, Estes C, Blach S, Razavi-Shearer K, Razavi H.* Global epidemiology and genotype distribution of the hepatitis C virus infection.. *J Hepatol. 2014 Nov; 61(1 Suppl):S45-57.*

[12] *Chevaliez S, Pawlotsky JM.* Hepatitis C virus: virology, diagnosis and management of antiviral therapy.. *World J Gastroenterol. 2007 May 7; 13(17):2461-6.*

[13] *Li HC, Ma HC, Yang CH, Lo SY.* Production and pathogenicity of hepatitis C virus core gene products.. *World J Gastroenterol. 2014 Jun 21; 20(23):7104-22.*

[14] Ekta Gupta, Meenu Bajpai, Aashish Choudhary. Hepatitis C virus: Screening, diagnosis, and interpretation of laboratory assays. Asian J Transfus Sci. 2014 Jan-Jun; 8(1): 19-25.

[15] Fabio Forghieri, Mario Luppi, Patrizia Barozzi, Rossana Maffei, Leonardo Potenza, Franco Narni, and Roberto Marasca. Pathogenetic Mechanisms of Hepatitis C Virus-Induced B-Cell Lymphomagenesis. Clin Dev Immunol. 2012; 2012: 807351.

[16] Siobhán B. Cashman, Brian D. Marsden, Lynn B. DustinThe Humoral Immune Response to HCV: Understanding is Key to Vaccine Development. Front Immunol. 2014; 5: 550.

[17] Maura O'Neil, Ivan Damjanov. Ryan M. Taylor. Basic Hepatopathology:

Terminology and Definition. Liver Pathology for Clinicians pp 23-44| Cite as

[18] Philippe J. Zamor, Andrew S. deLemos, Mark W. Russo. Viral hepatitis and hepatocellular carcinoma: etiology and management. J Gastrointest Oncol. 2017 Apr; 8(2): 229-242.

[19] *Rau M, Baur K, Geier A*Host genetic variants in the pathogenesis of hepatitis C.*Viruses. 2012 Dec; 4(12):3281-302.*

[20] Sheetal Trivedi, Satyapramod Murthy, Himanshu Sharma, Alex S. Hartlage, Arvind Kumar, Sashi Gadi, Peter Simmonds, Lokendra V. Chauhan, Troels K. H. Scheel, Eva Billerbeck, Peter D. Burbelo, Charles M. Rice, W. Ian Lipkin, Kurt Vandergrift, John M. Cullen, Amit Kapoor Viral persistence, liver disease and host response in **Hepatitis C**-like virus rat model. Hepatology. Author manuscript; available in PMC 2019 Aug 1.

[21] Shiu-Wan Chan. Establishment of chronic **hepatitis C** virus infection: Translational evasion of oxidative defence. World J Gastroenterol. 2014 Mar 21; 20(11): 2785-2800. Published online 2014 Mar 21. doi: 10.3748/wjg.v20.i11.2785

[22] Giuseppe Castello, Susan Costantini, Stefania Scala. Targeting the inflammation in **HCV**-associated hepatocellular **carcinoma**: a role in the prevention and treatment. J Transl Med. 2010; 8: 109. Published online 2010 Nov 3.

[23] *Chevaliez S, Pawlotsky JM.* How to use virological tools for optimal management of chronic hepatitis C.. *Liver Int. 2009 Jan; 29 Suppl 1():9-14.*

[24] Verónica Saludes, Victoria González, Ramon Planas, Lurdes Matas, Vicente Ausina, and Elisa Martró. Tools for the diagnosis of hepatitis C virus infection and hepatic fibrosis staging. World J Gastroenterol. 2014 Apr 7; 20(13): 3431-3442.

[25] Maria Alice Sant'ana Zarife, Eliana Almeida Gomes Reis, Mitermayer G. Reis. Indeterminate RIBA results were associated with the absence of hepatitis C virus RNA (HCV-RNA) in blood donors. Rev. Soc. Bras. Med. Trop. vol.47 no.1 Uberaba Jan./Feb. 2014

[26] *Campos-Outcalt D.* Hepatitis C: new CDC screening recommendations.*J Fam Pract. 2012 Dec; 61(12):744-6.*

[27] *Scalioni Lde P, Cruz HM, de Paula VS, Miguel JC, Marques VA, Villela-Nogueira CA, Milagres FA, Cruz MS, Bastos FI, Andrade TM, Motta-Castro AR, Lewis-Ximenez LL, Lampe E, Villar LM.* Performance of rapid hepatitis C virus antibody assays among high- and low-risk populations.. *J Clin Virol. 2014 Jul; 60(3):200-5.*

[28] *Martin P, Fabrizi F, Dixit V, Quan S, Brezina M, Kaufman E, Sra K, DiNello R, Polito A, Gitnick G* Automated RIBA hepatitis C virus (HCV) strip immunoblot assay for reproducible HCV diagnosis.. *J Clin Microbiol. 1998 Feb; 36(2):387-90.*

[29] *Chevaliez S, Pawlotsky JM.*How to use virological tools for optimal management of chronic hepatitis C.. *Liver Int. 2009 Jan; 29 Suppl 1():9-14.*

[30] Philippe Halfon, Marc Bourlière, Guillaume Pénaranda, Hacène Khiri, Denis Ouzan· Real-Time PCR Assays for Hepatitis C Virus (HCV) RNA Quantitation Are Adequate for Clinical Management of Patients with Chronic HCV Infection. J Clin Microbiol. 2006 Jul; 44(7): 2507-2511.

[31] Mel Krajden, Rainer Ziermann, Asphani Khan, Annie Mak, Kimmy Leung, David Hendricks,[2] and Lorraine Comanor. Qualitative Detection of Hepatitis C Virus RNA: Comparison of Analytical Sensitivity, Clinical Performance, and Workflow of the Cobas Amplicor HCV Test Version 2.0 and the HCV RNA

Transcription-Mediated Amplification Qualitative Assay. J Clin Microbiol. 2002 Aug; 40(8): 2903-2907.

[32] Adeel A. Butt, Liver Fibrosis Progression in Hepatitis C Virus Infection After Seroconversion. JAMA Intern Med. 2015 Feb; 175(2): 178-185.

[33] Butt AA, Wang X, Moore CM. Effect of HCV and its treatment upon survival. Hepatology. 2009;50(2):387-392.

[34] Julien Massard et al. Natural history and predictors of disease severity in chronic hepatitis C. Journal of Hepatology 44 (2006) S19–S24

[35] Siobhán B. Cashman, Brian D. Marsden, Lynn B. Dustin. The Humoral Immune Response to HCV: Understanding is Key to Vaccine Development. Front Immunol. 2014; 5: 550.

[36] Emmanuel Thomas, Jordan J. Feld,Qisheng Li, Zongyi Hu,Michael W. Fried, T. Jake Liang Ribavirin Potentiates Interferon Action by Augmenting Interferon-Stimulated Gene Induction in Hepatitis C Virus Cell Culture Models. Hepatology. 2011 Jan; 53(1): 32-41.

[37] Shalimar Et al. Hepatitis C Virus Genotype 3: Hope for Nonresponders and Patients With CirrhosisJ Clin Exp Hepatol. 2014 Jun; 4(2): 179-181.

[38] Laure Izquierdo, François Helle, Catherine François, Sandrine Castelain, Gilles Duverlie, Etienne Brochot **Simeprevir for the treatment of hepatitis C virus infection.** Pharmgenomics Pers Med. 2014; 7: 241-249.

[39] *Toshikuni N, Arisawa T, Tsutsumi M.* Hepatitis C-related liver cirrhosis - strategies for the prevention of hepatic decompensation, hepatocarcinogenesis, and mortality.. *World J Gastroenterol. 2014 Mar 21; 20(11):2876-87.*

[40] Emilio Palumbo, **Pegylated Interferon and Ribavirin Treatment for Hepatitis C Virus Infection.** Ther Adv Chronic Dis. 2011 Jan; 2(1): 39-45.

[41] Caroline M Perry. Telaprevir: A Review of its Use in the Management of Genotype 1 Chronic Hepatitis . March 2012. Drugs 72(5):619-41

[42] Megan H. Powdrill, Jean A. Bernatchez,Matthias Götte. Inhibitors of the Hepatitis C Virus RNA-Dependent RNA Polymerase NS5B. Viruses. 2010 Oct; 2(10): 2169-2195.

[43] *Alborino F, Burighel A, Tiller FW, van Helden J, Gabriel C, Raineri A, Catapano R, Stekel H.*Multicenter evaluation of a fully automated third-generation anti-HCV antibody screening test with excellent sensitivity and specificity.. *Med Microbiol Immunol. 2011 May; 200(2):77-83.*

[44] Hideki Fujii, et al. Comparison of peg-interferon, ribavirin plus telaprevir *vs* simeprevir by propensity score matching. World J Hepatol. 2015 Dec 8; 7(28): 2841-2848.

[45] Silvano Wendel. Primary screening of blood donors by nat testing for HCV-RNA: development of an "in-house" method and results. Rev. Inst. Med. trop. S. Paulo vol.49 no.3 São Paulo May/June 2007

Section 3

Extrahepatic Manifestations

Chapter 3

Extrahepatic Manifestations of Hepatitis C Infection

Alberto Frosi

Abstract

Chronic infection with the hepatitis C virus (HCV) is a major cause of liver disease worldwide and is also responsible for extrahepatic manifestations (EHM) involving many different organs and apparatus: skin, salivary glands, eyes, thyroid, kidneys, peripheral and central nervous system, and immune system. Mixed cryoglobulinemia is the most frequent, best known and strictly HCV-associated EHM. A significant association between HCV and B-cell Non-Hodgkin-Lymphoma is reported although the incidence of lymphoma among HCV-infected patients overall remains low. HCV-infected patients have increased rates of insulin resistance, diabetes, and atherosclerosis, which may lead to increased cardiovascular disorders. The mechanisms causing the extrahepatic effects of HCV infection are likely multifactorial and may include endocrine effects, HCV replication in extrahepatic cells, or a heightened immune reaction with systemic effects. Because of this associations, it is suggested testing for HCV infection the patients with a clinical condition described as linked to hepatitis C. Conversely, patients diagnosed with HCV infection should have evaluation for a possible EHM. EHM of HCV can be considered an established indication for antiviral treatment with direct acting antivirals, even in the absence of overt liver disease. Successful eradication of HCV can improve and in some cases cure EHM of HCV. B cell depleting agents may be considered to be the best biological target option for patients with more severe EHM in combination with the antivirals.

Keywords: HCV, chronic hepatitis C, cryoglobulinemia, B-cell lymphoma, thyroid dysfunction, type 2 diabetes, Sjögren's syndrome, porphyria cutanea tarda, lichen planus, glomerulonephritis, neuropathy, polyarthritis, extrahepatic manifestations

1. Introduction

Persistent infection with hepatitis C virus (HCV) is a leading cause of chronic liver disease, resulting in about 400000 deaths per year. The estimated global HCV prevalence is 1.0%, corresponding to 71 million individuals. Antiviral medicines can cure more than 95% of persons with hepatitis C infection, thereby reducing the risk of death from cirrhosis and liver cancer, but access to diagnosis and treatment is low. There is currently no effective vaccine against hepatitis C; however, research in this area is ongoing [1].

However, these data are underestimated do not taking into account the extrahepatic aspects that make this infection a systemic disease. Early after its discovery, it was shown that HCV is not only hepatotropic but also lymphotropic. It was also shown that several extrahepatic manifestations (EHM) can complicate HCV infection [2–4].

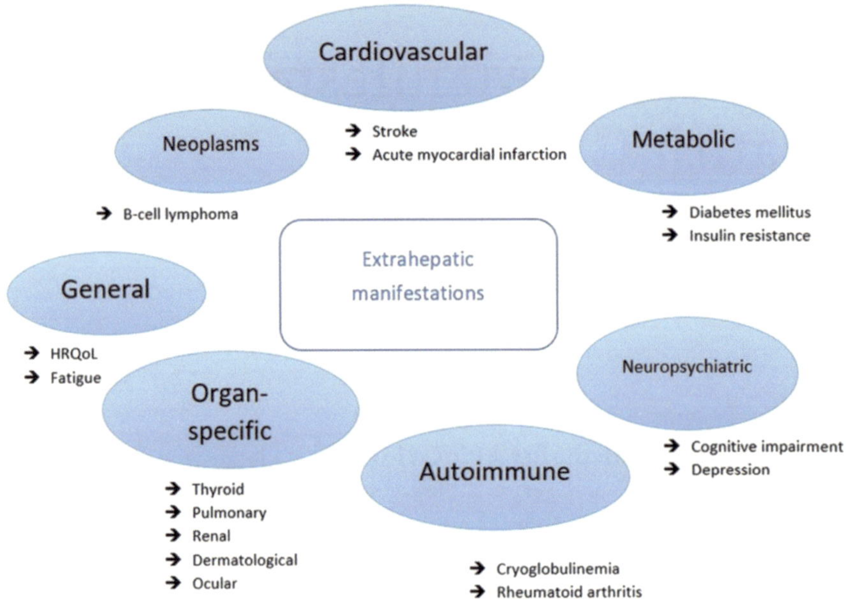

Figure 1.
The spectrum of extrahepatic manifestations of HCV [6].

Moreover, chronic HCV infection has been associated with numerous EHM and diseases, although a direct link is often difficult to establish.

Association should not be confused with causality. The association merely suggests a hypothesis, such as a common cause, but does not offer proof [5].

A causal relationship is easily acceptable if the strength of association is hight. Furthermore, according to the criterion of plausibility, the association ought to be biologically plausible.

The EHM described as linked to HCV hepatitis are numerous:

Mixed cryoglobulinemia (MC), sicca syndrome (SS), Non-Hodgkin Lymphoma (NHL), serum monoclonal gammopathy, thyroid disease, type 2 diabetes mellitus and glucose intolerance, many autoimmune disorders, renal disease, rheumatologic, neurological, cardiovascular and dermatological disorders [6] (**Figure 1**).

Here are described the most clinical important and best studied of these pathological conditions.

2. Biological plausibility and pathophysiology

The pathophysiology of EHM of HCV hepatitis is only in part understood and for some of them unexplained.

The mechanisms causing the extrahepatic effects of HCV infection are likely multifactorial and may include endocrine effects, HCV replication in extrahepatic cells, or a heightened immune reaction with systemic effects.

Due to the fact that HCV has been shown to infect both hepatocytes and lymphocytes, lymphoproliferative diseases such as lymphoma and MC are most closely linked to hepatitis C infection. These conditions are the most studied from the point of view of their pathophysiology. The primary mechanism of injury in cryoglobulinemia is a vasculitis triggered by immune complex deposition.

HCV has been shown to be a lymphotropic virus and associated with several lymphoproliferative disorders, including monoclonal gammopathies in addition to

MC and B-cell NHL. HCV infection of lymphocytes could play a direct role in cellular transformation, specifically in de novo large B-cell lymphoma. HCV infection of two B-cell lines can produce mutations in tumor suppressor and proto-oncogenes which were identified in HCV-associated B-cell lymphomas.

Two particulars although not mutually exclusive models of infection-driven malignant transformation were described.

Direct lymphocyte transformation by lymphotropic transforming viruses (Epstein–Barr virus, human herpesvirus, and human T-lymphotropic virus type) expressing viral oncogenes has been reported. A model of lymphocyte transformation finally leading to clonal expansion as an indirect mechanism of pathogenesis has been proposed. Sustained stimulation of lymphocyte receptors by viral antigens, viral replication in B-cells, and damage of B-cells have been also proposed as mechanisms of pathogenesis.

Expression of HCV viral proteins in B-cells of HCV-infected patients upregulates B-cell receptor signaling. Pro-inflammatory cytokines, such as the interleukins (IL-6, IL-17 and IL-10) and transforming growth factor-beta have also been reported to contribute to aberrant B-cell proliferation.

Glomerular injury in HCV-related glomerulonephritis is primary induced by a deposition of circulating immunocomplexes containing anti-HCV antibodies, HCV antigens and complement factors. Formation and deposition of such immunocomplexes occurs also in absence of cryoglobulins. Formation of glomerular antibodies is a further possible mechanism of HCV-related glomerular injury.

Peripheral nerves of patients with HCV-related peripheral neuropathy may show vasculitic changes involving the vasa nervorum, giving a possible explanation of nerve damage.

Studies have shown that dysthyroidism is mediated by immunological mechanisms rather than by direct HCV infection. The pathogenesis may involve changes in self-antigen expression and sustained stimulation of the immune system by HCV, bystander activation of autoreactive T-cells by cytokine release, infection of the lymphatic cells, chromosomal aberrations and abnormal expression of major histocompatibility complex class II molecules by thyrocytes, or cross-reactivity between viral antigens and thyroidal antigens.

Primary causation of dermatological EHM (apart the cryoglobulinaemic ones) results from direct infection of HCV in the skin, lymphocytes, dendritic antigen-presenting cells, and blood vessels. Secondary causation occurs when HCV infection manifests in the skin due to epiphenomena resulting from the disruption of immune responses [2–4, 6, 7].

The most common extrahepatic findings with which the relationship to HCV infection is more strongly established are cryoglobulinemia, autoimmune disorders (including autoantibodies and SS), porphyria cutanea tarda (PCT), and lichen planus (LP). There also appears to be a clear association with B-cell NHL (particularly in patients with underlying cryoglobulinemia), but the incidence of lymphoma among HCV-infected patients overall remains low.

3. Mixed cryoglobulinemia

MC is the most frequent, best known and strictly HCV-associated EHM (about 90% of MC patients tested positive for HCV antibodies in some studies) [7, 8].

MC may be defined a both autoimmune and B-lymphoproliferative disorder (LPD) that may evolve to a frank malignancy in about 8–10% of cases [9].

The definition of MC refers to the presence of serum Igs that reversibly precipitate at low temperatures (<37°C) and are represented by circulating immune complex typically consisting of an IgM rheumatoid factor (mono-oligoclonal in type II MC, or polyclonal in type III MC) and polyclonal Ig (most frequently IgG) including anti-HCV antibodies. MC has been generally reported, at least subclinical, in the majority of HCV patients, even if data may widely vary in different geographical areas (from 20 to >50%). Only a minority of MC patients (5 to >30%) shows a symptomatic MC or MC syndrome (usually women aged more than 50 years), but even asymptomatic patients might develop MC in the future [10].

Factors that seem to favor the development of MC are female sex, increasing age, alcohol consumption (> 50 g/day), advanced liver fibrosis and steatosis.

The clinical manifestations of MC are secondary to a systemic vasculitis characterized by the deposition of cryoglobulins in the vessels and can be classified as one of the circulating immune complexes mediated systemic vasculitis involving small and medium-sized blood vessels.

The classic syndrome of MC consists in the triad of purpura, fatigue and arthralgia, but the various involvement of different organs and tissues (mainly skin, joints, renal, peripheral nerves) leads to variable clinical presentation and evolution.

Palpable purpura (leukocytoclastic vasculitis) and petechiae most often affects the legs (**Figure 2**).

Papules, ulcers, and livedo can also occur and can affect any skin site.

Reynaud Syndrome can be present, with or without digital gangrene, in about one third of patients.

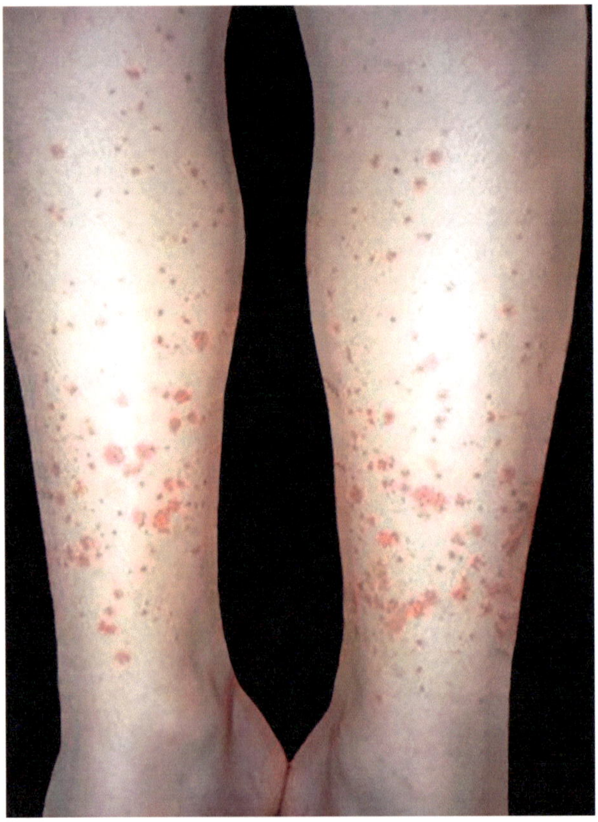

Figure 2.
Cutaneous manifestation of mixed cryoglobulinemia (see text).

Common manifestations of MC are arthralgias (polyarthralgia, but relatively rare is arthritis), renal disease, usually membranoproliferative glomerulonephritis (MPGN), and neurologic disease.

MPGN is characterized in most cases by proteinuria, mild haematuria and mild renal insufficiency. In the worst cases, a severe involvement of the kidney is observed (15% of cases).

The peripheral neuropathy including mixed neuropathies (prevalently sensitive, axonal) is common in MC (80–90% of cases), and also in HCV without MC (see below 9.).

HCV-related peripheral neuropathy is characterized by numbness, burning skin and pruritus.

Central nervous system involvement in patients with HCV-positive MC is rare (see below 9).

4. Sicca syndrome (secondary Sjögren syndrome)

Sjögren syndrome is described as a chronic, slowly progressive autoimmune disease characterized by lymphocytic infiltration of the exocrine glands and B-lymphocyte reactivity resulting in xerostomia and dry eyes. SS, to be differentiated from the primary Sjögren Syndrome, occurs in MC and also in HCV patients without MC [2–4]. In most instances the typical serological and histopathologic findings of Sjögren Syndrome are lacking. SS is more frequently reported in type II than in type III MC [2, 4].

Some studies showed an association between MC in HCV infected patients and severe liver damage [11].

However, discordant data exist. It is common clinical experience, including our own, to find patients with symptomatic HCV-related MC and a mild or moderate liver disease and conversely patients with the most severe form of chronic hepatitis C (advanced fibrosis, compensated and decompensated cirrhosis, hepatocellular carcinoma) without any symptom of MC (even when laboratory testing positive for MC).

5. Non-Hodgkin lymphoma and other hematological disorders

5.1 Non-Hodgkin lymphoma

The very close association between MC and HCV infection leads to the hypothesis that HCV may be involved in the pathogenesis of lymphoma as well.

A significant association between HCV and B-cell NHL was reported and confirmed in the large majority of studies [12].

This association involves different histopathological types of B-cell NHL, the most strictly associated being the lymphoplasmacytic, marginal zone and diffuse large B-cell lymphoma.

Some discordant data suggested the contribution of genetic factors and the incidence of lymphoma among HCV-infected patients overall remains low.

In an observational, prospective, multicenter, case–control study, the prevalence of HCV-antibodies was found of 0.16 among NHL and of 0.085 among controls and non-lymphoid malignancies patients [13].

Although the difference was statistically significant ($P < 0.001$), the odds ratio was 2.049 and its confidence intervals included the equality. NHL features

Feature (overall freq.)	HCV-positive NHL (48)		HCV-negative NHL (252)	
	Bearing feature	Freq. (conf. Int. 95%)	Bearing feature	Freq. (conf. Int. 95%)
Extranodal inv. (0.593)	30	0.625 (0.488–0.762)	148	0.587 (0.526–0.648)
Marrow inv. (0.283)	16	0.333 (0.200–0.466)	69	0.274 (0.219–0.329)
Stomach inv. (0.067)	2	0.042[a]	18	0.071 (0.039–0.103)
Liver inv. (0.030)	4	0.083 (0.005–0.161)	5	0.020 (0.003–0.037)
Cryoglobulinis (0.033)	3	0.063[a]	7	0.028 (0.026–0.030)
Age to 20 (0.007)	0	0	2	0.008[a]
Age 21–40 (0.090)	2	0.042[a]	25	0.099 (0.062–0.136)
Age 41–60 (0.300)	12	0.250 (0.128–0.372)	78	0.310 (0.253–0.367)
Age > 60 (0.603)	34	0.708 (0.579–0.837)	147	0.583 (0.522–0.643)
WF A, B, C[b] (0.286)	14	0.304 (0.071–0.437)	70	0.283 (0.227–0.339)
WF D, E, F[b] (0.248)	10	0.217 (0.098–0.336)	63	0.255 (0.201–0.309)
WF G, H, I, J[b] (0.464)	22	0.478 (0.334–0.622)	114	0.462 (0.400–0.524)
MALT (0.053)	3	0.062[a]	13	0.052 (0.022–0.088)

[a]*Lower confidence limit below.*
[b]*WF classification is available for 293.*

Table 1.
NHL features among HCV-positive and HCV-negative patients [13].

among HCV-positive and HCV-negative patients observed in this study are reported in the **Table 1**.

5.2 Serum monoclonal gammopathy and thrombocytopenia

A serum monoclonal gammopathy (MG), more frequently type IgMk and diagnosed as MG of uncertain significance (MGUS), was frequently observed in HCV patients, in most cases associated with a 2a/c genotype of the virus.

Available data suggest that HCV-related LPD are the result of multiple and cooperating mechanisms and events belonging to three principal categories: an important and sustained activation of the B-cell compartment; an inhibition of B-cell apoptosis; genetic/epigenetic and environmental factors (see also above 2.).

Thrombocytopenia is often observed in patients with chronic HCV hepatitis and sometimes it is disproportionally severe with respect of the stage of fibrosis-cirrhosis.

It is possible recognize as causal factors of thrombocytopenia in HCV chronic hepatitis the following: decrease of hepatic thrombopoietin, direct cytopathic involvement of HCV on megakaryocytes, production of platelets-associated immunoglobulins, hypersplenism.

6. Endocrine pathology and hepatitis C virus infection

6.1 Thyroid disease

The prevalence of thyroid disorders is generally high in HCV-positive patients and most frequently represented by antithyroid peroxidase antibodies in female subjects. Hypothyroidism has been frequently observed, especially in HCV MC, and an association with papillary thyroid carcinoma was also shown [14].

6.2 Type 2 diabetes mellitus and glucose intolerance

Several studies showed that HCV (especially genotype 3) could lead to the development of type 2 diabetes mellitus, possibly as a result of HCV-induced metabolic disturbances. However, discordant data exist. Insulin resistance was observed in 30–70% of HCV patients [3, 15].

The cause of the association of HCV with diabetes is unknown. In addition, the magnitude of the association may be overestimated because patients with diabetes have more parenteral exposures than the general population, placing them at increased risk for transmission of blood transmitted viruses. Furthermore, not all studies controlled for the presence of cirrhosis, which may be associated with impaired glucose tolerance.

7. Autoimmune and rheumatologic disorders

7.1 Autoantibodies

A number of autoimmune disorders have been associated with chronic HCV infection, including subclinical autoantibody formation, autoimmune thyroid disease, sialadenitis/SS, and autoimmune thrombocytopenic purpura.

Autoantibodies are common in patients with chronic HCV infection. Antinuclear antibodies, antibodies directed against the Fc portion of IgG (rheumatoid factor), anticardiolipin antibodies, smooth muscle antibodies, or antithyroid antibodies are detected in 40 to 65 percent of patients. While antibodies are often present in low titres, do not appear to influence the presentation or course of the infection.

Nevertheless, the presence of autoantibodies may result in diagnostic difficulties.

For example, an HCV-infected patient with arthralgias, arthritis, and rheumatoid factor positivity may be misdiagnosed initially as having rheumatoid arthritis. In this setting, testing for other rheumatoid-arthritis-associated autoantibodies that are observed infrequently in patients with HCV infection, such as anti-citrullinated peptide antibodies (anti-CCP), may be helpful diagnostically.

In other cases, a difficult differential diagnosis between hepatitis C and autoimmune hepatitis can rise. In these cases, the liver biopsy findings are decisive. In rare cases the two disease coexist in the same patient.

Making a precise diagnosis is crucial because the treatment is completely different.

7.2 Rheumatologic disorders

Polyarthralgia is the most common rheumatologic symptom described in HCV-infected patients. HCV arthritis could be part of the MC or be independent. HCV-associated oligoarticular or polyarticular non-erosive arthritis can clinically mimic rheumatoid arthritis, although anti-CCP antibodies and erosive joint changes are generally absent [2].

8. Renal disease

Several renal manifestations have been associated with HCV infection, the most common being MPGN. HCV-associated membranous or proliferative glomerulonephritis or focal segmental glomerulosclerosis have been also described. The strongest association was reported for cryoglobulinaemic MPGN. Microhaematuria and proteinuria are the most frequent clinical findings of MPGN. The presence of a renal involvement is one of the worst prognostic indices in the natural history of MC [16].

9. Neurological disorders

Peripheral neuropathy: see above, in the context of MC. Less frequently, peripheral neuropathy can be present without MC. Peripheral neuropathy can be sensory or sensorimotor.

Symptoms of fatigue and deficits in concentration and working memory are commonly reported in patients with chronic HCV infection. Some studies have suggested neurocognitive impairments associated with HCV, even after controlling for other comorbid conditions, such as substance abuse, affective disorders, and cirrhosis. Functional imaging studies have also identified metabolic changes in the central nervous system in the setting of HCV infection (not ascribable to hepatic encephalopathy) [3].

10. Dermatological manifestations

Apart the dermatological manifestations of MC (see above 3.) the are other dermatological conditions associated with HCV infection deserving to be discussed.

10.1 Lichen planus

Cutaneous LP is characterized by flat-topped, pink to violaceous, pruritic papules with a potentially generalized distribution. The papules appear

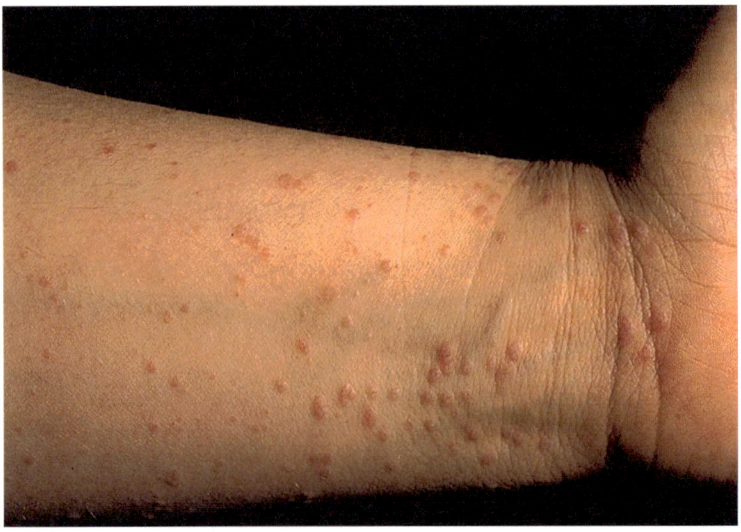

Figure 3.
Typical manifestation of lichen planus of the volar distal forearm and wrist in a hepatitis C patient (see text).

polygonal-shaped, translucent under incident light. They are 2–4 mm in diameter, with irregular margins and a hard-elastic consistency (**Figure 3**). LP can also involve mucus membranes, hair, and nails.

HCV infection has been reported frequently among patients with LP. In some studies, the prevalence of anti-HCV antibodies in patients with LP ranges from 10 to 40%.

Systematic reviews have reported that patients with oral LP planus are approximately two to six times more likely to have reactive anti-HCV antibodies compared with controls, although there is substantial geographical heterogeneity to the findings.

LP can be seen in patients with a variety of liver diseases, particularly advanced liver disease.

There is evidence of a genetic risk for HCV-associated LP. The most commonly used drugs in cutaneous LP are topical and systemic corticosteroids, for their immunosuppressive and anti-inflammatory effects [4, 17, 18].

10.2 Porphyria cutanea tarda

PCT is a disease caused by reduced activity of the enzyme uroporphyrinogen decarboxylase (UROD), causing the subsequent build-up of uroporphyrinogen in the blood and urine. PCT has both sporadic and inherited (autosomal dominant) forms that are indistinguishable clinically. A strong association between the sporadic form of PCT and HCV infection has been demonstrated in multiple studies (an overall prevalence of HCV of 50%). However, there was marked geographic variability; lowest prevalence rates (20 to 30%) were observed in reports from Australia, the Czech Republic, and France, while the highest rates (71 to 85%) were observed in Japan, Italy, and Spain. The prevalence in North America was 66%.

A central factor in the geographic variability appeared to be the baseline rates of HCV infection in the general population.

The skin and the liver are the two main sites affected in sporadic PCT. Skin disease is characterized by photosensitivity and skin fragility, with which exposure

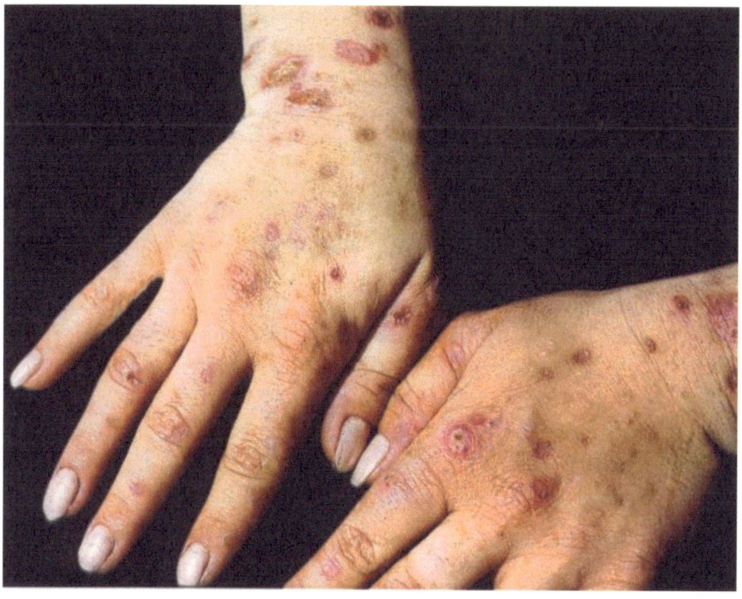

Figure 4.
Typical cutaneous manifestations of porphyria cutanea tarda (see text).

to the sun and/or minor trauma can lead to skin erythema and the development of vesicles and bullae that may become haemorrhagic.

Hyperpigmentation, hypopigmentation, hirsutism, and sclerodermatous changes may develop with the passage of time (**Figure 4**).

Chronic liver disease is common in sporadic PCT. Liver biopsy shows a wide range of changes, including steatosis, mild to severe inflammation, hepatic fibrosis, and cirrhosis. Environmental triggers are thought to be necessary to provoke an attack of PCT. Possible triggers of PCT include polyhalogenated hydrocarbons (such as hexachlorobenzene), oestrogens, but above all, iron overload and alcoholic beverages. The diagnosis of PCT is typically suspected on clinical grounds and is confirmed by the demonstration of markedly elevated urine uroporphyrin levels. The diagnosis can also be made directly by measuring hepatic UROD activity. All patients with PCT should be tested for HCV infection, as well as other potential disease associations, including HIV infection, iron overload, and hemochromatosis (with HFE mutation testing). Careful history of alcohol intake and testing of heavy alcohol intake markers are fundamental.

Management of PCT in patients with HCV infection includes avoiding precipitating factors (such as sun, alcohol, oestrogens, and polyhalogenated hydrocarbons), treating an underlying iron overload state, if present, and treating HCV infection.

PCT often, but not always, improves with clearance of HCV viremia. The currently used pharmacological protocol for PCT include the administration of a half tablet of chloroquine (125 mg) twice a week [19, 20].

11. Cardiovascular and respiratory diseases

Although data from individual cohorts have not been consistent, evidence overall suggests that chronic HCV infection is associated with adverse cardiovascular diseases and outcomes: dilated cardiomyopathy, hypertrophic cardiomyopathy and arrhythmogenic right ventricular cardiomyopathy, myocarditis, and aortic atherosclerosis. These associations are still object of debate. Because cardiovascular diseases are common and multifactorial, it is difficult to determine whether HCV is a major contributing factor in an individual patient [3].

Idiopathic pulmonary fibrosis is a serious condition described in association with HCV infection.

12. Clinical implications and laboratory tests

Because of the associations, it is suggested testing for HCV infection in patients with clinical condition described above and other suspected to be linked to HCV. Anti-HCV antibodies (an inexpensive test) must be checked and if positive, quantitative HCV-RNA, genotype and complete workup of hepatitis C performed.

Conversely, patients diagnosed with chronic HCV infection should have evaluation for EHM at the initial visit and routinely during follow-up. History of an HCV-infected patient should cover rheumatologic symptoms (e.g., arthritis/arthralgias, dry eyes or mouth) and the physical exam should include a skin exam to evaluate for findings of cryoglobulinemia, PCT, and other associated dermatologic features. Superficial lymph node sites must be checked. Abdominal ultrasound is part of the HCV patient evaluation. It is in addiction necessary to perform a chest x-ray with particular attention to the mediastinum.

Laboratory testing should include a complete blood count, an assessment of renal function, evaluation for proteinuria and haematuria, and thyroid function tests. Cryoglobulins and complement levels should be checked if there is evidence of renal disease or other compatible clinical findings. Testing for other EHM should be guided by symptoms or specific physical findings.

Mild serum amylase elevation is a common finding in HCV patients generally without any pancreatic involvement clinically detectable.

13. Treatment of extrahepatic manifestations of HCV infection

13.1 Antiviral treatment

The armamentarium against HCV has been expanded with the availability of molecules able to directly target non-structural proteins that play a key role in HCV replication. These agents, orally administrated for a relatively short period of time (2–3 months) have been called direct acting antivirals (DAA) and target some of the main molecular components of HCV, including NS3/4A protease (first and second-generation protease inhibitors), NS5B polymerase (nucleoside and non-nucleoside analogues) and NS5A protein.

DAA can cure more than 95% of persons with HCV infection, thereby reducing the risk of death from cirrhosis and liver cancer.

Antiviral treatment is recommended for all patients with EHM.

Because of their not negligible rate of contraindications, important side effects, scarce tolerability, low compliance and adherence, length course of treatment, parenteral route of administration, and the insufficient rate of sustained virological response (SVR) obtainable (not more than 60%), the interferon (IFN) based therapies for HCV hepatitis must be considered obsolete.

Moreover, IFN, with its immunological stimulating properties, could be contraindicated and possibly worsen or elicit some EHM (for example thyroid disfunction, autoimmune EHM). A caution attitude could be suggested also in MC, exacerbated in some cases treated with IFN alone (without glucocorticoids).

The antiviral drug ribavirin maintains a very marginal role in this context. Ribavirin common side effects are dermatologic and require caution if used in cutaneous EHM of HCV hepatitis.

DAA-based, IFN-free regimens should be considered the standard antiviral therapeutic approach in HCV-related EHM [21].

At the present, DAA-based, IFN-free regimens should be used following the recommendations for individuals with HCV mono-infection in the current international guidelines.

Detailed assessment of drug–drug interactions is crucial since some medications are contraindicated or not recommended during DAA therapy [22, 23].

The vast majority of studies on the use of antiviral therapies in EHM - HCV diseases have been carried out in patients with MC vasculitis, which is considered the prototype of systemic autoimmune disease associated with HCV, both for their frequency and potential life-threatening involvement. All reported studies show that vasculitic manifestations largely improve after antiviral treatment (even in patients with partial virological responses) and often disappear, especially in patients with SVR.

Treatment of low-grade lymphomas only with DAAs antiviral therapies may be recommended whereas more aggressive lymphomas would require the addition of chemotherapy/rituximab.

IFN-free antiviral regimens might be less effective than IFN-containing regimens in some patients with B cell lymphoma, possibly due to the lack of additional anti-proliferative activity of IFN, while the association of rituximab with DAA regimens could be more effective than isolated antiviral therapies.

At the present there is little data on the response of other EHM to DAAs antiviral therapies for HCV hepatitis.

13.2 Non antiviral treatment of HCV-extrahepatic manifestations

Non-antiviral therapeutic approaches should be evaluated according to the type of EHM and the severity of the clinical presentation. The non-antiviral therapeutic approaches mainly used in EHM patients include glucocorticosteroids, immunosuppressant agents, plasma exchange and biological therapies.

Non-antiviral therapeutic approaches are recommended for moderate and, especially, for severe organ-specific involvements. Patients with moderate to severe vasculitic manifestations may be treated with short-term glucocorticoid regimens to control inflammation rapidly. Regimens of methylprednisolone (0.5–1.0 g/day) for three days followed by prednisone (not exceeding 1 mg/kg/day) may be appropriate in the setting of skin ulceration, sensorimotor neuropathy, glomerulonephritis, and other severe vasculitic manifestations.

For aggressive B cell NHL, the therapy remains based on immunochemotherapy with anthracycline-containing regimens in combination with rituximab as in HCV-negative patients.

Plasma exchange may be added to other therapies, especially in patients with severe/life-threatening cryoglobulinaemic vasculitis. Such intervention is useful in patients with immediately life-threatening involvements and for those with hyperviscosity syndrome. Apheresis techniques should always be used as a complementary therapy in combination with other strategies (antiviral therapies, B cell depleting agents).

B cell depleting agents may currently be considered to be the best biological target option for patients with the more severe EHM, always with a reasonable individualized assessment of the benefits and risks. The most promising non-antiviral therapeutic approach to HCV-related cryoglobulinemia is rituximab.

The use of antiviral therapies in combination with immunosuppressant/biological agents should normally be made sequentially (first, use immunosuppressant/biological agents and, once the major end-organ effects have been controlled, use antiviral therapy), or concomitantly. It seems reasonable to carry out the combination on a case by-case basis [21].

The orally active thrombopoietin-receptor agonist elthrombopag may be used in severe thrombocytopenic HCV patients.

Appropriate local and systemic treatments are needed for cutaneous and ocular EHM of HCV (see above 10.) [18, 20].

14. Prevention of extrahepatic manifestations treating HCV hepatitis with DAAs

In a large population study, it was found that successful DAA treatment resulting in SVR was associated with significant reductions in the future risk of several EHM of HCV, including MC, glomerulonephritis and LP but not NHL or diabetes. The magnitude of risk reductions ranged between 0.23 and 0.61.

SVR was associated with a reduction in risk of PCT, but it was only marginally statistically significant [24].

15. Conclusions

Chronic HCV infection can cause significant EHM and should be considered as a systemic disease rather than a disease affecting only the liver.

EHM of HCV can affect virtually every organ via a variety of mechanisms.

It is important to emphasize that the severity of these disorders does not necessarily correlate with the severity of hepatic disease.

Some investigations have shown that therapy of chronic HCV infection can result in resolution or improvement of extrahepatic diseases linked to HCV and even prevent their onset.

Awareness on the part of the clinician is necessary to recognize these numerous and heterogeneous pathological conditions. This in turn can lead to appropriate screening, early treatment and improved outcomes [4, 6].

Acknowledgements

The author acknowledges Prof. Alberto Giannetti for the permission of reproducing **Figure 3**.

Author details

Alberto Frosi
Multimedica Hospital and Scientific Institute, Sesto San Giovanni, (Milano), Italy

*Address all correspondence to: albertofrosi21@gmail.com

References

[1] Spearman CW, Dusheiko GM, Hellard M, Sonderup M. Hepatitis C. Lancet 2019; 394:1451-1466.

[2] Zignego AL, Ferri C, Pileri SA, Caini P, Bianchi FB. Extrahepatic manifestations of Hepatitis C Virus infection: a general overview and guidelines for a clinical approach. Dig Liver Dis 2007; 39:2-17.

[3] Negro F, Forton D, Craxì, Sulkowski MS, Feld JJ, Manns. Extrahepatic morbidity and mortality of chronic hepatitis C. Gastroenterology 2015; 149:1345-1360.

[4] Gill K, Ghazinian H, Manch R, Gish R. Hepatitis C virus as a systemic disease: reaching beyond the liver. Hepatol Int 2016; 10:415-423.

[5] Altman N, Krzywinski M. Association, correlation and causation. Nature Methods 2015; 12: 899-900.

[6] Kuna L, Jakab J, Smolic R, Wu GY, Smolic M. HCV Extrahepatic Manifestations. Journal of Clinical and Translational Hepatology 2019;7: 172-182.

[7] Schamberg NJ, Lake-Bakaar GV. Hepatitis C Virus-related Mixed Cryoglobulinemia: Pathogenesis, Clinical Manifestations, and New Therapies. Gastroenterology and Hepatology 2007; 3: 695-703.

[8] Ferri C, Monti M, La Civita L, Longombardo G, Greco F, Pasero G, Gentilini P, Bombardieri S, Zignego AL. Infection of peripheral blood mononuclear cells by hepatitis C virus in mixed cryoglobulinemia. Blood 1993; 82:3701-3704.

[9] Morra E. Cryoglobulinemia. Hematology 2005;1: 368-372.

[10] Lunel F, Musset L, Cacoub P, Frangeul L, Cresta P, Perrin M, Grippon P, Hoang C, Piette JC, Hureaux JM, Opolon. Cryoglobulinemia in chronic liver diseases: role of hepatitis C virus and liver damage. Gastroenterology 1994; 106:1291-1300.

[11] Kayali Z, Buckwold VE, Zimmerman B, Schmidt WN. Hepatitis C, cryoglobulinemia, and cirrhosis: a meta-analysis. Hepatology 2002; 36:978-985.

[12] Giordano TP, Henderson L, Landgren O, Chiao EY, Kramer JR, El-Serag H, Engels EA. Risk of non-Hodgkin lymphoma and lymphoproliferative precursor diseases in US veterans with hepatitis C virus. JAMA 2007; 297:2010-2017.

[13] Pioltelli P , Gargantini L, Cassi E, Santoleri E, Bellati G, Magliano EM, Morra E. Hepatitis C virus in non-Hodgkin's lymphoma. A reappraisal after a prospective case-control study of 300 patients. Lombard Study Group of HCV-Lymphoma (Frosi A. and others). Am J Hematol 2000; 64:95-100.

[14] Antonelli A, Ferri C, Pampana A, Fallahi P, Nesti C, Pasquini M, Marchi S, Ferrannini E. Thyroid disorders in chronic hepatitis C. Am J Med 2004;117:10-13.

[15] White DL, Ratziu V, El-Serag HB. Hepatitis C infection and risk of diabetes: a systematic review and meta-analysis. J Hepatol 2008; 49:831-844.

[16] Martin P, Fabrizi F. Hepatitis C virus and kidney disease. Journal of Hepatology 2008; 49: 613-624.

[17] Mignogna MD, Lo Muzio L, Lo Russo L, Fedele S, Ruoppo E, Bucci E. Oral lichen planus: different clinical features in HCV-positive and HCV-negative patients. Int J Dermatol 2000; 39:134-139.

[18] Cottoni F, Montesu MA. Lichen Planus, Lichen Nitidus. In:

Giannetti A, Del Forno C, editors. Textbook of Dermatology and Sexual Transmitted Diseases. Piccin; 2013. p. 1225-1244.

[19] Gisbert JP, García-Buey L, Pajares JM, Moreno-Otero R. Prevalence of hepatitis C virus infection in porphyria cutanea tarda: systematic review and meta-analysis. J Hepat 2003; 39: 620-627.

[20] Biolcati G. Porphyrias. In: Giannetti A, Del Forno C, editors. Textbook of Dermatology and Sexual Transmitted Diseases. Piccin; 2013. p. 2021-2044.

[21] Ramos-Casals M, Zignego AL , Ferri C, Brito-Zerón P, Retamozo S, Casato M, Lamprecht P, Mangia A, Saadoun D, Tzioufas AG, Younossi ZM, Cacoub P, on behalf of the International Study Group of Extrahepatic Manifestations related to HCV (ISG-EHCV). Evidence-based recommendations on the management of extrahepatic manifestations of chronic hepatitis C virus infection. J Hepat 2017; 66:1282-1299.

[22] AASLD-IDSA Hepatitis C Guidance Panel. Hepatitis C Guidance 2019 Update: American Association for the Study of Liver Diseases–Infectious Diseases Society of America Recommendations for Testing, Managing, and Treating Hepatitis C Virus Infection. Hepatology 2020;71: 686-721.

[23] European Association for the Study of the Liver. EASL recommendations on treatment of hepatitis C: Final update of the series. J Hepatol 2020;73: 1170-1218.

[24] El-Serag HB, Christie IC, Puenpatom A, Castillo D, Kanwal F, Kramer JR. The effects of directly acting antiviral-related sustained virological response on the risk of extrahepatic manifestations of hepatitis C infection. Aliment Pharmacol Ther 2019; 49:1442-1447.

Section 4

Antiviral Treatments

Chapter 4

Host-Targeting Antivirals for Treatment of Hepatitis C

Bouchra Kitab, Michinori Kohara and Kyoko Tsukiyama-Kohara

Abstract

Treatment of chronic hepatitis C virus (HCV) infection has been revolutionized during last years with the development of highly potent direct-acting antivirals (DAAs) specifically targeting HCV proteins. DAAs are the current standard of care for patients with chronic hepatitis C, leading to high cure rates. However, some hurdles exist including the high cost of these therapies restricting access to patients, their inability to protect against the risk of developing hepatocellular carcinoma in patients with advanced fibrosis, and emergence of resistant variants resulting in treatment failure. New therapeutic options should be essential to overcome DAAs limitations and improve survival. By targeting host-cell factors involved in HCV life cycle, host-targeting antivirals (HTAs) offer opportunity for promising anti-HCV therapy with low mutational rate and may act in a synergistic manner with DAAs to prevent viral resistance and reduce viral replication. Moreover, HTAs could be effective in difficult-to-cure patients by acting through complementary mechanisms. In this chapter, we will focus on the latest and most relevant studies regarding the host-cell factors required in HCV infection and explored as targets of antiviral therapy, we will also discuss the HTAs evaluated in preclinical and clinical development and their potential role as alternative or complementary therapeutic strategies.

Keywords: chronic hepatitis C, direct-acting antivirals, cell factors, host-targeting antivirals, antiviral therapy

1. Introduction

Hepatitis C virus (HCV) is a major causative agent of chronic liver diseases. Globally, it is estimated that 71 million people have chronic HCV infection, defined as the persistence of HCV genome in the blood for at least six months after the onset of acute infection [1, 2]. Patients with chronic HCV infection are at high risk of developing liver cirrhosis, hepatic decompensation, and hepatocellular carcinoma (HCC), which are the most common indications for liver transplantation [3]. Until 2011, the standard-of-care therapy for HCV infection consisted on pegylated-interferon alpha in combination with the nucleotide analogue ribavirin (peg-IFNα/RBV) leading to sustained virologic response (SVR) in 54–63% of patients with substantial side effects [4, 5]. The great advances in HCV research allowed the development of direct-acting antivirals (DAAs) which have dramatically improved the standard-of-care for HCV-infected patients [6, 7]. As their name suggests, DAAs are class of antivirals that directly target viral proteins required in HCV replication.

IntechOpen

The first-generation DAAs used in combination with peg-IFNα/RBV improve SVR rates by approximately 70% [8, 9]. Subsequently, IFN-free DAAs regimens, based on the use of highly potent and well-tolerated DAAs combinations were introduced and currently used for treatment, providing SVR in more than 95% of patients, with minimal side effects [10, 11].

Although DAAs offer the chance of viral cure for most of HCV patients, there are some limitations that restrain their full potential, including their high cost limiting access to treatment, the high mutation rate of HCV which may lead to the selection of DAA-resistant HCV variants resulting in treatment failure, and the low SVR rate in difficult-to-treat patients such as those with advanced liver cirrhosis [12–14]. Recent studies reported the inability of DAAs to protect against the risk of HCV re-infection of liver graft in transplanted patients, or the risk of developing HCC in patients with advanced liver fibrosis [15, 16]. Consequently, there is a need for other therapeutic options with better affordability, high rate of viral cure, and fewer cases of viral resistance. HCV requires host-cell factors to establish productive infection and propagation, thus development of host-targeting antivirals (HTAs) that interfere with these factors provides promising antiviral candidates, which may help to improve the current landscape of hepatitis C therapy [14, 17]. Several HTAs have been evaluated for preclinical and clinical development with some of them showing promising results. In this chapter, we provide an overview on recent advances in antiviral therapies against HCV and highlight the most important host factors explored as therapeutic targets. We also discuss the different HTAs evaluated in preclinical and clinical development and their potential impact as alternative or complementary therapeutic options to cure HCV infection and associated liver diseases.

2. Molecular virology of HCV

HCV is an enveloped, positive-sense single-stranded RNA virus, classified in the *hepacivirus* genus of *Flaviviridae* family [18]. HCV genomic RNA (~9.6 kb in length) contains highly structured 5′- and 3′-untranslated regions (UTRs) flanking a single open reading frame [19, 20]. The 5'-UTR is highly conserved and contains an internal ribosome entry site (IRES) essential to initiate viral RNA translation [21]. The high error prone of HCV NS5B RNA-dependent RNA polymerase leads to frequent mutations across the viral genome, resulting in high intra-patient variability (1–5%) represented in the form of quasispecies, and high inter-patient variability manifested by the existence of 7 genotypes, and 67 confirmed subtypes [22, 23]. HCV genotypes differ from each other by 31–33% at nucleotide level, compared with 15–25% between subtypes within a given genotype [24]. A global survey showed that HCV genotypes 1 and 3 are the most prevalent worldwide accounting for 46% and 30% of global HCV cases, respectively. Genotypes 2, 4, 5, and 6 are responsible for the majority of remaining HCV cases: 9%, 8%, <1%, and 5.4%, respectively [25]. Genotype 7 has been identified in Canada in few patients originating from Central Africa [26]. HCV genotypes have distinct geographic distributions throughout the world, which reflect differences in mode of transmission and ethnic variability. While genotype 1a is predominant in USA, genotype 1b dominated in Europe and Japan, genotype 2 dominated in West Africa and parts of South America, genotype 3 in south Asia, genotype 4 in middle East and Central/North Africa, genotype 5 in South Africa, and genotype 6 in Southeast Asia [25].

HCV replication cycle initiates through viral attachment and entry into the hepatocyte by clathrin-mediated endocytosis [27, 28]. The acidic pH of the early endosomes is essential to trigger fusion leading to nucleocapsid uncoating and release of the viral RNA genome in the cytosol [29]. At the rough endoplasmic reticulum (ER), HCV genomic RNA is translated via an HCV-IRES mediated mechanism to produce a single polyprotein of ~3010 amino acids [30]. This polyprotein is cleaved by cellular and viral proteases into three structural proteins that build up the HCV particle (Core and envelope glycoproteins E1 and E2) and seven nonstructural (NS) proteins permitting viral RNA replication, and viral particle assembly (p7, NS2, NS3, NS4A, NS4B, NS5A, and NS5B) [31]. The viroporin p7 and the cysteine protease NS2 are involved in viral particle assembly. NS3, NS4A, NS4B, NS5A, NS5B and HCV genomic RNA template form the viral replicase complex for HCV RNA replication [31, 32]. As all positive-strand RNA viruses, HCV induces massive rearrangements of cytoplasmic membranes in the host cell to generate a replication-favorable compartment called "the membranous web" in the case of HCV [33]. The membranous web is mainly composed of double membrane vesicles (DMVs) derived from the ER and may serve to increase the local concentration of viral proteins and relevant host cell factors required for efficient viral RNA replication [33, 34]. Within the replicase complex, the plus-strand RNA genome is replicated into a minus-strand RNA intermediate, which then gives rise to multiple plus-stranded HCV RNA copies [35]. The importance of specific lipids in HCV RNA replication has been highlighted. Indeed, HCV infection induces synthesis of specific sphingolipids that enhance NS5B-mediated RNA replication [36].

The newly progeny plus-strand RNAs can either be used for translation, therefore production of new viral proteins, or synthesis of new minus-strand RNAs, or packaged into viral particles. It has been shown that HCV assembly initiates at the ER membrane in close proximity to lipid droplets where the viral RNA is packaged into capsids [37]. HCV proteins NS5A and core have been reported as key players in the translocation of viral structures from the replication complex to lipid droplets [38]. The nascent nucleocapsids bud into the ER thereby acquiring a ER-derived lipid bilayer envelope in which the viral glycoproteins E1 and E2 are anchored as heterodimers [39]. Interestingly, a peculiar feature of HCV is its association with host lipoproteins and apolipoproteins such as ApoE, ApoB, and ApoA1, leading to the formation of lipo-viroparticles (LVPs) [40, 41]. Incorporation of host lipoproteins into HCV virions plays an essential role in virus infectivity and immune escape [40]. Next, LVPs traffic through the Golgi secretory pathway for final egress [42]. Several key components of the endosomal transport system are necessary for the egress of HCV LVPs, including the endosomal-sorting complex required for transport (ESCRT) pathway and Rab proteins [43, 44]. Estimations showed that approximatively 1.3×10^{12} HCV virions are produced per day in each infected patient [45].

3. Impact of current antiviral therapies in the clinical outcome of hepatitis C

There are three critical points in the natural history of HCV infection including development of chronic hepatitis C, development of liver cirrhosis, and development of cirrhosis-related complications including portal hypertension and hepatocellular carcinoma (HCC) [46]. Chronic hepatitis C is a slowly progressive disease. It is estimated that 20–30% of chronic HCV patients develop liver cirrhosis over a 20 years period [46]. A deep inter-individual variability exists in the progression of hepatitis C and response to antiviral treatment, mainly related to viral factors such as HCV genotype, viral load, or coinfection with hepatitis B virus (HBV) or human immunodeficiency virus (HIV), and host factors such as patient's genetic background including interleukin-28B (IL-28B) polymorphism, age, gender, and obesity [47, 48].

The ultimate aim of antiviral treatment is to cure chronic HCV infection, in order to prevent the progression to liver cirrhosis and severe hepatic events (decompensation and HCC), and thereby improve patient survival and prevent

HCV transmission. Viral cure, known as sustained virological response (SVR) is defined as undetectable HCV RNA in blood 12–24 weeks after completing antiviral treatment [49, 50]. Current anti-HCV treatment consists on all-oral, IFN-free regimens combining highly potent, and well tolerated DAAs achieving SVR rates over 95% [11, 50]. DAAs specifically target HCV nonstructural proteins resulting in disruption of HCV replication (**Figure 1**). According to the therapeutic target and mechanism of action, DAAs are divided into four categories: NS3/4A protease inhibitors (e.g. simeprevir, paritaprevir, glecaprevir), NS5A protein inhibitors (e.g. velpatasvir, daclatasvir, pibrentasvir), NS5B nucleoside polymerase inhibitors and NS5B non-nucleoside polymerase inhibitors (e.g. sofosbuvir and dasabuvir, respectively) [11, 49, 50] (**Figure 1**). Combination of DAAs targeting different viral proteins regularly each of them with high potency and high genetic barrier, allows a high success of treatment regimens. Also, combination regimens comprising two drugs are preferred to triple combination regimens, to minimize the risk of side-effects and drug–drug interactions [11, 49, 50].

The introduction of DAAs has many positive impacts, through decreasing the incidence of severe hepatic complications and extra-hepatic diseases and reducing hepatitis C-related mortality [51, 52]. However, the high cost of DAAs still a barrier to access to therapy [12, 53]. According to recent estimations, the overall access to DAA is less than 10% of the HCV-infected patients on a global level [54]. Moreover, the potency of DAAs can be impaired by the emergence of specific amino acid substitutions designated resistance-associated substitutions (RASs). As an RNA virus, HCV easily develops a resistance to antiviral treatments due to its error-prone replication property and drug pressure. Risk of treatment failure is low in patients receiving 2 different categories of highly potent DAAs [13]. NS3/4A protease inhibitors are generally unaffected earlier by RASs, but many NS5A inhibitors continue to have overlapping resistance profiles. Furthermore, large studies have shown that a higher proportion of patients failed by an NS5A inhibitor-based regimen developed RASs than patients failed by NS3/4A protease inhibitor-based regimens [14, 55, 56]. The prevalence of RASs varied among HCV genotypes. HCV genotype 3 exhibits the

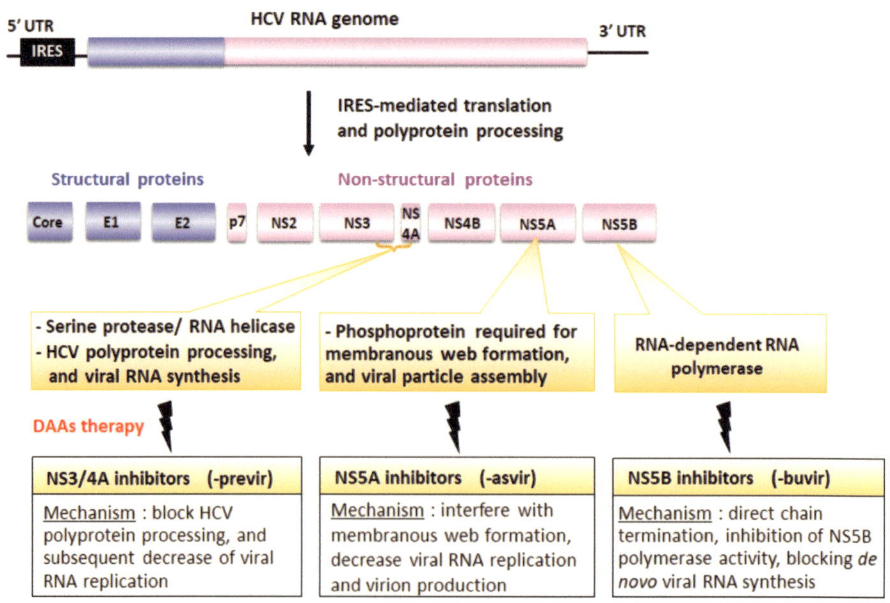

Figure 1.
HCV genomic RNA and encoded viral proteins; virological functions of targeted non-structural proteins for direct-acting antivirals (DAAs) therapy. UTR, untranslated region; IRES, internal ribosome entry site.

highest resistance to DAAs therapy, with lower SVR rates compared to other genotypes [57]. Moreover, the debate continues about DAAs treatment and development of HCC. Some studies have shown that DAAs treatment was not associated with an increase in the development of HCC [58, 59]. Other studies have shown conflicting results, indicating that DAAs therapy is associated with an increase in the recurrence of HCC in patients previously cured by liver transplantation [60]. Collectively, these findings indicate that surveillance for HCC should be continued especially for patients with advanced fibrosis and cirrhosis. Interestingly, the persisting risk for HCC development following SVR in patients treated with DAAs raises questions about the mechanisms that maintain HCC risk in these patients after viral cure.

4. Role of host-targeting antivirals in therapy of HCV infection

HCV exploits the host cell extensively to complete replication cycle and establish persistent infection. The unveiling of HCV-host cell interactions at both structural and functional levels has been investigated intensely, in relation with great progress in HCV cell culture systems and experimental animal models, and also advances in functional genomics screening, including genome-wide small interfering RNA (siRNA) screens and genome-scale CRISPR–Cas screens [61–63]. These tools paved the way for the identification of host-encoded factors involved in each step of HCV life cycle [63, 64]. Characterization of these factors, also known as host dependencies factors, provides not only critical insights into mechanisms of HCV pathogenesis, but also novel candidates for antiviral therapy.

To cure HCV infection, a therapeutic drug should combine a potent antiviral activity and a high genetic barrier to viral resistance. Unlike DAAs, which target viral proteins of high variability, most of host-targeting antivirals (HTAs) are expected to have a high genetic barrier to viral resistance since host factors are less prone to mutations [65]. In addition, HTAs are usually genotype-independent and thus exhibit a pan-genotypic antiviral activity. Nonetheless, a major concern in the usage of HTAs is their interference with physiological functions of targeted host factors, which may induce cellular toxicity and side effects mutations [65, 66]. In the following sections, we discuss recent advances in HTAs against HCV that have potential as new therapeutic options and are in preclinical/clinical development. We also discuss their potential to overcome the current challenges of anti-HCV treatment. **Table 1** summarizes the different HTAs evaluated against HCV with their targeted host-cell factors and current development phase.

4.1 HTAs involved in HCV entry

HCV entry is the first step of virus–host cell interactions required for spread and maintenance of infection. HCV enters the hepatocyte through a highly orchestrated process involving HCV envelope glycoproteins E1 and E2 and four main host-cell receptors: the scavenger receptor class B type I (SR-BI), the human cluster of differentiation 81 (CD81) and the tight-junction proteins Claudin-1 (CLDN-1) and Occludin (OCLN) [67–69]. A genome-scale CRISPR/Cas9 knockout screening in human cells demonstrated that cellular receptors CD81, CLDN1, and OCLN are particularly critical for HCV infection *in vitro*, and thus determine the tropism of HCV for human cells [63]. HTAs targeting HCV entry offer the advantage of blocking HCV life cycle before the beginning of viral genome translation and replication, which might block cell–cell transmission, virus spread, and thus persistent infection [70]. Interestingly, because viral entry plays an important role during HCV re-infection of the graft in end-stage patients undergoing liver transplantation,

Host factor	Host-targeting antiviral	HCV life cycle step	Phase of development	References
Scavenger receptor BI (SR-BI)	ITX-5061	Entry	Phase 2	[73, 74]
Human cluster of differentiation 81 (CD81)	Anti-CD81 mAbs	Entry	Preclinical	[75]
Claudin-1 (CLDN1)	Anti-CLDN1 mAbs (OM-7D3-B3, H3L3)	Entry	Preclinical	[76–79]
Occludin (OCLN)	Anti-OCLN mAbs (Xi 1-3, Xi 37-5)	Entry	Preclinical	[80]
Epidermal growth factor receptor (EGFR)	Erlotinib	Entry	Preclinical	[82]
Nieman-Pick C1-Like 1 (NPC1L1)	Ezetimibe	Entry	Phase 1	[81, 83]
Cyclophilin A	- Alisporivir	RNA replication	Phase 3 (halted)	[87, 90–93]
	- NIM811	RNA replication	Phase 2	[88]
	- SCY-635	RNA replication	Phase 2a	[89, 94]
micoRNA-122	-Miravirsen/ SPC3649	RNA replication	Phase 2a	[102–105]
	-RG-101	RNA replication	Phase 1b	[106–108]
Diglyceride acyltransferase I (DGAT-I)	-siRNA	Assembly	Preclinical	[109]
	-Quercetin	Assembly	Phase 1	[110, 111]
	-LCQ908/Pradigastat	Assembly	Phase 2	[112]
Acyl coenzyme A:cholesterol acyltransferase (ACAT)	Avasimibe	Assembly/Egress	Preclinical	[114, 115]
Adaptor-associated kinase 1 (AAK1)	Sunitinib	Assembly/Egress	Preclinical	[116]
Cyclin-associated kinase (GAK)	-Erlotinib	Assembly/Egress	Preclinical	[117]
	-Isothiazolo [5,4-b] pyridine	Assembly/Egress	Preclinical	[118]

Table 1.
Host-targeting antivirals against HCV with their targeted host-cell factors and current phase of clinical development.

entry inhibitors represent an interesting strategy to prevent graft reinfection [71]. Numerous compounds have been evaluated, the most advanced was ITX-5061, an antagonist of SR-BI that reduces SR-BI-mediated HDL lipid transfer [72]. SR-BI binds HDL and delivers lipids into the cell membrane. The lipid transfer activities of SR-BI play an important role in HCV entry, thus reducing cholesterol transfer into the cell membrane may be one possible mechanism by which ITX-5061 reduces HCV entry [72]. An *in vitro* study indicated that ITX-5061 functions synergistically with the protease inhibitor telaprevir, and no cross-resistance is expected between ITX-5061 and HCV polymerase or protease inhibitors [73]. ITX-5061 completed a clinical phase 1b study. Oral ITX-5061 was safe and well tolerated over 28 days of dosing in noncirrhotic adults with chronic HCV infection [74]. This compound is undergoing phase II clinical trials in HCV-positive patients and appears to be a promising option for treatment [74]. Antibodies targeting CD81 have also been investigated and demonstrated potent antiviral effects in preclinical mouse studies [75]. In the case of CLDN1-targeting inhibitors, a rodent anti-CLDN1 mAb (OM-7D3-B3) demonstrated antiviral potential against HCV infection in primary human hepatocytes (PHHs) and human liver-chimeric mice [76, 77]. Towards a clinical development, Colpitts and colleagues [78] successfully humanized anti-CLDN1 mAb (OM-7D3-B3) into human IgG4 isotype, designed as H3L3. This antibody exhibits pan-genotypic activity against HCV entry without viral escape both *in vitro* and in mouse model [78]. Furthermore, H3L3 demonstrated a synergy with DAAs sofosbuvir and daclatasvir. Such synergy could allow shortening of treatment duration, thus reducing costs and side effects [79]. OCLN may also be considered as a potential target. To date, two successful human-rat chimeric mAbs have been developed against OCLN, and completely inhibit HCV infection *in vitro* and in human liver-chimeric mice without side effects [80]. Other inhibitors of kinases and host-cell pathways involved in HCV entry have been evaluated *in vitro* and significant results have been obtained in mouse models including Nieman-Pick C1-Like 1 (NPC1L1) and epidermal growth factor receptor (EGFR) [81, 82]. The clinically approved EGFR inhibitor Erlotinib, that prevents the formation of CLDN1-CD81 complex, and NPC1L1 inhibitor Ezetimibe, that decreases systemic cholesterol in patients, markedly impaired the establishment of HCV infection in the uPA-SCID mouse model [81, 82]. However, in a phase I clinical trial that enrolled, Ezetimibe elicits only minor effects on HCV viral loads in patients undergoing liver transplantation [83].

4.2 HTAs involved in HCV RNA replication

Targeting HCV RNA replication is a promising approach to eradicate HCV from infected liver cells in patients. The most advanced HTAs against HCV RNA replication are the inhibitors of Cyclophilin A (CypA) and antagomirs of microRNA-122 (miR-122). Cyclophilin A (CypA) is an essential proviral factor for HCV replication, and interacts with HCV NS5A protein to initiate the formation of the replicase complex, and thereby promote viral RNA replication [84, 85]. Specific inhibition of CypA by cyclosporine A destroys the CypA/NS5A complex and suppresses HCV RNA replication *in vitro* [86]. Because cyclosporine A exhibits both antiviral and immunosuppressive activities, non-immunosuppressive antiviral derivatives of cyclosporine A were developed, including Alisporivir/Debio-025, N-methyl-4-isoleucine-cyclosporin (NIM811), and SCY-635 [87–89]. The comparison of CsA-resistant mutants for resistance to Alisporivir and NIM811 demonstrated that Alisporivir has the highest resistant activity against the adaptive mutations [90]. The antiviral effect of Alisporivir on HCV genotypes 1a or 1b has been confirmed in chimeric mice with human hepatocytes [87]. Alisporivir is the most advanced in clinical development. In a phase II clinical trial, administration of Alisporivir in combination with pegIFN-α/RBV to treatment-naïve HCV genotype 1 patients, resulted in SVR rates of 69–76% compared to 55% in the group receiving only pegIFN-α/RBV [91]. Recently, Alisporivir was explored as an interferon-free combination regimen with DAAs in HCV genotype 2 and 3 infected patients, resulting into SVR rates of 80–85% [92]. However, the development of Debio-025 was halted following the report of seven cases of acute pancreatitis [93]. For CypA inhibitor SCY-635, a clinical phase 2a study demonstrated that SCY-635 reduces HCV viral load and increases plasma levels of type I and III IFNs and IFN-stimulated genes, thereby contributes to the activation of innate antiviral immunity [94].

Another important host factor is the liver-specific microRNA-122 (miR-122). microRNAs are small (~22 nucleotides) endogenous noncoding RNAs, which bind to the 3′-untranslated region of the messenger RNAs (mRNAs), resulting in gene silencing through mRNA degradation or translational repression [95]. The replication of HCV in hepatocytes has been shown to be critically dependent on miR-122, as the sequestration of miR-122 in liver cells results in marked loss of replicating HCV RNAs [96]. Several mechanisms by which miR-122 promotes HCV replication have been reported. miR-122 promotes HCV genome replication by direct binding with two adjacent sites in the 5'-UTR of the HCV RNA [97]. miR-122 protects HCV RNA genome from degradation by host 5′-3′ exonucleases Xrn1 and Xrn2, and phosphatases DOM3Z and DUSP11 [98–101]. Therapeutic approaches based on inhibition of miR-122 using modified anti-sense oligonucleotides have been generated. Miravirsen/SPC3649 is a locked nucleic acid-modified DNA antisense oligonucleotide that sequesters mature miR-122 in a highly stable heteroduplex, thereby inhibiting its function. Miravirsen demonstrated antiviral activity against all HCV genotypes *in vitro* [102]. In a phase 2a study, the safety and efficacy of miravirsen were evaluated in 36 patients with chronic HCV genotype 1 infection. The results showed a prolonged and dose-dependent decrease in HCV RNA levels without evidence of viral resistance and serious adverse effects [103]. Miravirsen treatment results in a prolonged reduction in cholesterol levels in line with the effects of miR-122 on cholesterol metabolism [103, 104]. In addition, Miravirsen demonstrated a potent antiviral activity when tested against DAA-resistant HCV variants [105]. Another antimir-122 molecule is RG-101, a hepatocyte targeted N-acetylgalactosamine conjugated oligonucleotide that antagonizes miR-122 [106]. Van der Ree and colleagues [106] performed a phase 1B study that assessed the safety, tolerability and antiviral effect of RG-101 in 32 patients chronically infected with HCV genotypes 1, 3, or 4. The results showed that RG-101 was well tolerated and resulted in substantial decrease in viral load in all treated patients within 4 weeks, and sustained virological response in 3 patients at week 76 of follow-up. However, viral rebound between weeks 5 and weeks 12 was observed in six patients with HCV genotype 1 [106]. Another phase 1B study assessed the effects of dosing RG-101 on antiviral immunity in chronic HCV patients and showed that a single dose of RG-101 led to a decrease in HCV RNA levels in all patients and SVR >76 weeks in 3 patients [107]. The combination of a highly potent DAAs with miravirsen or RG-101 could potentially shorten HCV treatment duration. Recently, two clinical studies were performed to evaluate the potential of combining a NS5B inhibitor (GSK2878175) and RG-101 as a single- visit curative regimen for chronic hepatitis C [108]. GSK2878175 molecule demonstrated acceptable safety, tolerability and pan-genotypic antiviral activity, especially for HCV genotype 3 that is considered difficult to treat. The results showed that daily oral administration of GSK2878175 with a single dose of RG- 101 results in high cure rates if the treatment duration is >9 weeks in noncirrhotic, treatment-naïve patients with HCV genotype 1 and 3 infections [108]. Altogether, these findings highlight the clinical potential of miR-122 inhibitors as complementary therapeutic strategy that especially may be valuable for difficult-to-cure patients with current DAAs.

4.3 HTAs involved in HCV assembly and egress

There is a close relationship between HCV particle biogenesis and host-cell lipid metabolism. HCV circulates as lipo-viralparticles (LVPs) in the blood of infected patients, thus targeting the host-cell factors involved in the lipid metabolism may provide potential therapeutic options. An essential cellular enzyme involved in this process is the diglyceride acyltransferase I (DGAT-I) which directly interacts with the HCV core protein, and is required for the trafficking of core to lipid droplets [109]. Inhibition of DGAT1 activity or RNAi-mediated knockdown of DGAT1 severely impairs infectious viral particles production *in vitro*, implicating DGAT-1 as a new target for antiviral therapy [109]. Interestingly, quercetin, a natural flavonoid that inhibits DGAT-I, was reported to have anti-HCV properties [110]. In a phase I study, quercetin exhibited high safety and potent antiviral activity in patients with chronic HCV infection [111]. Moreover, the antiviral efficacy of the DGAT-I inhibitor LCQ908/pradigastat was assessed in phase II clinical trials in patients with HCV infection, but no significant decrease in HCV viral load was observed in treated patients [112]. Further studies are needed to determine whether the DGAT-I inhibitor could be used in combination with DAAs.

Apolipoproteins (e.g. ApoE, ApoB, and ApoA1) are essential to the formation of infectious HCV particles during viral assembly, and highly infectious HCV particles are usually associated with more lipoproteins [40, 113]. Mechanistic studies demonstrated that Avasimibe, an inhibitor of acyl coenzyme A:cholesterol acyltransferase (ACAT), induced downregulation of microsomal triglyceride transfer protein expression, resulting in reduced ApoE and ApoB secretion [114]. Avasimibe significantly impairs the assembly of infectious HCV virions and exhibits significant pan-genotypic antiviral activity and great potential for combination therapy with DAAs [115]. Furthermore, the adaptor-associated kinase 1 (AAK1) and the cyclin-associated kinase (GAK) are known to regulate core-AP2M1 interaction [116]. Accordingly, Neveu and colleagues showed that AAK1 and GAK inhibitors, including the approved anti-cancer drugs sunitinib and erlotinib, can block HCV assembly [116, 117]. However, these compounds could induce adverse effects due to their lack of specificity. To overcome this limitation, a specific GAK inhibitor, isothiazolo [5,4-b]pyridine was developed [118]. This drug efficiently impairs HCV entry and assembly *in vitro* with limited off-target effects [118].

5. Conclusion and prospects

The great advances in hepatitis C treatment through the development of highly potent DAAs define the intense efforts towards a global eradication of HCV infection. However, most infected people live in low resource countries, which may limit access to treatment and restrain the impact of DAAs on the global burden of HCV infection and associated diseases. Another principal challenge is viral resistance, subsequent treatment failure and emergence of DAA-resistant variants. HTAs against host-cell factors required for HCV pathogenesis are promising candidates for development as alternative or complementary therapeutic options. Intense research on HTAs is needed to develop highly effective drugs with the least side effects. Several HTAs are at different stages of preclinical and clinical development, which promise for enlarged therapeutic arsenal against chronic HCV infection in the future.

Acknowledgements

This work was supported by grants from the Japan Agency for Medical Research and Development; the Tokyo Metropolitan Government; the Ministry of Health and Welfare of Japan; and the Ministry of Education, Culture, Sports, Science, and Technology of Japan.

Conflict of interest

The authors declare no conflict of interest.

Author details

Bouchra Kitab[1], Michinori Kohara[2] and Kyoko Tsukiyama-Kohara[1*]

1 Transboundary Animal Diseases Centre, Joint Faculty of Veterinary Medicine, Kagoshima University, Kagoshima, Japan

2 The Tokyo Metropolitan Institute of Medical Science, Japan

*Address all correspondence to: kkohara@vet.kagoshima-u.ac.jp

References

[1] World Health Organization. Global Hepatitis Report 2017; World Health Organization: Geneva, Switzerland,2017.

[2] Polaris Observatory HCV Collaborators. Global prevalence and genotype distribution of hepatitis C virus infection in 2015: a modelling study. Lancet Gastroenterol Hepatol. 2017;2:161-176. doi: 10.1016/S2468-1253(16)30181-9

[3] Brown RS. Hepatitis C and liver transplantation. Nature. 2005;436:973-978. doi: 10.1002/cld.62

[4] Hadziyannis SJ, Sette H Jr, Morgan TR, Balan V, Diago M, Marcellin P, Ramadori G, Bodenheimer H Jr, Bernstein D, Rizzetto M, Zeuzem S, Pockros PJ, Lin A, Ackrill AM; PEGASYS International Study Group. Peginterferon-alpha2a and ribavirin combination therapy in chronic hepatitis C: a randomized study of treatment duration and ribavirin dose. Ann Intern Med. 2004;140:346-355. doi: 10.7326/0003-4819-140-5-200403020-00010

[5] Heim MH. 25 years of interferon-based treatment of chronic hepatitis C: an epoch coming to an end. Nat Rev Immunol. 2013;13:535-542. doi: 10.1038/nri3463

[6] Aghemo A, De Francesco R. New horizons in hepatitis C antiviral therapy with direct acting antivirals. Hepatology. 2013;58:428-438. doi: 10.1002/hep.26371

[7] Spengler U. Direct antiviral agents (DAAs)—A new age in the treatment of hepatitis C virus infection. Pharmacol Ther. 2018;183:118-126. doi: 10.1016/j.pharmthera.2017.10.009

[8] Tungol, A., Rademacher, K., Schafer, J.A., 2011. Formulary management of the protease inhibitors boceprevir and telaprevir for chronic hepatitis C virus. J Manag Care Pharm. 2011;17:685-694. doi: 10.18553/jmcp.2011.17.9.685

[9] Lawitz E, Lalezari JP, Hassanein T, Kowdley KV, Poordad FF, Sheikh AM, Afdhal NH, Bernstein DE, Dejesus E, Freilich B, Nelson DR, Dieterich DT, Jacobson IM, Jensen D, Abrams GA, Darling JM, Rodriguez-Torres M, Reddy KR, Sulkowski MS, Bzowej NH, Hyland RH, Mo H, Lin M, Mader M, Hindes R, Albanis E, Symonds WT, Berrey MM, Muir A. Sofosbuvir in combination with peginterferon alfa-2a and ribavirin for non-cirrhotic, treatment-naive patients with genotypes 1, 2, and 3 hepatitis C infection: a randomised, double-blind, phase 2 trial. Lancet Infect Dis. 2013;13:401-408. doi: 10.1016/S1473-3099(13)70033-1

[10] Asahina Y, Izumi N, Hiromitsu K, Kurosaki M, Koike K, Suzuki F, Takikawa H, Tanaka A, Tanaka E, Tanaka Y, Tsubouchi H, Hayashi N, Hiramatsu N, Yotsuyanagi H. JSH Guidelines for the Management of Hepatitis C Virus Infection: A 2016 update for genotype 1 and 2. Hepatol Res. 2016;46:129-165. doi: 10.1111/hepr.12645

[11] Pawlotsky JM. Interferon-Free Hepatitis C Virus Therapy. Cold Spring Harb Perspect Med. 2020;10:a036855. doi: 10.1101/cshperspect.a036855

[12] Dusheiko G, Gore C. Antiviral treatment for hepatitis C: rebalancing cost, affordability, and availability. Lancet Glob Health. 2019;7:e1150-e1151. doi: 10.1016/S2214-109X(19)30313-4

[13] Sarrazin C. The importance of resistance to direct antiviral drugs in HCV infection in clinical practice. J Hepatol. 2016;64:486-504. doi: 10.1016/j.jhep.2015.09.011

[14] Hayes CN, Chayama K. Why highly effective drugs are not enough: the need for an affordable solution to eliminating HCV. Expert Rev Clin Pharmacol. 2017;10:583-594. doi: 10.1080/17512433.2017.1313111

[15] Torres HA, Vauthey JN, Economides MP, Mahale P, Kaseb A. Hepatocellular carcinoma recurrence after treatment with direct-acting antivirals: First, do no harm by withdrawing treatment. J Hepatol. 2016;65:862-864. doi:10.1016/j.jhep.2016.05.034

[16] Lim N, Singh D, Jackson S, Lake JR. Recurrence of Hepatocellular Carcinoma in Hepatitis C Virus (HCV) Liver Transplant Recipients Treated with Pretransplant Direct-Acting Antiviral (DAA) Therapy. Gastrointest Tumors. 2020;7:134-143. doi: 10.1159/000510341

[17] Crouchet E, Wrensch F, Schuster C, Zeisel MB, Baumert TF. Host-targeting therapies for hepatitis C virus infection: Current developments and future applications. Therap Adv Gastroenterol. 2018. doi: 10.1177/1756284818759483

[18] Simmonds P, Becher P, Bukh J, Gould EA, Meyers G, Monath T, Muerhoff S, Pletnev A, Rico-Hesse R, Smith DB, Stapleton JT, Ictv Report Consortium. ICTV Virus Taxonomy Profile: Flaviviridae. J Gen Virol. 2017;98:2-3. doi: 10.1099/jgv.0.000672

[19] Choo QL, Kuo G, Weiner AJ, Overby LR, Bradley DW, Houghton M. Isolation of a cDNA clone derived from a blood-borne non-A, non-B viral hepatitis genome. Science. 1989;244:359-362. doi: 10.1126/science.2523562

[20] Kato N, Hijikata M, Ootsuyama Y, Nakagawa M, Ohkoshi S, Sugimura T, Shimotohno K. Molecular cloning of the human hepatitis C virus genome from Japanese patients with non-A, non-B hepatitis. Proc Natl Acad Sci USA. 1990;87:9524-9528. doi: 10.1073/pnas.87.24.9524

[21] Tsukiyama-Kohara K, Iizuka N, Kohara M, Nomoto A. Internal ribosome entry site within hepatitis C virus RNA. J Virol. 1992;66:1476-1483. doi: 10.1128/JVI.66.3.1476-1483.1992

[22] Smith DB, Bukh J, Kuiken C, Muerhoff AS, Rice CM, Stapleton JT, Simmonds P. Expanded classification of hepatitis C virus into 7 genotypes and 67 subtypes: updated criteria and genotype assignment web resource. Hepatology. 2014; 59:318-327. doi: 10.1002/hep.26744

[23] Tsukiyama-Kohara K, Kohara M. Hepatitis C Virus: Viral Quasispecies and Genotypes. Int J Mol Sci. 2017;19:23. doi: 10.3390/ijms19010023

[24] Simmonds P, Bukh J, Combet C, Deléage G, Enomoto N, Feinstone S, Halfon P, Inchauspé G, Kuiken C, Maertens G, Mizokami M, Murphy DG, Okamoto H, Pawlotsky JM, Penin F, Sablon E, Shin-I T, Stuyver LJ, Thiel HJ, Viazov S, Weiner AJ, Widell A. Consensus proposals for a unified system of nomenclature of hepatitis C virus genotypes. Hepatology. 2005;42:962-973. doi: 10.1002/hep.26744

[25] Messina JP, Humphreys I, Flaxman A, Brown A, Cooke GS, Pybus OG, Barnes E. Global distribution and prevalence of hepatitis C virus genotypes. Hepatology. 2015;61:77-87. doi: 10.1002/hep.27259

[26] Murphy DG, Sablon E, Chamberland J, Fournier E, Dandavino R, Tremblay CL. Hepatitis C virus genotype 7, a new genotype originating from central Africa. J Clin Microbiol. 2015; 53:967-972. doi: 10.1128/JCM.02831-14

[27] Blanchard E, Belouzard S, Goueslain L, Wakita T,

Dubuisson J, Wychowski C, Rouillé Y. Hepatitis C virus entry depends on clathrin-mediated endocytosis. J Virol. 2006;80:6964-6972. doi: 10.1128/JVI.00024-06

[28] Burlone ME, Budkowska A. Hepatitis C virus cell entry: role of lipoproteins and cellular receptors. J Gen Virol. 2009;90:1055-1070. doi: 10.1099/vir.0.008300-0

[29] Tscherne DM, Jones CT, Evans M.J, Lindenbach BD, McKeating JA, and Rice CM. Time- and temperature-dependent activation of hepatitis C virus for low-pH-triggered entry. J. Virol. 2006;80:1734-1741. doi: 10.1128/JVI.80.4.1734-1741.2006

[30] Niepmann M. Hepatitis C virus RNA translation. Curr Top Microbiol Immunol. 2013;369:143-66. doi: 10.1007/978-3-642-27340-7_6

[31] Moradpour D, Penin F. Hepatitis C virus proteins: from structure to function. Curr Top Microbiol Immunol.2013; 369:113-142. doi: 10.1007/978-3-642-27340-7_5

[32] Lohmann KF, Koch JO, Herian U, Theilmann L, and Batenschlager R. Replication of subgenomic hepatitis C virus RNAs in a hepatoma cell line. Science. 1999;285:110-113. doi: 10.1126/science.285.5424.110

[33] Romero-Brey I, Merz A, Chiramel A, Lee JY, Chlanda P, Haselman U, Santarella-Mellwig R, Habermann A, Hoppe S, Kallis S, Walther P, Antony C, Krijnse-Locker J, Bartenschlager. Three-dimensional architecture and biogenesis of membrane structures associated with hepatitis C virus replication. PLoS Pathog. 2012;8:e1003056. doi: 10.1371/journal.ppat.1003056

[34] Paul D, Hoppe S, Saher G, Krijnse-Locker J, Bartenschlager R. Morphological and biochemical characterization of the membranous hepatitis C virus replication compartment. J Virol; 2013;87:10612-10627. doi: 10.1128/JVI.01370-13

[35] Lohmann V. Hepatitis C virus RNA replication. Curr Top Microbiol Immunol. 2013;369:167-198. doi: 10.1007/978-3-642-27340-7_7

[36] Hirata Y, Ikeda K, Sudoh M, Tokunaga Y, Suzuki A, Weng L, Ohta M, Tobita Y, Okano K, Ozeki K, Kawasaki K, Tsukuda T, Katsume A, Aoki Y, Umehara T, Sekiguchi S, Toyoda T, Shimotohno K, Soga T, Nishijima M, Taguchi R, Kohara M. Self-enhancement of hepatitis C virus replication by promotion of specific sphingolipid biosynthesis. PLoS Pathog. 2012;8: e1002860. doi: 10.1371/journal.ppat.1002860

[37] Paul D, Madan V, Bartenschlager R. Hepatitis C virus RNA replication and assembly: living on the fat of the land. Cell Host Microbe. 2014;16:569-579. doi: 10.1016/j.chom.2014.10.008

[38] Masaki T, Suzuki R, Murakami K, Aizaki H, Ishii K, Murayama A, Date T, Matsuura Y, Miyamura T, Wakita T, Suzuki T. Interaction of hepatitis C virus nonstructural protein 5A with core protein is critical for the production of infectious virus particles. J Virol. 2008;82:7964-7976. doi: 10.1128/JVI.00826-08

[39] Miyanari Y, Atsuzawa K, Usuda N, Watashi K, Hishiki T, Zayas M, Bartenschlager R, Wakita T, Hijikata M, Shimotohno K. The lipid droplet is an important organelle for hepatitis C virus production. Nat Cell Biol. 2007;9:1089-1097. doi: 10.1038/ncb1631

[40] Bankwitz D, Doepke M, HuegingK,WellerR,BrueningJ,BehrendtP, Lee JY, Vondran FWR, Manns, MP, Bartenschlager R, Pietschmann T. Maturation of secreted HCV particles by incorporation of secreted ApoE protects from antibodies by enhancing

infectivity. J Hepatol. 2017;67:480-489. doi: 10.1016/j.jhep.2017.04.010

[41] Andre P, Komurian-Pradel F, Deforges S, Perret M, Berland JL, Sodoyer M, Pol S, Brechot C, Paranhos-Baccala G, Lotteau V. Characterization of low- and very-low-density hepatitis C virus RNAcontaining particles. J Virol. 2002;76:6919-6928. doi: 10.1128/jvi.76.14.6919-6928.2002

[42] Syed GH, Khan M, Yang S, Siddiqui A. Hepatitis C Virus Lipoviroparticles Assemble in the Endoplasmic Reticulum (ER) and Bud off from the ER to the Golgi Compartment in COPII Vesicles. J Virol. 2017;91:e00499-17. doi: 10.1128/JVI.00499-17

[43] Corless L, Crump CM, Griffin SD, Harris M. Vps4 and the ESCRT-III complex are required for the release of infectious hepatitis C virus particles. J Gen Virol. 2010; 91:362-372. doi: 10.1099/vir.0.017285-0

[44] Takacs CN, Andreo U, Dao Thi VL, Wu X, Gleason CE, Itano MS, Spitz-Becker GS, Belote RL, Hedin BR, Scull MA, Rice CM, Simon SM. Differential Regulation of Lipoprotein and Hepatitis C Virus Secretion by Rab1b. Cell Rep. 2017;21:431-441. doi: 10.1016/j.celrep.2017.09.053

[45] Neumann AU, Lam NP, Dahari H, Gretch DR, Wiley TE, Layden TJ, Perelson AS. Hepatitis C viral dynamics in vivo and the antiviral efficacy of interferon-alpha therapy. Science. 1998 ;282:103-107. doi: 10.1126/science.282.5386.103

[46] Seeff LB. Natural history of chronic hepatitis C. Hepatology. 2002;36:35-46. doi: 10.1053/jhep.2002.36806

[47] Ghany MG, Strader DB, Thomas DL, Seeff LB. Diagnosis, management, and treatment of hepatitis C: an update. American Association for the Study of Liver Diseases. Hepatology. 2009;49:1335-1374. doi: 10.1002/hep.22759

[48] Ge D, Fellay J, Thompson AJ, Simon JS, Shianna KV, Urban TJ, Heinzen EL, Qiu P, Bertelsen AH, Muir AJ, Sulkowski M, McHutchison JG, Goldstein DB. Genetic variation in IL28B predicts hepatitis C treatment-induced viral clearance. Nature. 2009;461:399-401. doi: 10.1038/nature08309

[49] European Association for the Study of the Liver. EASL Recommendations on Treatment of Hepatitis C 2018. J Hepatol. 2018;69:461-511. doi: 10.1016/j.jhep.2018.03.026

[50] Hayes CN, Imamura M, Chayama K. Management of HCV patients in cases of direct-acting antiviral failure. Expert Rev Gastroenterol Hepatol. 2019;13:839-848. doi: 10.1080/17474124.2019.1651642

[51] Colussi G, Donnini D, Brizzi RF, Maier S, Valenti L, Catena C, Cavarape A, Sechi LA, Soardo G. Sustained virologic response to direct-acting antiviral agents predicts better outcomes in hepatitis C virus-infected patients: A retrospective study. World J Gastroenterol. 2019;25: 6094-6106. doi: 10.3748/wjg.v25.i40.6094

[52] Mohanty A, Salameh S, Butt AA. Impact of Direct Acting Antiviral Agent Therapy upon Extrahepatic Manifestations of Hepatitis C Virus Infection. Curr HIV/AIDS Rep. 2019;16:389-394. doi: 10.1007/s11904-019-00466-1

[53] Zhuo Y, Hayashi T, Chen Q, Aggarwal R, Hutin Y, Chhatwal J. Estimating the price at which hepatitis C treatment with direct-acting antivirals would be cost-saving in Japan. Sci Rep. 2020;10:4089. doi: 10.1038/s41598-020-60986-4

[54] https://www.who.int/news/item/31-10-2017-close-to-3-million-people-access-hepatitis-c-cure [Accessed: 2019-7-7]

[55] Di Maio VC, Cento V, Aragri M, Paolucci S, Pollicino T, Coppola N, Bruzzone B, Ghisetti V, Zazzi M, Brunetto M, Bertoli A, Barbaliscia S, Galli S, Gennari W, Baldanti F, Raimondo G, Perno CF, Ceccherini-Silberstein F; HCV Virology Italian Resistance Network (VIRONET-C). Frequent NS5A and multiclass resistance in almost all HCV genotypes at DAA failures: What are the chances for second-line regimens?. J Hepatol. 2018;68:597-600. doi: 10.1016/j.jhep.2017.09.008

[56] Mawatari S, Oda K, Kumagai K, Tabu K, Ijuin S, Fujisaki K, Inada Y, Uto H, Saisyoji A, Hiramine Y, Hori T, Taniyama O, Toyodome A, Sakae H, Hashiguchi M, Kure T, Sakurai K, Tamai T, Moriuchi A, Ido A. Viral and host factors are associated with retreatment failure in hepatitis C patients receiving all-oral direct antiviral therapy. Hepatol Res. 2020;50:453-465. doi: 10.1111/hepr.13474

[57] Smith D, Magri A, Bonsall D, Ip CLC, Trebes A, Brown A, Piazza P, Bowden R, Nguyen D, Ansari MA, Simmonds P, Barnes E; STOP-HCV Consortium. Resistance analysis of genotype 3 hepatitis C virus indicates subtypes inherently resistant to nonstructural protein 5A inhibitors. Hepatology. 2019;69:1861-1872. doi: 10.1002/hep.29837

[58] Waziry R, Hajarizadeh B, Grebely J, Amin J, Law M, Danta M, George J, Dore GJ. Hepatocellular carcinoma risk following direct-acting antiviral HCV therapy: A systematic review, meta-analyses, and meta-regression. J Hepatol. 2017;67:1204-1212. doi: 10.1016/j.jhep.2017.07.025

[59] Ogawa E, Nomura H, Nakamuta M, Furusyo N, Kajiwara E, Dohmen K, Kawano A, Ooho A, Azuma K, Takahashi K, Satoh T, Koyanagi T, Ichiki Y, Kuniyoshi M, Yanagita K, Amagase H, Morita C, Sugimoto R, Kato M, Shimoda S, Hayashi J. Incidence of Hepatocellular Carcinoma after Treatment with Sofosbuvir-Based or Sofosbuvir-Free Regimens in Patients with Chronic Hepatitis C. Cancers (Basel). 2020;12:2602. doi: 10.3390/cancers12092602

[60] Kanwal F, Kramer J, Asch SM, Chayanupatkul M, Cao Y, El-Serag HB. Risk of Hepatocellular Cancer in HCV Patients Treated With Direct-Acting Antiviral Agents. Gastroenterology. 2017;153:996-1005. doi: 10.1053/j.gastro.2017.06.012

[61] Randall G, Panis M, Cooper JD, Tellinghuisen TL, Sukhodolets KE, Pfeffer S, Landthaler M, Landgraf P, Kan S, Lindenbach BD, Chien M, Weir DB, Russo JJ, Ju J, Brownstein MJ, Sheridan R, Sander C, Zavolan M, Tuschl T, Rice CM. Cellular cofactors affecting hepatitis C virus infection and replication. Proc Natl Acad Sci U S A. 2007;104:12884-12889. doi: 10.1073/pnas.0704894104

[62] Puschnik AS, Majzoub K, Ooi YS, Carette JE. A CRISPR toolbox to study virus-host interactions. Nat Rev Microbiol. 2017;15:351-364. doi: 10.1038/nrmicro.2017.29

[63] Marceau CD, Puschnik AS, Majzoub K, Ooi YS, Brewer SM, Fuchs G, Swaminathan K, Mata MA, Elias JE, Sarnow P, Carette JE. Genetic dissection of Flaviviridae host factors through genome-scale CRISPR screens. Nature. 2016;535:159-163. doi: 10.1038/nature18631

[64] Li Q, Zhang YY, Chiu S, Hu Z, Lan KH, Cha H, Sodroski C, Zhang F, Hsu CS, Thomas E, Liang TJ. Integrative functional genomics of hepatitis C virus infection identifies host dependencies in complete viral replication cycle. PLoS Pathog. 2014;10:e1004163. doi: 10.1371/journal.ppat.1004163

[65] Delang L, Vliegen I, Froeyen M, Neyts J. Comparative study of the

genetic barriers and pathways towards resistance of selective inhibitors of hepatitis C virus replication. Antimicrob Agents Chemother 2011;55:4103-4113. doi: 10.1128/AAC.00294-11

[66] Pawlotsky JM .What are the pros and cons of the use of host-targeted agents against hepatitis C?. Antiviral Res. 2014;105:22-25. doi: 10.1016/j.antiviral.2014.02.008 26

[67] Evans MJ, von Hahn T, Tscherne DM, Syder AJ, Panis M, Wölk B, Hatziioannou T, McKeating JA, Bieniasz PD, Rice CM. Claudin-1 is a hepatitis C virus co-receptor required for a late step in entry. Nature. 2007;446:801-805. doi: 10.1038/nature05654

[68] Ploss A, Evans MJ, Gaysinskaya VA, Panis M, You H, de Jong YP, Rice CM. Human occludin is a hepatitis C virus entry factor required for infection of mouse cells. Nature. 2009;457:882-886. doi: 10.1038/nature07684

[69] Da Costa D, Turek M, Felmlee DJ, Girardi E, Pfeffer S, Long G, Bartenschlager R, Zeisel MB, Baumert TF. Reconstitution of the entire hepatitis C virus life cycle in nonhepatic cells. J Virol. 2012;86:11919-11925. doi: 10.1128/JVI.01066-12

[70] Xiao F, Fofana I, Heydmann L, Barth H, Soulier E, Habersetzer F, Doffoël M, Bukh J, Patel AH, Zeisel MB, Baumert TF. Hepatitis C virus cell-cell transmission and resistance to direct-acting antiviral agents. PLoS Pathog. 2014;10:e1004128. doi: 10.1371/journal.ppat.1004128

[71] Colpitts CC, Chung RT, Baumert TF. Entry Inhibitors: A Perspective for Prevention of Hepatitis C Virus Infection in Organ Transplantation. ACS Infect Dis. 2017;3:620-623. doi: 10.1021/acsinfecdis.7b00091

[72] Syder AJ, Lee H, Zeisel MB, Grove J, Soulier E, Macdonald J, Chow S, Chang J, Baumert TF, McKeating JA, McKelvy J, Wong-Staal F. Small molecule scavenger receptor BI antagonists are potent HCV entry inhibitors. J Hepatol. 2011;54:48-55. doi: 10.1016/j.jhep.2010.06.024

[73] Zhu H, Wong-Staal F, Lee H, Syder A, McKelvy J, Schooley RT, Wyles DL. Evaluation of ITX 5061, a scavenger receptor B1 antagonist: resistance selection and activity in combination with other hepatitis C virus antivirals. J Infect Dis. 2012;205:656-662. doi: 10.1093/infdis/jir802

[74] Sulkowski MS, Kang M, Matining R, Wyles D, Johnson VA, Morse GD, Amorosa V, Bhattacharya D, Coughlin K, Wong-Staal F, Glesby MJ; AIDS Clinical Trials Group A5277 Protocol Team. Safety and antiviral activity of the HCV entry inhibitor ITX5061 in treatment-naive HCV-infected adults: a randomized, double-blind, phase 1b study. J Infect Dis. 2014;209:658-667. doi: 10.1093/infdis/jit503

[75] Meuleman P, Hesselgesser J, PaulsonM,VanwolleghemT,DesomberеI, Reiser H, Leroux-Roels G. Anti-CD81 antibodies can prevent a hepatitis C virus infection in vivo. Hepatology. 2008;48:1761-1768. doi: 10.1002/hep.22547

[76] Fofana I, Krieger SE, Grunert F, Glauben S, Xiao F, Fafi-Kremer S, Soulier E, Royer C, Thumann C, Mee CJ, McKeating JA, Dragic T, Pessaux P, Stoll-Keller F, Schuster C, Thompson J, Baumert TF. Monoclonal anti-claudin 1 antibodies prevent hepatitis C virus infection of primary human hepatocytes. Gastroenterology. 2010;139:953-964. doi: 10.1053/j.gastro.2010.05.073

[77] Mailly L, Xiao F, Lupberger J, Wilson GK, Aubert P, Duong FHT, Calabrese D, Leboeuf C, Fofana I, Thumann C, Bandiera S, Lütgehetmann M, Volz T, Davis C, Harris HJ, Mee CJ, Girardi E, Chane-Woon-Ming B, Ericsson M, Fletcher N, Bartenschlager R, Pessaux P, Vercauteren K, Meuleman P, Villa P, Kaderali L, Pfeffer S, Heim MH, Neunlist M, Zeisel MB, Dandri M, McKeating JA, Robinet E, Baumert TF. Clearance of persistent hepatitis C virus infection in humanized mice using a claudin-1-targeting monoclonal antibody. Nat Biotechnol. 2015;33:549-554. doi: 10.1038/nbt.3179

[78] Colpitts CC, Tawar RG, Mailly L, Thumann C, Heydmann L, Durand SC, Xiao F, Robinet E, Pessaux P, Zeisel MB, Baumert TF. Humanisation of a claudin-1-specific monoclonal antibody for clinical prevention and cure of HCV infection without escape. Gut. 2018;67:736-745. doi: 10.1136/gutjnl-2016-312577

[79] Mailly L, Wrensch F, Heydmann L, Fauvelle C, Brignon N, Zeisel MB, Pessaux P, Keck ZY, Schuster C, Fuerst TR, Foung SKH, Baumert TF. In vivo combination of human anti-envelope glycoprotein E2 and -Claudin-1 monoclonal antibodies for prevention of hepatitis C virus infection. Antiviral Res. 2019;162:136-141. doi: 10.1016/j.antiviral.2018.12.018

[80] Shimizu Y, Yoneda K, Shirasago Y, Suzuki T, Tada M, Ishii-Watabe A, Sugiyama K, Suzuki T, Wakita T, Yagi K, Kondoh M, Fukasawa M. Human-rat chimeric anti-occludin monoclonal antibodies inhibit hepatitis C virus infection. Biochem Biophys Res Commun. 2019;514:785-790. doi: 10.1016/j.bbrc.2019.05.019

[81] Sainz B Jr, Barretto N, Martin DN, Hiraga N, Imamura M, Hussain S, Marsh KA, Yu X, Chayama K, Alrefai WA, Uprichard SL. Identification of the Niemann-Pick C1-like 1 cholesterol absorption receptor as a new hepatitis C virus entry factor. Nat Med. 2012;18:281-285. doi: 10.1038/nm.2581.

[82] Lupberger J, Zeisel MB, Xiao F, Thumann C, Fofana I, Zona L, Davis C, Mee CJ, Turek M, Gorke S, Royer C, Fischer B, Zahid MN, Lavillette D, Fresquet J, Cosset FL, Rothenberg SM, Pietschmann T, Patel AH, Pessaux P, Doffoël M, Raffelsberger W, Poch O, McKeating JA, Brino L, Baumert TF. EGFR and EphA2 are host factors for hepatitis C virus entry and possible targets for antiviral therapy. Nat Med. 2011;17:589-595. doi: 10.1038/nm.2341

[83] Monrroy-Bravo H, Angulo J, Pino K, Labbé P, López-Lastra M, Soza A. Effect of ezetimibe in HCV viral load after liver transplantation. Ann Hepatol. 2016;15:803-805. doi: 10.5604/16652681.1212623

[84] Kaul A, Stauffer S, Berger C, Pertel T, Schmitt J, Kallis S, Zayas M, Lohmann V, Luban J, Bartenschlager R. Essential role of cyclophilin A for hepatitis C virus replication and virus production and possible link to polyprotein cleavage kinetics. PLoS Pathog. 2009;5:e1000546. doi: 10.1371/journal.ppat.1000546

[85] Coelmont L, Hanoulle X, Chatterji U, Berger C, Snoeck J, Bobardt M, Lim P, Vliegen I, Paeshuyse J, Vuagniaux G, Vandamme AM, Bartenschlager R, Gallay P, Lippens G, Neyts J. DEB025 (Alisporivir) inhibits hepatitis C virus replication by preventing a cyclophilin A induced cis-trans isomerisation in domain II of NS5A. PLoS One. 2010;5:e13687. doi: 10.1371/journal.pone.0013687

[86] Watashi K, Hijikata M, Hosaka M, Yamaji M, Shimotohno K. Cyclosporin A suppresses replication of hepatitis C virus genome in cultured hepatocytes.

Hepatology. 2003;38:1282-1288. doi: 10.1053/jhep.2003.50449

[87] Inoue K, Umehara T, Ruegg UT, Yasui F, Watanabe T, Yasuda H, Dumont JM, Scalfaro P, Yoshiba M, Kohara M. Evaluation of a cyclophilin inhibitor in hepatitis C virus-infected chimeric mice in vivo. Hepatology. 2007;45:921-928. doi: 10.1002/hep.21587

[88] Lawitz E, Godofsky E, Rouzier R, Marbury T, Nguyen T, Ke J, Huang M, Praestgaard J, Serra D, Evans TG. Safety, pharmacokinetics, and antiviral activity of the cyclophilin inhibitor NIM811 alone or in combination with pegylated interferon in HCV-infected patients receiving 14 days of therapy. Antiviral Res. 2011;89:238-245. doi: 10.1016/j.antiviral.2011.01.003

[89] Hopkins S, Scorneaux B, Huang Z, Murray MG, Wring S, Smitley C, Harris R, Erdmann F, Fischer G, Ribeill Y. SCY-635, a novel nonimmunosuppressive analog of cyclosporine that exhibits potent inhibition of hepatitis C virus RNA replication in vitro. Antimicrob Agents Chemother. 2010;54:660-672. doi: 10.1128/AAC.00660-09

[90] Arai M, Tsukiyama-Kohara K, Takagi A, Tobita Y, Inoue K, Kohara M. Resistance to cyclosporin A derives from mutations in hepatitis C virus nonstructural proteins. Biochem Biophys Res Commun. 2014;448:56-62. doi: 10.1016/j.bbrc.2014.04.053

[91] Flisiak R, Pawlotsky JM, Crabbe R, Callistru PI, Kryczka W, Häussinger D. Once daily alisporivir (Debio025) plus pegIFNalfa2a/ribavirin results in superior sustained virologic response (SVR) in chronic hepatitis C genotype 1 treatment naive patients. J Hepatol 2011;54:24.

[92] Pawlotsky JM, Flisiak R, Sarin SK, Rasenack J, Piratvisuth T, Chuang WL, Peng CY, Foster GR, Shah S, Wedemeyer H, Hézode C, Zhang W, Wong KA, Li B, Avila C, Naoumov NV; VITAL-1 study team. Alisporivir plus ribavirin, interferon free or in combination with pegylated interferon, for hepatitis C virus genotype 2 or 3 infection. Hepatology 2015;62:1013-1023. doi: 10.1002/hep.27960

[93] Zeuzem S, Flisiak R, Vierling JM, Mazur W, Mazzella G, Thongsawat S, Abdurakhmanov D, Van Kinh N, Calistru P, Heo J, Stanciu C, Gould M, Makara M, Hsu SJ, Buggisch P, Samuel D, Mutimer D, Nault B, Merz M, Bao W, Griffel LH, Brass C, Naoumov NV. Randomised clinical trial: alisporivir combined with peginterferon and ribavirin in treatment-naïve patients with chronic HCV genotype 1 infection (ESSENTIAL II). Aliment Pharmacol Ther 2015;42:829-844. doi: 10.1111/apt.13342

[94] Hopkins S, DiMassimo B, Rusnak P, Heuman D, Lalezari J, Sluder A, Scorneaux B, Mosier S, Kowalczyk P, Ribeill Y, Baugh J, Gallay P. The cyclophilin inhibitor SCY-635 suppresses viral replication and induces endogenous interferons in patients with chronic HCV genotype 1 infection. J Hepatol. 2012;57:47-54. doi: 10.1016/j.jhep.2012.02.024

[95] Bartel DP. MicroRNAs: target recognition and regulatory functions. Cell. 2009;136:215-233. doi: 10.1016/j.cell.2009.01.002

[96] Jopling CL, Yi M, Lancaster AM, Lemon SM, Sarnow P. Modulation of hepatitis C virus RNA abundance by a liver-specific MicroRNA. Science. 2005;309:1577-1581. doi: 10.1126/science.1113329

[97] Jopling CL, Schutz S, Sarnow P. Position-dependent function for a tandem microRNA miR-122 binding site located in the hepatitis C virus RNA genome. Cell host

microbe. 2008;4:77-85. doi: 10.1016/j.chom.2008.05.013.

[98] Li Y, Masaki T, Yamane D, McGivern DR, Lemon SM. Competing and noncompeting activities of miR-122 and the 5' exonuclease Xrn1 in regulation of hepatitis C virus replication. Proc Natl Acad Sci U S A. 2013;110:1881-1886. doi: 10.1073/pnas.1213515110

[99] Masaki T, Arend KC, Li Y, Yamane D, McGivern DR, Kato T, Wakita T, Moorman NJ, Lemon SM. miR-122 stimulates hepatitis C virus RNA synthesis by altering the balance of viral RNAs engaged in replication versus translation. Cell Host Microbe. 2015;17:217-228. doi: 10.1016/j.chom.2014.12.014

[100] Shimakami T, Yamane D, Jangra RK, Kempf BJ, Spaniel C, Barton DJ, Lemon SM. Stabilization of hepatitis C virus RNA by an Ago2-miR-122 complex. Proc Natl Acad Sci U S A. 2012;109:941-946. doi: 10.1073/pnas.1112263109

[101] Henke JI, Goergen D, Zheng J, Song Y, Schüttler CG, Fehr C, Jünemann C, Niepmann M.EMBO J. microRNA-122 stimulates translation of hepatitis C virus RNA. 2008;27:3300-3310. doi: 10.1038/emboj.2008.244

[102] Li YP, Gottwein JM, Scheel TK, Jensen TB, Bukh J. MicroRNA-122 antagonism against hepatitis C virus genotypes 1-6 and reduced efficacy by host RNA insertion or mutations in the HCV 5' UTR. Proc Natl Acad Sci U S A. 2011;108:4991-4996. doi: 10.1073/pnas.1016606108

[103] Janssen HL, Reesink HW, Lawitz EJ, Zeuzem S, Rodriguez-Torres M, Patel K, van der Meer AJ, Patick AK, Chen A, Zhou Y, Persson R, King BD, Kauppinen S, Levin AA, Hodges MR. Treatment of HCV infection by targeting microRNA. N Engl J Med. 2013;368:1685-1694. doi: 10.1056/NEJMoa1209026

[104] Tsai WC, Hsu SD, Hsu CS, Lai TC, Chen SJ, Shen R, Huang Y, Chen HC, Lee CH, Tsai TF, Hsu MT, Wu JC, Huang HD, Shiao MS, Hsiao M, Tsou AP. MicroRNA-122 plays a critical role in liver homeostasis and hepatocarcinogenesis. J Clin Invest. 2012;122:2884-2897. doi: 10.1172/JCI63455

[105] Liu F, Shimakami T, Murai K, Shirasaki T, Funaki M, Honda M, Murakami S, Yi M, Tang H, Kaneko S. Efficient Suppression of Hepatitis C Virus Replication by Combination Treatment with miR-122 Antagonism and Direct-acting Antivirals in Cell Culture Systems. Sci Rep. 2016;6:30939. doi: 10.1038/srep30939

[106] van der Ree MH, de Vree JM, Stelma F, Willemse S, van der Valk M, Rietdijk S, Molenkamp R, Schinkel J, van Nuenen AC, Beuers U, Hadi S, Harbers M, van der Veer E, Liu K, Grundy J, Patick AK, Pavlicek A, Blem J, Huang M, Grint P, Neben S, Gibson NW, Kootstra NA, Reesink HW. Safety, tolerability, and antiviral effect of RG-101 in patients with chronic hepatitis C: a phase 1B, double-blind, randomised controlled trial. Lancet. 2017;389:709-717. doi: 10.1016/S0140-6736(16)31715-9

[107] Stelma F, van der Ree MH, Sinnige MJ, Brown A, Swadling L, de Vree JML, Willemse SB, van der Valk M, Grint P, Neben S, Klenerman P, Barnes E, Kootstra NA, Reesink HW. Immune phenotype and function of natural killer and T cells in chronic hepatitis C patients who received a single dose of anti-MicroRNA-122, RG-101. Hepatology. 2017;66:57-68. doi: 10.1002/hep.29148

[108] Deng Y, Campbell F, Han K, Theodore D, Deeg M, Huang M, Hamatake R, Lahiri S,

Chen S, Horvath G, Manolakopoulos S, Dalekos GN, Papatheodoridis G, Goulis I, Banyai T, Jilma B, Leivers M. Randomized clinical trials towards a single-visit cure for chronic hepatitis C: Oral GSK2878175 and injectable RG-101 in chronic hepatitis C patients and long-acting injectable GSK2878175 in healthy participants. J Viral Hepat. 2020;27:699-708. doi: 10.1111/jvh.13282

[109] Herker E, Harris C, Hernandez C, Carpentier A, Kaehlcke K, Rosenberg AR, Farese RV Jr, Ott M. Efficient hepatitis C virus particle formation requires diacylglycerol acyltransferase-1. Nat Med. 2010;16:1295-1298. doi: 10.1038/nm.2238

[110] Rojas Á, Del Campo JA, Clement S, Lemasson M, García-Valdecasas M, Gil-Gómez A, Ranchal I, Bartosch B, Bautista JD, Rosenberg AR, Negro F, Romero-Gómez M. Effect of Quercetin on Hepatitis C Virus Life Cycle: From Viral to Host Targets. Sci Rep. 2016;6:31777. doi: 10.1038/srep31777

[111] Lu NT, Crespi CM, Liu NM, Vu JQ, Ahmadieh Y, Wu S, Lin S, McClune A, Durazo F, Saab S, Han S, Neiman DC, Beaven S, French SW. A Phase I Dose Escalation Study Demonstrates Quercetin Safety and Explores Potential for Bioflavonoid Antivirals in Patients with Chronic Hepatitis C. Phytother Res. 2016;30:160-168. doi: 10.1002/ptr.5518

[112] Gane E, Stedman C, Dole K, Chen J, Meyers CD, Wiedmann B, Zhang J, Raman P, Colvin RA. A Diacylglycerol Transferase 1 Inhibitor Is a Potent Hepatitis C Antiviral in Vitro but Not in Patients in a Randomized Clinical Trial. ACS Infect Dis. 2017;3:144-151. doi: 10.1021/acsinfecdis.6b00138

[113] Falcón V, Acosta-Rivero N, González S, Dueñas-Carrera S, Martinez-Donato G, Menéndez I, Garateix R, Silva JA, Acosta E, Kourı J. Ultrastructural and biochemical basis for hepatitis C virus morphogenesis. Virus Genes. 2017;53:151-164. doi: 10.1007/s11262-017-1426-2

[114] Insull W Jr, Koren M, Davignon J, Sprecher D, Schrott H, Keilson LM, Brown AS, Dujovne CA, Davidson MH, McLain R, Heinonen T. Efficacy and short-term safety of a new ACAT inhibitor, avasimibe, on lipids, lipoproteins, and apolipoproteins, in patients with combined hyperlipidemia. Atherosclerosis. 2001;157:137-144. doi: 10.1016/s0021-9150(00)00615-8

[115] Hu L, Li J, Cai H, Yao W, Xiao J, Li YP, Qiu X, Xia H, Peng T. Avasimibe: A novel hepatitis C virus inhibitor that targets the assembly of infectious viral particles. Antiviral Res. 2017;148:5-14. doi: 10.1016/j.antiviral.2017.10.016

[116] Neveu G, Barouch-Bentov R, Ziv-Av A, Gerber D, Jacob Y, Einav S. Identification and targeting of an interaction between a tyrosine motif within hepatitis C virus core protein and AP2M1 essential for viral assembly. PLoS Pathog. 2012;8:e1002845. doi: 10.1371/journal.ppat.1002845

[117] Neveu G, Ziv-Av A, Barouch-Bentov R, Berkerman E, Mulholland J, Einav S. AP-2-associated protein kinase 1 and cyclin G-associated kinase regulate hepatitis C virus entry and are potential drug targets. J Virol. 2015;89:4387-404. doi: 10.1128/JVI.02705-14

[118] Kovackova S, Chang L, Bekerman E, Neveu G, Barouch-Bentov R, Chaikuad A, Heroven C, Šála M, De Jonghe S, Knapp S, Einav S, Herdewijn P. Selective Inhibitors of Cyclin G Associated Kinase (GAK) as Anti-Hepatitis C Agents. J Med Chem. 2015 23;58:3393-3410. doi: 10.1021/jm501759m

Chapter 5

The Influence of Protease Inhibitors on the Evolution of Hepatitis C in Patients with HIV and HCV Co-Infection

Elena Dumea and Simona Claudia Cambrea

Abstract

Prevalence of hepatitis C in HIV infected patients is much higher than in the general population. There is the possibility of viral clearance HCV, in some patients co-infected HIV and HCV, in the phase of immune reconstruction after antiretroviral treatment (ART). There are patients' anti-HCV positive who initially did not show HCV viral load detected and after the start of ART becomes HCV viral load detectable. There are studies that described that immune restoration with increase in CD4+ and CD8+ T cells, from ART, was important in control of HCV viremia. Has been proposed hypothesis that direct or indirect effect of ART on HCV replication play a role in spontaneous resolution of HCV infection. We evaluated the co-infected patients with HIV and HCV under combined antiretroviral treatment, containing PI boosted with ritonavir in terms of immunological and virological status (for both infection) and also liver disease. Patients were evaluated for liver damage by non-invasive methods. We have shown that a small percentage of patients have severe liver damage. We demonstrated the negative role of HCV on immunological status and in liver fibrosis in co-infected patients. A high proportion of these HIV and HCV co-infected patients had no detectable viremia, higher than other studies published.

Keywords: protease inhibitors, HCV, HIV, co-infection, non invasive liver fibrosis test, seroclearence

1. Introduction

Approximate 1/3 of HIV infected patients are also infected with hepatitis C virus (HCV) due to shared routes of transmission.

The clinical implications of this crossroad are important and challenging issues regarding the evaluation and management of the co-infected patient.

Patients with HIV and HCV infection have higher risk for developing cirrhosis, hepatic decompensation, increased rates of end-stage liver diseases, hepatocellular carcinoma and shortened lifespan after hepatic decompensation.

2. Virology

There are similarities by virological point of view for these two viruses: HIV and HCV. Although both HIV and HCV are single-stranded RNA viruses with worldwide distribution, that can result in chronic, subclinical infection, they differ with regard to several important characteristics. HCV is a *flavivirus*, which does not replicate through a DNA-intermediate, as retroviruses do. This allows the possibility of eradication of HCV. HIV viral production rates are approximate 10^{10} virions per day with half life less than 6 hours and this production is even greater for HCV with production of 10^{12} virions per day and average virirons half-life 27 hours [1]. Details of the HCV replicative process are still not well known.

In chronic mono-infection with hepatitis C virus or HIV is maintained a viral load relatively stable as a "set point" over long periods of time. Virus specific T-cell responses play a role in the control of virus during chronic HCV.

In co-infection HIV and HCV, HCV RNA levels increase after HIV seroconversion, and continue to increase over time, different from HCV mono-infection. Quantitative loss of memory lymphocytes that occurs in HIV infection could potentially be responsible for the elevated HCV RNA levels, observed in co-infected patients [2]. In combined infection, HCV viral load is related with level of immunosuppression (inversely correlated with CD4 counts), and can increase with heavy alcohol use and transient with the antiretroviral therapy initiation [3]. HIV by himself can increase HCV replication due to gp120 protein (HIV envelope protein) through engagement of cellular co-receptors of HIV (ie, CXCR4 or CCR5) [4].

In addition to quantitative changes of T-cells, HIV may induce qualitative defects in immune responses through alteration of cytokine secretion profiles, and/or dendritic cell function. Innate effectors, such as natural killer (NK) cells and natural killer T (NKT) cells, also mediate antiviral defenses. Disruption of NK cell function such as increased activation or decreased cytokine secretion induced by HIV-1 could also be responsible for the development of chronic HCV [5, 6].

HIV replicates in CD4+ T-cells as well in many cell types. There are controversial data regarding HCV replicates in extrahepatic sites, a study suggests peripheral blood mononuclear cells (PBMCs) [7]. Some studies have suggested that HCV RNA replication in PBMCs may occur in patients with HIV/HCV co-infection, but not in those with HCV alone [8]. The mechanism for the relapse of HCV viral load after HIV treatment discontinuation can be HCV replication in dendritic cells or PBMCs [9].

The higher rates of perinatal HCV transmission in co-infected patients can be explained by the fact that HCV has been isolated from the cervico-vaginal lavage fluid in HIV HCV positive women (not in HCV positive alone) [10].

After introduction of directly acting agents against HCV (DAA) it was demonstrated the potential drug resistance for HCV parallels as in HIV, resistance mutation to specific polymerase and protease HCV inhibitors [11].

3. Epidemiology

Since both infections have similar routes of transmission, co-infection HIV and HCV is common. The prevalence of co-infection varies by geographic areas, across risk groups, by route of transmission. Also the sequence of infection depends by transmission route.

HCV infection is transmitted by **percutaneous route** with highest rates in people who inject drugs (PWID) and hemophiliacs. The risk of **post-transfusion** HCV infection deeply decreases. Injection drug use is the most important route of HCV transmission, approximately 80% of HIV persons with history of injection drug use are infected with HCV, and they usually acquire HCV before HIV infection while men who have sex with men (MSM) typically are infected with HIV before HCV infection [12].

HIV is much easily transmissible via **sexual intercourse** than HCV. In heterosexual partners the prevalence of HCV co-infection is estimated as 4% in persons whose main HIV exposure risk is heterosexual sex with multiple partners. Globally, is estimated a 6.4% of HCV/HIV co-infection prevalence among MSM, with variations depending on the geographic region [13]. In MSM, HCV acquisition is associated with unprotected anal intercourse, group sex, fisting and recreational drugs [14]. HCV transmission may be increased by mucosal injury and/or concomitant other sexually transmitted diseases [15]. Ongoing HCV transmission is occurring in MSM with declining after DAAs but high rate of reinfection.

Regarding **perinatal** transmission of HCV, vertical transmission of HCV seems to be facilitated by HIV co-infection. Maternal co-infection increases the risk of vertical HCV transmission to their infants with about 2.82 fold more than for women who are infected with HCV alone [16].

There are rare reported cases of acquisition HIV and HCV via percutaneous exposure in **health care workers**.

4. Pathophysiology

Patients with co-infection HIV/HCV have higher rates of liver fibrosis progression compared with patients with HCV alone.

In patients with HIV, liver fibrosis progression is linked to week cellular immune responses to HCV antigens. The cellular immune response to viral infection is linked to CD8+ T-cell responses and in HIV infection there is a decreases number of CD4 cells, functional impairment of CD4 and CD8 cells and a down-regulation of a co-stimulatory molecule necessary for lymphocyte activation CD28. These observations explain the link between liver progression and advanced immunosuppression.

Also, liver progression can be determined by chronic immune activation through increased levels of pro-inflammatory cytokines, secondary to HIV infection. Kupffer cell depletion is associated with CD4 cell decline and may be related to development of fibrosis [17].

In HCV related liver fibrosis, activated hepatic stellate cells (HSCs) mediate collagen formation. There levels were associated with T cell immune activation and increased gene expression of interleukin-15. In HIV/HCV patients IL-15 play a pathogenic role in mediating liver fibrosis [18].

In normal hepatocytes apoptosis is mediated by tumor necrosis factor-related apoptosis-inducing ligand (TRAIL). Glycoproteins of HIV (gp120) through upregulation of TRAIL-mediated apoptosis triggered to hepatocytes death [19].

HCV-associated proinflammatory cytokines may contribute to liver fibrosis progression and these may have a damaging effect on HIV disease [18].

In acute HCV infection, patients with HIV, especially those with low CD4 counts, have lower rates of spontaneous virologic clearance.

In co-infected patients there is a much more rapid rate of progression to cirrhosis than in HCV alone [20]. The prevalence of extensive liver fibrosis was higher in coinfected patients [21]. Non-invasive assessments of liver fibrosis can be used more frequently and these also suggested more rapid fibrosis progression in coinfection but this can be related with the degree of HIV-immunosuppression.

In coinfection, as in monoinfection, some patients clinical characteristics: older age, diabetes, alcohol consumption, diabetes, obesity, elevated liver enzymes, have been associated with fibrosis progression [22].

5. Effect of antiretroviral treatment (ART) on HCV progression

There are studies that suggested a decline in liver-related mortality associated with a potent ART introduction which also slows the rates of fibrosis progression, due to immune reconstruction [23]. A cross-sectional study demonstrated a lower necroinflammatory activity on liver biopsy in HIV viral suppressed ART patients and another study showed an increased risk of fibrosis progression in those patients with ART interruption [24, 25]. There is a decrease in AIDS and non-AIDS related morbidity and mortality in HIV patients with early ART initiation and this approach is important especially in HIV/HCV patients. There is evidence that use of ART partially restores T-cell responses to core HCV peptides. Successful response to ART among HIV/HCV patients is associated with increased cellular immune responses to HCV infection, long-term reduction in HCV RNA levels and with HCV clearance [26].

Drug induced liver injury (DILI) is more common in HIV/HCV coinfection following ART. Even liver toxicity is more common in patients with chronic viral hepatitis the benefit of ART exceeds the risk of liver injury. Some studies found an increased risk not for all ART regimens, only for some antiretroviral agents, such as ritonavir or nevirapine [27, 28].

The role of particular drug or antiretroviral class in liver progression rates is questionable, there are conflicting data. In a retrospective analysis, the authors observed that along with young age at infection, heavy alcohol use, and a low CD4 count, patients whose ART regimen did not contain a protease inhibitor (PI) had higher inflammation and fibrosis scores when compared to those who took a PI as part of their ART regimen [29]. In another retrospective analysis of coinfected patients, no significant differences in the proportion of severe fibrosis (approximately 25%) were observed between those on an non-nucleoside reverse transcriptase inhibitors (NNRTI), a PI, or both [30]. Therefore, specific PI or NNRTI use may not be associated with evident histological benefit or obvious histological worsening of HCV disease.

There are conflicting studies regarding the role of HCV in clinical progression of HIV disease. Some studies have suggested that co-infected patients have an increased progression to AIDS, as well as a decrease in survival from the time of diagnosis of HIV and AIDS [31, 32].

6. Treatment of chronic hepatitis C virus infection in the patient with HIV

The goal of HCV antiviral treatment is to cure the infection, characterized by achievement of a sustained virological response (SVR) defined as an undetectable HCV RNA at week 12 to 24 after the end of treatment. Thus, an effective cure is associated with substantial reduction in liver-related mortality and morbidity and reduced incidence of hepatocellular carcinoma.

HIV/HCV coinfected patients had lower response rates to HCV treatment with peginterferon and ribavirin regimens compared with individuals without HIV. They have comparable SVR rates with DAA-regimens as HCV-monoinfected patients. Eradication of HCV infection may reduce the antiretrovirus-associated DILI.

The decision of optimal regimen and timing vary based upon: genotype, the stage of liver disease, prior treatment history, drug interaction and some medical and social priorities.

Because of the more rapid progression of liver fibrosis in the settings of HIV infection, coinfected patients should be prioritized for HCV antiviral therapy and

DOI: http://dx.doi.org/10.5772/intechopen.96282

another reason to prioritize HCV treatment is cirrhosis and bridging fibrosis. With highly effective interferon-free regimens (DAA), curative all-oral treatment is possible also for those patients with coinfection. There is a low incidence of adverse events and high efficacy and that means that almost all patients can benefit from HCV treatment.

All HIV patients should be evaluated for chronic HCV infection using a third generation enzyme immunoassay. Patients found to be HCV positive should undergo quantitative HCV RNA testing to confirm the presence of viremia. HIV patients who are found to be HCV seronegative but if they are with advanced immnuosuppression (CD4 counts<100 cells/mm^3), risk factors for HCV acquisition or elevated liver enzymes should undergo HCV-RNA testing.

Evaluation for coinfected patients for HCV treatment, by the point of view of HCV infection, is similar to those monoinfected. Prior to treatment evaluation should focus on these factors: HCV genotype, viral resistance testing for certain populations, history of prior treatment, assessment of liver fibrosis stage using noninvasive tests for fibrosis or liver biopsy, history, physical and basic laboratory tests, evaluation for conditions that might affect the therapy.

6.1 Management of antiretroviral treatment in coinfected patients

Timing of HCV therapy in relation to ART initiation in ART-naïve patients is important and that it will be discussed below. For special population, such as those with decompensate liver diseases, the treatment should be established only in specialized center with expertise in managing HIV/HCV coinfection.

For HIV/HCV coinfected patients whom are considered to receive HCV treatment, the appropriate antiretroviral treatment regimen used should not have serious drug interaction with HCV antiviral agents. Another management issue in coinfected patients is the timing of antiretroviral therapy initiation or regimen switch. It is not recommended an ART interruption to allow HCV antiviral therapy [33].

In ART-naive HIV/HCV patients is preferable to start ART first and begin HCV treatment later. HIV/HCV patients should be initiated on ART for HIV disease without taking into account their CD4 cell count [34]. In selection of ART regimen should be taken into account the potential drug–drug interactions with HCV antivirals. It is recommended to initiate ART approximately 4 to 6 weeks before starting HCV therapy for two reasons: initiation of ART first allows assessment of tolerability and adverse effects of ART alone and the second reasons is an improved HCV outcome, by suppression HIV viral load by ART treatment through restoration of immune response or other effects [35].

In ART-experienced HIV/HCV patients, who achieved HIV viral suppression on an ART well tolerate regimen, should continue the regimen, if it does not have significant drug interactions with the HCV treatment selected. A regimen switch may be necessary if ART regimen components cannot be used with HCV antiviral drugs. In failure to suppress HIV or adverse effects or intolerance to an ART regimen, the regimen switch should be indicated. In this case should be taken into account in selection of a new ART regimen potential drug interaction with HCV-antivirals, in addition to all specific recommendations that appeared in the choice of ART regimen in treatment-experienced patients. In ART regimen switches, prior antiretroviral history drugs and resistance profiles should be studied, to ensure that the new regimen is active, with two or three fully active antiretroviral drugs. The treatment should be initiated after 4 to 6 weeks after ART regimen switch by the same reasons as in ART-naive patients. Additionally, HIV RNA should be determined at 4 to 6 weeks after the switch to ensure that the new regimen maintains HIV viral suppression. If it is wished to switch back, the new ART regimen to the original ART regimen, following completion of HCV treatment, this should be delayed until at least two weeks after completion of HCV treatment, to ensure clearance of the HCV antivirals [34].

6.2 HCV regimen selection in coinfected patients

The efficacy of DAA regimens among HIV/HCV coinfected patients it seems to be comparable to that in HCV monoinfected patients, the regimen selection decisions are similar for these two groups.

The HCV selection regimen is based on genotype, prior HCV treatment, the stage of liver fibrosis and in rare cases by the presence of baseline NS5A inhibitor resistance associated substitutions. In co-infected patients, the HCV regimen drug interaction with HIV antiretroviral is the major consideration in selection of HCV regimen.

The regimen options for coinfected patients with a particular genotype are the same as those for HCV monoinfected patients with the same genotype. Potential drug interactions with antiretroviral regimen is the major consideration factor that decide between the several regimens available for a specific genotype. There are regimens that have been studied in coinfected patients.

6.2.1 Genotype 1 HCV infection

- Elbasvir-grazoprevir- high efficacy of this regimen in HIV/HCV patients. Analysis in monoinfected patients has suggested an association between lower SVR rates and pre-existing variations in the genotype's 1 NS5A inhibitor sequence. In genotype-1a infected patients is recommended testing for these resistance-associated substitution, and, if present, adding ribavirin and extended to 16 weeks the duration of treatment [35, 36].

- Sofosbuvir- velpatasvir- is a highly effective pangenotypic regimen, for 12 weeks, the SVR rates are high regardless cirrhosis or treatment history [37].

    - Sofosbuvir-velpatasvir-voxilaprevir, a regimen reserved for patients who failed on certain DAA-regimen, can be used also for 8 weeks in naïve patients, has not been studied in coinfected patients but is thought to be the same efficient as in monoinfected patients

- Glecaprevir-pibrentasvir, is also a potent effective pangenotypic regimen, with high efficiency in coinfected patients treatment for 8 or 12 weeks [38].

- Ledipasvir-sofosbuvir- is highly effective in several studies in coinfected patients treatment naive or experienced, for 12 weeks, with high SVR overall even in patients with cirrhosis or prior treatment failure [39].

- Ombitasvir- paritaprevir- ritonavir plus dasabuvir- this regimen with or without ribavirin is highly effective for coinfected patients with genotype1, given for 12 to 24 weeks (depending on the infection subtype and the presence of cirrhosis) [40].

- Simeprevir and sofosbuvir – effective in HIV/HCV patients with cirrhosis who had failed to a prior regimen, given 16 or 24 weeks. (telaprevir plus peginterferon and ribavirin) [41]. The SVR rates in real-life are higher in patients without these negative predictors of response.

DOI: http://dx.doi.org/10.5772/intechopen.96282

- Daclatasvir combinations
  - Daclatasvir plus sofosbuvir is highly effective for genotype 1, 12 weeks of treatment in naïve or experienced- coinfected patients. For these regimens, allowed ART agents included darunavir, atazanavir, or lovinavir, each ritonavir-boosted, efavirenz, rilpivirine, raltegravir and dolutegravir. When it is used with specific asntiretrovirals, the dose adjustment of daclatasvir is needed.
  - Daclatasvir plus asunaprevir is available in Japan for genotype 1b infection.

6.2.2 Genotype 2 infection: highly effective options, formally evaluated for coinfected patients

- Sofosbuvir-velpatasvir 12 weeks [37].
- Glecaprevir-pibrentasvir 8 weeks in non-cirrothic patients, 12 weeks for patients with compensated cirrhosis [38]. The choice between them depends on drug interaction.
- Sofosbuvir- velpatasvir-voxilaprevir – reserved for patients who previously failed on an certain DAA regimen, 8 weeks treatment, has not been studied for HIV/HCV patients

Administration and dosing of these regimens in coinfected patients are similar to monoinfection.

6.2.3 Genotype 3 infection

- Glecaprevir-pibrentasvir for 8 to 16 weeks depending on treatment history and presence of cirrhosis
- Sofosbuvir-velpatasvir with or without ribavirin for 12 weeks.
- Daclatasvir plus sofosbuvir
- Sofosbuvir- velpatasvir-voxilaprevir – reserved for patients who previously failed on an certain DAA regimen,, has not been studied for HIV/HCV patients

The choice between them depends on drug interaction. The studies are in a limited number of coinfected patients [37, 38].

6.2.4 Genotype 4, 5 and 6 infection

Studies in limited numbers of coinfected patients have demonstrated good efficacy with various regimens as those recommended for HCV-monoinfected patients.

- Ledipasvir-sofosbuvir
- Elbasvir-grazoprevir
- Glecaprevir-pibrentasvir

6.3 Potential drug interaction with ART

When assessing a HIV/HCV patient for HCV treatment there some important drug interactions to be considered.

- ribavirin. The interaction between it and antiretroviral agents include direct interaction but also a combination that potentiate adverse effects (with atazanavir- containing ART, patients may develop jaundice).

- sofosbuvir. Have few drug interactions with antiretroviral agents. In clinical studies was used in combination with tenofovir disoproxil fumarate- emtricitabine (TDF-EMT), efavirenz, darunavir or atazanavir boosted with ritonavir, raltegravir and rilpivirine, without any evidence of decreased efficacyor adverse events.

- ledipasvir- sofosbuvir. It is available only as a fixed-dose combination. Co-administration with tenofovir disoproxil fumarate (TDF), increased levels of tenofovir. Co-admistration with tenofovir alafenamide (TAF) does not elevate plasma levels of tenofovir, that's why we can switch patients from TDF to TAF containing regimen when planning a treatment with ledipasvir- sofosbuvir. There are specific options for different TDF-containing antiretrovirals in combination with ledipasvir-sofosbuvir.

- sofosbuvir –velpatasvir is only available in fixed-dose combination. There are no evidence of interaction or adverse events in combination with abacavir, atazanavir, darunavir, ritonavir, cobicistat, elvitegravir, raltegravir, lamivudine, emtricitabine, TAF, rilpivirine.

- glecaprevir-pibrentasvir is available in fixed-dose combination. It was used in studies in combination with tenofovor, abacavirm, lamivudine, emtricitabine, raltegravir, dolutegravir, evitegravir with cobicistat and rilpivirine without clinical relevant interactions.

- elbasvir-grazoprevir- is available in fixed-dose combination. Both are primarly metabolized through CYP3A metabolism, thus, coadminsitration with several antiretrovirals is not advised. It can be used in combination with tenofovir, lamivudine, abacavir, emtricitabine, rilpivirine and dolutegravir, raltegravir.

- Ombitasvir-paritaprevir-ritonavir plus dasabuvir. Drug –interactions are expected since all of these agents are substrates and inhibitors of major metabolic enzymes. It was used safely with TDF-FTC and raltegravir, or in combination with atazanavir, when ritonavir boosting was served by ritonavir contained in HCV regimen.

- voxilaprevir, is available in fixed-dose combination pills with sofosbuvir and velpatasvir. Voxilaprevir is a substrate and inhibitor of P-glycoprotein, slowly metabolized by CYP34A. Coadministration with several antiretrovirals is not advised.

- daclatasvir is metabolized by CYP3A, thus inducers or inhibitors of these enzyme are expected to modify daclatasvir concentration.

- simeprevir is oxidatively metabolized by CYP3A. Inducers or inhibitors of CYP3A are expected to modify simeprevir concentration.

Patients should be monitored for side effects and adherence, viral loads responses on therapy and also depending on ART regimen all the tests needed for evaluate side effects or toxicity.

7. Personal contribution

In our hospital, we are treating patients with HIV infection for about 20 years, with a history of long-term antiretroviral regimens which include protease inhibitors (PI). The newly regimens for HCV treatment with direct-acting antivirals contains protease inhibitors (PI) and ritonavir for HCV infection, like in HIV infection.

In our clinic there are 4.33% patients HIV/HCV coinfected, this incidence is similar to HCV in general population in Romania. In a previous study using noninvasive methods FibroScan (transient elasthography) we demonstrated that 84.6% of HIV patients had mild or no fibrosis, 15.4% had moderate–severe fibrosis, and no cirrhosis [42]. We also demonstrated the concordance between noninvasive fibrosis evaluation methods Fibroscan, APRI and FIB-4 score for HIV [43, 44] and in literature these are used in coinfected HIV/HCV patients monitoring.

We evaluated the patients HIV/HCV coinfected under combined antiretroviral treatment containing PI boosted with ritonavir in terms of immunological and virological status (for both HIV and HCV infection) and also liver disease. Patients were evaluated for liver damage by non-invasive methods, APRI score and FIB-4.

By immunological HIV status 64.5% have CD4 ≥ 500cells/mm3, 29.03% have CD4 = 200-499cells/mm^3, and 6.45% CD4 ≤ 200cells/mm3. HIV viral load was <40 copies/ml in 70% of cases, 11% presented less than 100 copies/ml, and 19% of patients, noncompliant to ART treatment, with detectable HIV viral load.

Using APRI score 69% of HIV/HCV patients have APRI < 0.5, representing mild or no fibrosis, 24% moderate or severe fibrosis and 7%, APRI > 1.5 corresponding to cirrhosis. The same results are when we used FIB-4 score: 77% no/mild fibrosis, (FIB4 < 1.45), 16% moderate/severe fibrosis, 7% cirrhosis (FIB-4 > 3.25. We have shown that a small percentage of patients have severe liver damage but significantly higher in HIV HCV co-infection than in mono HIV infected persons (**Table 1**).

In another study on these cohort 34% of coinfected patients have undetectable HCV viral load without any HCV regimen only the same exposure to PI, (ritonavir-boosted lopinavir majority or other PI) [45]. This seroclearence can be explained by immune reconstruction induced by antiretroviral treatment or by direct antiviral effect of PIs on HCV infection.

A high proportion of these HIV/HCV co-infected patients had no detectable viremia, higher than other studies published which may be explained by the fact that these patients have had HCV clearance, spontaneous or induced by the antiretroviral therapy.

Infection	Non-invasive liver fibrosis tests	Fibrosis		
		No/mild (%)	Moderate/severe (%)	Cirrhosis (%)
HIV	APRI	84.6	15.4	0
	FIB-4	82.0	18.0	0
HIV/HCV	APRI	69	24	7
	FIB-4	77	16	7

Table 1.
Liver fibrosis.

The immunological and virological HIV status of these undetectable HCV viral load patients was better than in those with detectabile HCV viral load. There are also diferencies regarding PI regimens and duration between these two groups. We have limited experience on DAA treatment in HIV/HCV coinfected patients.

8. Conclusion

With the growing availability and diversity of direct-acting antiviral combination regimen for HCV treatment, a curative treatment will be possible for majority patients, even those with HIV.

The sustained virologic response rates in coinfected patients treated with DAA are similar with monoinfected patients, with almost the same regimens. These are associated with substantial reductions in liver-related morbidity and mortality. A testing algorithm based on primary care screening (e.g. with APRI, FIB-4) followed by referral for specialty confirmatory testing (e.g, transient elastography) would best fit most practice models.

There are some management issues in HIV/HCV coinfection regarding appropriate antiretroviral regimens and drug interactions with HCV treatment.

With these DAA regimens, as in HIV preexposure prophylaxis (PrEP), maybe we can limit the extension of HCV infections in some risk group of HIV patients.

Conflict of interest

“The authors declare no conflict of interest.”

Author details

Elena Dumea[1,2] and Simona Claudia Cambrea[1,2]*

1 Faculty of Medicine, “Ovidius” University, Constanta, Romania

2 Infectious Diseases Clinical Hospital, Constanta, Romania

*Address all correspondence to: cambrea.claudia@gmail.com

References

[1] Neumann AU, Lam NP, Dahari H, Gretch D R, Wiley T E, Layden T J, Perelson A S. Hepatitis C viral dynamics in vivo and the antiviral efficacy of interferon-alpha therapy. Science 1998; 282:103. DOI:10.1126/science.282.5386.103

[2] Thein HH, Yi Q, Dore GJ, et al. Natural history of hepatitis C virus infection in HIV infected individuals and the impact of HIV in the era of highly active antiretroviral therapy: a meta-analysis. AIDS. 2008;22:1979-1991 DOI:10.1097/QAD.0b013e32830e6d51

[3] Netski DM, Mao Q, Ray SC, Klein RS. Genetic divergence of hepatitis C virus: the role of HIV-related immunosuppression. J Acquir Immune Defic Syndr 2008; 49:136. DOI:10.1097/QAI.0b013e3181869a6f

[4] Lin W, Weinberg EM, Tai AW, et al. HIV increases HCV replication in a TGF-beta1-dependent manner. Gastroenterology 2008; 134:803. DOI:https://doi.org/10.1053/j.gastro.2008.01.005

[5] Khakoo SI, Thio CL, Martin MP, et al. HLA and NK cell inhibitory receptor genes in resolving hepatitis C virus infection. Science. 2004; 305:872-874. DOI:10.1126/science.1097670

[6] Iannello A, Debbeche O, Samarani S, et al. Antiviral NK cell responses in HIV infection: viral strategies for evasion and lessons for immunotherapy and vaccination. J Leukoc Biol. 2008;84:27-49 DOI: 10.1189/jlb.0907649

[7] Blackard JT, Kemmer N, Sherman KE. Extrahepatic replication of HCV: insights into clinical manifestations and biological consequences. Hepatology 2006; 44:15. DOI:10.1002/hep.21283

[8] Laskus T, Radkowski M, Piasek A, et al. Hepatitis C virus in lymphoid cells of patients coinfected with human immunodeficiency virus type 1: evidence of active replication in monocytes/macrophages and lymphocytes. J Infect Dis 2000; 181:442. DOI: 10.1086/315283

[9] Blackard JT, Smeaton L, Hiasa Y, et al. Detection of hepatitis C virus (HCV) in serum and peripheral-blood mononuclear cells from HCV-monoinfected and HIV/HCV-coinfected persons. J Infect Dis 2005; 192:258. DOI: 10.1086/430949

[10] Minosse C, Calcaterra S, Abbate I, et al. Possible compartmentalization of hepatitis C viral replication in the genital tract of HIV-1-coinfected women. J Infect Dis 2006; 194:1529. DOI: 10.1086/508889

[11] Gaudieri S, Rauch A, Pfafferott K, et al. Hepatitis C virus drug resistance and immune-driven adaptations: relevance to new antiviral therapy. Hepatology 2009; 49:1069. DOI: 10.1002/hep.22773

[12] Kim AY, Chung RT. Coinfection with HIV-1 and HCV--a one-two punch. Gastroenterology 2009; 137:795. DOI: 10.1053/j.gastro.2009.06.040

[13] Platt L, Easterbrook P, Gower E, et al. Prevalence and burden of HCV co-infection in people living with HIV: a global systematic review and meta-analysis. Lancet Infect Dis 2016; 16:797. DOI: 10.1016/S1473-3099(15)00485-5

[14] Urbanus AT, van de Laar TJ, Stolte IG, et al. Hepatitis C virus infections among HIV-infected men who have sex with men: an expanding epidemic. AIDS 2009; 23:F1. DOI: 10.1097/QAD.0b013e32832e5631

[15] Tohme RA, Holmberg SD. Is sexual contact a major mode of hepatitis C virus transmission? Hepatology 2010; 52:1497. DOI: 10.1002/hep.23808

[16] Polis CB, Shah SN, Johnson KE, Gupta A. Impact of maternal HIV coinfection on the vertical transmission of hepatitis C virus: a meta-analysis. Clin Infect Dis 2007; 44:1123 DOI: 10.1086/512815

[17] Balagopal A, Ray SC, De Oca RM, et al. Kupffer cells are depleted with HIV immunodeficiency and partially recovered with antiretroviral immune reconstitution. AIDS 2009; 23:2397. DOI: 10.1097/QAD.0b013e3283324344

[18] Allison RD, Katsounas A, Koziol DE, et al. Association of interleukin-15-induced peripheral immune activation with hepatic stellate cell activation in persons coinfected with hepatitis C virus and HIV. J Infect Dis 2009; 200:619. DOI: 10.1086/600107

[19] Volkmann X, Fischer U, Bahr MJ, et al. Increased hepatotoxicity of tumor necrosis factor-related apoptosis-inducing ligand in diseased human liver. Hepatology 2007; 46:1498. DOI: 10.1002/hep.21846

[20] Fierer DS, Dieterich DT, Fiel MI, et al. Rapid progression to decompensated cirrhosis, liver transplant, and death in HIV-infected men after primary hepatitis C virus infection. Clin Infect Dis 2013; 56:1038. DOI: 10.1093/cid/cis1206

[21] Benhamou Y, Bochet M, Di Martino V, et al. Liver fibrosis progression in human immunodeficiency virus and hepatitis C virus coinfected patients. The Multivirc Group. Hepatology 1999; 30:1054. DOI: 10.1002/hep.510300409

[22] Sulkowski MS, Mehta SH, Torbenson MS, et al. Rapid fibrosis progression among HIV/hepatitis C virus-co-infected adults. AIDS 2007; 21:2209. DOI: 10.1097/QAD.0b013e3282f10de9

[23] Klein MB, Althoff KN, Jing Y, et al. Risk of End-Stage Liver Disease in HIV-Viral Hepatitis Coinfected Persons in North America From the Early to Modern Antiretroviral Therapy Eras. Clin Infect Dis 2016; 63:1160. DOI: 10.1093/cid/ciw531

[24] Pascual-Pareja JF, Caminoa A, Larrauri C, et al. HAART is associated with lower hepatic necroinflammatory activity in HIV-hepatitis C virus-coinfected patients with CD4 cell count of more than 350 cells/microl at the time of liver biopsy. AIDS 2009; 23:971. DOI: 10.1097/qad.0b013e328329f994

[25] Thorpe J, Saeed S, Moodie EE, et al. Antiretroviral treatment interruption leads to progression of liver fibrosis in HIV-hepatitis C virus co-infection. AIDS 2011; 25:967. DOI: 10.1097/QAD.0b013e3283455e4b

[26] Thein HH, Yi Q, Dore GJ, et al. Natural history of hepatitis C virus infection in HIV infected individuals and the impact of HIV in the era of highly active antiretroviral therapy: a meta-analysis. AIDS. 2008;22: 1979-1991. DOI: 10.1097/QAD.0b013e32830e6d51

[27] Bonfanti P, Valsecchi L, Parazzini F, et al. Incidence of adverse reactions in HIV patients treated with protease inhibitors: a cohort study. Coordinamento Italiano Studio Allergia e Infezione da HIV (CISAI) Group. J Acquir Immune Defic Syndr 2000; 23:236. DOI: 10.1097/00126334-200003010-00004

[28] den Brinker M, Wit FW, Wertheim-van Dillen PM, et al. Hepatitis B and C virus coinfection and the risk for hepatotoxicity of highly active antiretroviral therapy in HIV-1 infection. AIDS 2000; 14:2895 DOI: 10.1097/00002030-200012220-00011

[29] Benhamou Y, Di MV, Bochet M, et al. Factors affecting liver fibrosis in human immunodeficiency virus-and hepatitis C virus-coinfected patients: impact of protease inhibitor therapy.

Hepatology. 2001;34: 283-287. DOI: 10.1053/jhep.2001.26517

[30] Sterling RK, Lissen E, Clumerk N, et al. Effect of protease inhibitors and non-nucleoside reverse transcriptase inhibitors on liver histology in HIV/HCV co-infection. Analysis of patients enrolled in the AIDS Pegasys Ribabirin International Co-infection Trial (APRICOT); 12th Conference on Retroviruses and Opportunisitic Infections (CROI); Feb 22-25; Boston, MA. 2005. Abstract 951.

[31] Anderson KB, Guest JL, Rimland D. Hepatitis C virus coinfection increases mortality in HIV-infected patients in the highly active antiretroviral therapy era: data from the HIV Atlanta VA Cohort Study. Clin Infect Dis. 2004; 39:1507-1513 DOI: 10.1086/425360

[32] Greub G, Ledergerber B, Battegay M, et al. Clinical progression, survival, and immune recovery during antiretroviral therapy in patients with HIV-1 and hepatitis C virus coinfection: the Swiss HIV Cohort Study. Lancet. 2000;356:1800-1805 DOI: 10.1016/s0140-6736(00)03232-3

[33] HCV Guidance: Recommendations for Testing, Managing, and Treating Hepatitis C. Joint panel from the American Association of the Study of Liver Diseases and the Infectious Diseases Society of America. http://www.hcvguidelines.org/ (Accessed on January 10, 2021).

[34] Panel on Antiretroviral Guidelines for Adults and Adolescents. Guidelines for the use of antiretroviral agents in HIV-1-inf ected adults and adolescents. Department of Health and Human Services. Available at http://aidsinfo.nih.gov/contentfil es/lvguidelines/AdultandAdolescentGL.pdf. (Accessed on January 10, 2021).

[35] Balagopal A, Kandathil AJ, Higgins YH, et al. Antiretroviral therapy, interferon sensitivity, and virologic setpoint in human immunodeficiency virus/hepatitis C virus coinfected patients. Hepatology 2014; 60:477. DOI: 10.1002/hep.27158

[36] Braun DL, Hampel B, Kouyos R, et al. High Cure Rates With Grazoprevir-Elbasvir With or Without Ribavirin Guided by Genotypic Resistance Testing Among Human Immunodeficiency Virus/Hepatitis C Virus-coinfected Men Who Have Sex With Men. Clin Infect Dis 2019; 68:569. DOI: 10.1093/cid/ciy547

[37] Wyles D, Bräu N, Kottilil S, et al. Sofosbuvir and Velpatasvir for the Treatment of Hepatitis C Virus in Patients Coinfected With Human Immunodeficiency Virus Type 1: An Open-Label, Phase 3 Study. Clin Infect Dis 2017; 65:6 DOI: 10.1093/cid/cix260

[38] Rockstroh JK, Lacombe K, Viani RM, et al. Efficacy and Safety of Glecaprevir/Pibrentasvir in Patients Coinfected With Hepatitis C Virus and Human Immunodeficiency Virus Type 1: The EXPEDITION-2 Study. Clin Infect Dis 2018; 67:1010. DOI: 10.1093/cid/ciy220

[39] Naggie S, Cooper C, Saag M, et al. Ledipasvir and Sofosbuvir for HCV in Patients Coinfected with HIV-1. N Engl J Med 2015; 373:705. DOI: 10.1056/NEJMoa1501315

[40] Rockstroh JK, Orkin C, Viani RM, et al. Safety and Efficacy of Ombitasvir, Paritaprevir With Ritonavir ± Dasabuvir With or Without Ribavirin in Patients With Human Immunodeficiency Virus-1 and Hepatitis C Virus Genotype 1 or Genotype 4 Coinfection: TURQUOISE-I Part 2. Open Forum Infect Dis 2017; 4:ofx154. DOI: 10.1093/ofid/ofx154

[41] Basu P, Shah N, Aloysius M. Simeprevir and sofosbuvir with modified doses of ribavirin therapy on telaprevir-experience coinfeced

(with HIV) cirrhotics with chronic hepatitis C: A randomized open label clinical pilot study: STOP C. Presented a t the American Association for the Study of Liver Diseases Liver Meeting, Boston MA, November 7-11, 2014. Abstract #9 93.

[42] Dumea E, Cambrea CS, Petcu LC, Streinu Cercel A. Evaluation of liver diseases through transient elastography in patients with HIV infection. Archives of the Balkan Medical Union, 2013 vol 48, no 4:354-359.

[43] Dumea E, Streinu-Cercel A., Rugină S, Petcu L.C., Halichidis S., Cambrea S.C. Noninvasive assessments (APRI, FIB-4, transient elastography) of fibrosis in patients with HIV and HIV/HBV infection. Proceedings of the 12th Edition of the Scientific Days of the National Institute for Infectious Diseases "Prof Dr Matei Bals", BMC Infectious Diseases 2016, 16(Suppl 4): A52,

[44] Dumea E, Cambrea S.C, Ilie M.M, Petcu L.C, Streinu Cercel A. Evolution of patients coinfected with HIV and hepatitis B: virologic, immunologic, hepatic, regimens. Romanian Journal of Infectious Diseases 2013, vol XVI, no. 4: 218-226. DOI: 10.37897/RJID

[45] Dumitru I., Rugina S., Alexandrescu L, Dumitru E. Increased rates of spontaneous clearance of hepatitis C virus in patients infected with HIV. J Gastrointestin Liver Dis., December 2014, vol.23, no.4:461-462

Section 5

Liver Transplantation

Chapter 6

Liver Transplantation and HCV Genotype 4

Saad Alghamdi and Waleed Al-hamoudi

Abstract

End-stage liver disease secondary to hepatitis C virus (HCV) infection is a major indication for liver transplantation (LT) worldwide. Previous studies have shown a negative impact of HCV on patient and graft survival leading to an inferior transplant outcome when compared to other liver transplant indications. The percentage of HCV patients infected with genotype 4 (G4) among recipients of OLT varies depending on geographic location. In the Middle East HCV-G4 infection is the most common genotype among transplant recipients. Direct antiviral agents (DAAs) have revolutionized the management of HCV infection in the pre- and post-transplant setting. Recent clinical trials have shown high sustained virologic response rates, shorter durations of treatment, and decreased adverse events when compared with the previous treatment of pegylated interferon (PEG-IFN)-based therapy. However, most of these studies were performed in HCV-G1-infected patients. Due to the low prevalence of HCV-G4 in Europe and the USA, this genotype has not been adequately studied in prospective trials evaluating treatment outcomes. The aim of this chapter is to summarize the natural history and treatment outcome of HCV-G4 in the liver transplant setting, with particular attention to new HCV therapies.

Keywords: cirrhosis, direct antiviral agents, genotype 4, hepatitis C, liver transplantation

1. Introduction

Hepatitis C virus (HCV) infection is one of the main indications for liver transplantation (LT) and is a major cause of liver related mortality [1, 2]. Patients transplanted for HCV-related cirrhosis have a worse 5-year survival than those with other indications [3, 4]. HCV eradication prior to LT will likely improve the outcome by eliminating the risk of post-transplant recurrence. Over the last decade, the development of highly effectively DAA agents has allowed for the safe and successful treatment of HCV, shrinking the number of recipients with chronic HCV and improving the post-transplant outcome [5].

Hepatitis C genotype 4 (HCV-G4) is the most prevalent genotype in the Middle East, and Northern Africa [6–9]. Egypt is the most affected nation by HCV and HCV-G4 accounted for 94. 1% of infections. More than 90% of liver transplants in Egypt are for HCV –G4 [10]. Earlier studies from Saudi Arabia also demonstrated that HCV-G4 is the leading indication for liver transplantation [11]. On the other hand, HCV-G4 is a rare indication for liver transplantation in other parts of the world [12, 13].

The frequency of infection with HCV-G4 is also increasing in European countries, particularly among intravenous drug users and immigrants [14–17]. HCV-G4 has not been adequately studied in prospective trials evaluating treatment outcomes and remains the least studied variant. However, over the past five years' data on treatment outcomes of HCV-G4 in the DAA era has been accumulating.

The treatment outcome of HCV-G4 in the interferon era has been reported in multiple studies [18–23]. A higher rate of spontaneous resolution after acute HCV-G4 infection has been reported [24, 25]. Other studies associated HCV-G4 infection with hepatic steatosis [26, 27]. These observations may have an impact on the natural history and treatment outcomes of HCV-G4.

Direct antiviral agents (DAAs) represent a breakthrough in the management of HCV. First generation DAAs (telaprevir, boceprevir) in post-liver transplant patients resulted in sustained virological response of up to 60% with telaprevir in HCV-G1. However, significant side effects including severe anemia, skin complications and significant drug interactions resulted in major concerns [28]. These agents are currently contraindicated and are not used anymore. Second line direct-acting antiviral DAAs have emerged with better safety and efficacy profiles, leading to dramatic changes in the practice of HCV management [29–36]. An international, multicenter, long-term follow-up study of 530 patients with chronic HCV infection who received interferon based therapy demonstrated that among patients with advanced hepatic fibrosis, sustained virological response was associated with lower all-cause mortality [37]. The revolutionary discovery of DAAs makes chronic HCV infection a curable disease in patients with advanced liver disease. Liver function may improve after antiviral therapy in patients on the waiting list and could result in patient delisting. Following liver transplantation, DAA treatment is also highly effective so that postponing antiviral treatment to the post-transplant setting may be of benefit for certain patients. The, aim of this Chapter is to examine the natural history and treatment outcomes of HCV-G4 following liver transplantation. This review includes all published studies and abstracts involving HCV-G4 patients.

2. Natural history of HCV-G4 after liver transplantation

The introduction of DAAs is a significant therapeutic breakthrough in the management of HCV infection. With a very high cure rate, a large proportion of LT candidates and recipients can be cured of HCV infection by DAA therapies that are safe and well-tolerated. Due to the high efficacy of these drugs, a major decline was observed in the number of LT performed both in patients with decompensated cirrhosis with HCV and in those with hepatocellular carcinoma associated with HCV worldwide [38–40]. Furthermore, the survival of LT recipients with HCV-related liver disease has clearly improved because of treatment for HCV recurrence. The advent of efficacious DAA therapy to treat HCV recurrence, resulted in an increasing trend to use HCV seropositive donors for both HCV seropositive and seronegative recipients with excellent outcome [41].

Re-infection of the graft is universal after liver transplantation regardless of genotype and has a negative impact on medium and long-term outcomes [42]. Western studies evaluating the natural history of HCV- G4 in the pre DAA era suggested a worse outcome compared to other genotypes. Zekry et al. analyzed factors that predicted outcome of HCV-liver transplant recipients in the Australian and New Zealand communities. Among 182 patient transplanted for HCV including 16 patients infected with HCV-G4 and a median follow-up of 4 years. HCV-G4 was associated with an increased risk of re-transplantation and death in univariate and multivariate analyses [43]. Whether this difference in outcomes was related to the pathogenicity of HCV-G4 or to other factors not examined in this study, including donor age, immunosuppression, and compliance with medications, is not clear (**Table 1**). Furthermore, patients infected with HCV-G4 in this study were older and more likely to have coexisting hepatocellular carcinoma. In a larger study Gane *et al.* investigated the impact of persistent HCV infection after liver transplantation on patient and graft survival and the effects of the HCV genotype on the severity of recurrent hepatitis. 149 patients with HCV including 14 patients with HCV-G4 infection were followed for a median of 36 months; 623 patients without HCV infection who underwent liver transplantation for end-stage chronic liver disease were used as a control group. Approximately 50% of HCV-G4 had progressive liver disease (moderate hepatitis or cirrhosis) during the follow-up period [44]. In the same study, patients infected with G1b had the worst outcome, whereas patients infected with G2 and G3 had less severe disease recurrence. A more detailed single center study from the UK aimed at studying the impact of HCV-G4 on transplant outcome. The study group included 128 patients who underwent transplantation for HCV infection: 28 patients, genotype 1; 11 patients, genotype 2; 19 patients, genotype 3; and 32 Middle Eastern patients with genotype 4 [45]. A significantly higher fibrosis progression rate was observed in HCV-G4 patients compared with non-G4 patients, although their rates of survival were similar. The five-year cumulative rates for the development of cirrhosis or severe fibrosis were 84% in HCV-G4-infected patients and 24% in patients infected with other genotypes. In the United Kingdom, those Middle Eastern patients maybe the recipients of donated organs only when available organs are declined by all UK transplant centers for UK-born patients. Thus, genotype-4 patients are more likely to receive marginal livers or livers from an older donor. This policy may have led to the selection of inferior grafts for the HCV-G4 patients, who were predominantly non-UK citizens, leading to inferior results in these patients. It has been clearly shown that advanced donor age has a negative impact on the transplant outcome including rapid progression to fibrosis and cirrhosis [46–48].

On the other hand, studies from the Middle East show a more favorable outcome. According to reports from Saudi Arabia and Egypt, overall graft and patient survival for HCV-G4 are comparable to rates reported in the international literature. Reports from Saudi Arabia reveal an overall three-year graft and patient survival rates of 90% and 80%, respectively [11, 49–53]. Similarly, in Egypt, where many

Factors affecting transplant outcome
Viral load
Genotype
Coinfections
Alcohol consumption
Compliance
Chronic kidney disease
Sarcopenia
Steatosis
Donor Age
Immunosuppression
Rejection

Table 1.
Factors affecting the outcome of HCV-related transplantation

active living–related liver transplant programs exist and HCV-G4 represents more than 90% of cases, graft and patient survival rates are approximately 86% [10].

Multiple recent studies from the Middle east evaluated the natural history of HCV-G4 following liver transplantation. A study from Saudi Arabia reported the results of patients who had biopsy-proven recurrent hepatitis C infection and made a comparison between patients with HCV-4 and non-HCV-4 genotype. They clearly demonstrated no significant differences between these two groups in terms of clinical, epidemiological, and histological factors and outcome. They found that in the initial liver biopsy, which was performed after a mean time from transplantation of more than 2 years, there were only four patients who had fibrosis scores greater than stage 3. Two of these patients progressed to cirrhosis on subsequent biopsies [54]. Among many factors included in that analysis, the only factor predictive of an advanced histological score was the HCV RNA level at the time of biopsy.

In studies published from Egypt reporting on living donor related liver (LDLT) transplantation of HCV-G4 patients, similar favorable outcomes were observed. Yosry et al. investigated the outcome of 74 Egyptian patients transplanted for HCV-G4. 31. 1% of patients developed HCV recurrence during a follow up period of 36 months. The majority of patients had mild recurrence, and 91% of the subjects had a fibrosis score of < or = F2. None of the transplanted patients developed cirrhosis or clinical decompensation. Recurrent hepatitis C virus infection was associated with a high pre and post-transplant viral load. The presence of antibodies to hepatitis B core antigen were also associated with disease recurrence [55]. In another study, recurrence was evaluated in 38 Egyptian patients infected with HCV-G4. Patient and graft survivals were 86.6% at the end of the 16 +/− 8.18 months (range, 4-35 months) follow-up period. Clinical HCV recurrence was observed in 10/38 patients (26. 3%). Similar to the previous study, none of the recipients developed cirrhosis or decompensation during the follow-up period [10]. Allam et al. compared the outcomes of Middle Eastern patients who received liver transplantation either in China or locally in Saudi Arabia, respective one- and three-year cumulative survival rates were 81% and 59% in patients transplanted in China compared with 90% and 84% for patients transplanted locally. The incidence of complications was significantly higher especially biliary complications, sepsis, metastasis and acquired HBV infection post-transplant in patients transplanted in China. Patients transplanted in Chine were more likely to undergo postoperative interventions and hospital admissions. This could be explained by the liberal recipient selection criteria, the use of donations after cardiac death, and to the limited post-transplant medical care [56].

HCV-G4 exhibits significant genetic diversity, and there are a number of viral subtypes. The impacts of the various subtypes have been demonstrated in recent studies; for example, HCV G1 subtype 1b patients were more likely to have a better post-transplant outcome compared with subtype 1a [57]. Studies performed in Egypt, where HCV-G4 subtypes 4a and 4b predominate, reveal a better antiviral treatment outcome compared with Saudi Arabia [58–60]. In a retrospective analysis of HCV-G4 patients, Roulot *et al.* reported better sustained virological response (SVR) in 4a subtype- compared with 4d subtype-infected individuals [61]. It is very important to point out the that the negative transplant outcome of HCV-G4 infected patients in the west is not accurate. The majority of recruited patients in these studies are older Egyptians, who have received marginal donor grafts. Co-morbidities, such as infection with schistosomiasis, and other unstudied variables may also have affected outcomes in these patients, leading to an impression that HCV-G4 is an aggressive virus. However, data originating from the Middle East, where HCV-G4 predominates, have revealed no significant difference in outcomes between G1 and G4.

More importantly the recent introduction of DAAs have changed the outlook for HCV-infected patients. The use of DAA agents in the liver transplantation setting has eliminated post-transplant HCV recurrence and improved graft and patient survival irrespective of many other factors including viral genotype.

3. Treatment of HCV in the peritransplant period

3.1 Pegylated interferon and ribavirin (RBV)

Viral eradication or suppression prior to liver transplantation reduces post-transplant recurrence rates [62]. Interferon-based therapy was the only treatment option for HCV prior to the DAA era, however, interferon was contraindicated in patients with advanced liver cirrhosis. This negatively impacted the HCV outcome in cirrhotic and organ transplant patients [63–65].

The limited treatment options lead multiple groups to carefully evaluate Interferon based therapy in the pre transplant setting. Everson *et al.* evaluated the effectiveness, tolerability, and outcome of a low accelerating dose regimen (LADR) of pegylated interferon (PEG-IFN) therapy in the treatment of patients with advanced HCV. This approach was poorly tolerated especially in patients with decompensated disease. One hundred twenty-four patients were treated with LADR, Sustained virological response was achieved in less than 25% and only 12/15 patients who became HCV-RNA negative prior to transplantation remained HCV-RNA negative 6 months after transplantation [64]. In a more recent study patient with various genotypes were randomized 2: 1 to treatment (n = 31) or untreated control (n = 16). Of the patients who were treated, 23 underwent liver transplantation, and 22% achieved a post-transplantation virological response. Although pre-transplant treatment prevented post-transplant recurrence in 25% of cases, including patients infected with HCV-G4, this approach was poorly tolerated and resulted in life-threatening complications [66]. With the introduction of DAA all trials and evaluating interferon based therapies were discontinued and interferon use in this setting is currently contraindicated.

Previously treatment options for patients with recurrent HCV after transplantation were limited. IFN based therapy for patients with post-transplant recurrence were the only available option in the past, these regimens are difficult to tolerate and have disappointing efficacy with hard-to-manage drug interactions. Reported SVR rates for PEG-IFN combination therapy following liver transplantation are lower than those in the nontransplant population. Treatment regimens have been hindered by a high incidence of adverse effects, leading to treatment withdrawal.

Dabbous *et al.* evaluated 243 patients transplanted for HCV-G4-related cirrhosis. Patients with proven histological recurrence received PEG-IFN and ribavirin. Repeated liver biopsies were performed at 3, 6, and 12 months during treatment for the detection of immune-mediated rejection induced by interferon. Histopathological disease recurrence was high 56 (23%), and 42 patients completed the treatment. Five patients were excluded due to fibrosing cholestatic hepatitis; therefore, 37 patients were included in the study. Erythropoietin and granulocyte colony-stimulating factor were used in 70% of patients. SVR was achieved in 29 (78%) patients [67]. Ponziani *et al.* evaluated treatment responses in 17 Italian patients with HCV-G4 recurrence following liver transplantation. The observed overall survival after LT was 100% at 1 year and 83. 3% at 5 years. Thirty-five percent of patients achieved SVR. This study included patients treated with conventional interferon; the lack of aggressive management of hematological side effects and the inclusion of patients with advanced liver disease contributed to the low response rate [68].

Al-hamoudi et al. assessed the safety and efficacy of PEG-IFN alpha-2a in combination with RBV in the treatment of recurrent HCV genotype 4 after LT. Pretreatment liver biopsies were obtained from all patients. Five patients had advanced pretreatment liver fibrosis. Only 14 (56%) patients achieved SVR. The most common adverse effects were flu-like symptoms and cytopenia. One patient developed severe rejection complicated by sepsis, renal failure, and death. Other adverse effects included depression, mild rejection, impotence, itching, and vitiligo [69].

4. Treatment of advanced disease in the new era

The treatment of chronic hepatitis C has been revolutionized with the introduction of DAAs. New oral DAAs have emerged with better safety and efficacy profiles, leading to dramatic changes in the practice of HCV management. The goal of HCV treatment is to reduce mortality and liver complications through virologic cure. The end point is sustained virological response (SVR), which is an undetectable viral load at least 12 weeks after completing treatment. The DAAs target various proteins throughout the HCV replication cycle [70]. These choices include sofosbuvir based therapy plus weight-adjusted RBV, ombitasvir/paritaprevir/ritonavir, elbasvir-grazoprevir and glecaprevir/pibrentasvir. The choice between them depends primarily on potential for drug interactions, availability, and cost. Data on the use of these new agents in cirrhotic G4 patients awaiting liver transplantation are limited. Up-to-date studies evaluating the safety and efficacy of these agents in HCV-G4 patients are summarized below.

4.1 Sofosbuvir and ribavirin

Sofosbuvir (SOF) is a novel pangenotypic nucleotide analog inhibitor that inhibits HCV RNA replication. SOF is administered orally and inhibits the HCV NS5B polymerase. SOF exerts potent antiviral activity against all HCV genotypes [71–75].

Curry et al. conducted a trial to determine whether sofosbuvir and RBV treatment before liver transplantation could prevent HCV recurrence afterward. They included 61 patients with child A cirrhosis and HCV of any genotype. All involved patients were on waitlists for liver transplantation for hepatocellular carcinoma and received up to 48 weeks of sofosbuvir (400 mg) and RBV before liver transplantation. Of 46 patients who were transplanted, 43 had HCV-RNA levels of less than 25 IU/ml at the time of transplantation. Of these 43 patients, 30 (70%) exhibited a post-transplantation virological response at 12 weeks [76]. Another study evaluated the efficacy and safety of SOF in combination with RBV in HCV-G4 patients in patients of Egyptian ancestry. 60 patients were included and half of them were treatment-naïve. Patients were treated for 12 weeks (n = 31) or 24 weeks (n = 29). Overall, 23% of patients had cirrhosis. SVR was achieved by 68% of patients in the 12-week group, and by 93% of patients in the 24-week group. Treatment was well tolerated and none of the patients discontinued treatment due to an adverse event [77]. Doss et al. evaluated the efficacy and safety of SOF in combination with ribavirin in HCV-G4 patients in Egypt. 103 patients were included and received a combination of SOF and weight-adjusted RBV. 17% of the study population were cirrhotic. Patients with cirrhosis at baseline had lower rates of SVR (63% at 12 weeks, 78% at 24 weeks) than those without cirrhosis (80% at 12 weeks, 93% at 24 weeks). The most common adverse events were fatigue, headache, insomnia, and anemia. Two patients experienced serious adverse events. No adverse events resulted in treatment discontinuation [78]. In a more recent study, 2400 Egyptian patients with liver cirrhosis due to chronic HCV infection were treated with SOF and RBV for 24 weeks. The majority of included patients were treatment-naive. The overall SVR rate was 71. 2%. The most common adverse events were fatigue, myalgia, headache, insomnia, and anemia. Only 5.6% of patients discontinued treatment due to the appearance of significant complications [79]. In another study 14 409 patients received either dual therapy, SOF/RBV for 6 months (group1) or triple therapy with SOF/peg-IFN-alfa-2a/RBV for 3 months (group 2), in a cohort of patients treated in National Treatment Programme affiliated centres in Egypt. In group 1, the SVR at week 12 was 94% and in group 2 the SVR was 78.7% [80].

The efficacy of this combination following LDLT was also evaluated in Saudi Arabia. Ajlan et al. reported the safety and efficacy data on 36 post liver transplant patients who received SOF and RBV ± peg-IFN. All patients were infected with HCV-G4, mean age was 56 years, and the cohort included 24 males and one patient had cirrhosis. The majority of patients had advanced fibrosis. 28 patients were treated with PEG-IFN and RBV in addition to SOF for 12 weeks and the remaining were treated with SOF and RBV only for 24 weeks. By week 4, only four (11. 1%) patients had detectable HCV RNA [81]. In another study 39 Egyptian liver transplant recipients were treated for recurrent HCV-G4 after transplantation with SOF and ribavirin for 6 months. SVR was achieved in 76% of recipients. SVR was significantly higher in treatment-naïve patients and in recipients with a low stage of fibrosis [82]. A prospective multicenter study enrolled 40 patients with compensated recurrent HCV infection of any genotype following liver transplantation. All patients received 24 weeks of SOF 400 mg daily and RBV. Of the 40 patients enrolled and treated, 40% had biopsy proven cirrhosis, and 88% received prior interferon treatment. SVR was achieved by 28 of 40 patients. Relapse accounted for all cases of virological failure, including the only patient with HCV-G4. No deaths, graft losses, or episodes of rejection occurred. No interactions with any concomitant immunosuppressive agents were reported [83]. Forns et al. conducted a post-transplantation study in which SOF and RBV were provided on a compassionate-use basis to patients with severe recurrent HCV, including those with fibrosing cholestatic hepatitis (FCH) and decompensated liver cirrhosis with a life expectancy of less than one year. Patients received SOF and RBV for 24–48 weeks, PEG-IFN was added in some patients. The study population included patients infected with HCV- G4. The overall SVR rate was 59% and was higher (73%) in those with early severe recurrence. 123 serious adverse events occurred in 49 patients (47%). Severe adverse events associated with hepatic decompensation were the most frequent, with 26 adverse events occurring in 19 patients (18%) [84]. However, with the emergence of other treatment options this combination is not considered the best treatment option (**Table 2**).

4.2 Sofosbuvir/ledipasvir (LDV)

Colombo et al. evalaluated the safety and efficacy of LDV-SOF in kidney transplant recipients with chronic genotype 1 or 4 HCV infection and included patients with cirrhosis. Ten patients in this trial were infected with HCV-G4 and all included patients achieved SVR. Treatment with LDV-SOF for 12 or 24 weeks was well-tolerated and seemed to have an acceptable safety profile among kidney transplant recipients with HCV genotype 4 infection [85]. In a recently published study real-world effectiveness of LDV-SOF was evaluated. 135 patients infected with G4 were included, the overall SVR rate was 89.6% including treatment experienced and cirrhotic patients [86]. Charlton et al. (SOLAR-1) assessed treatment with LDV, SOF, and RBV in patients infected with HCV-G1 or HCV-G4. This study included a cohort of patients with cirrhosis who had not undergone liver transplantation. The SVR rate in the cirrhotic group was 86–89% [87]. Kohli et al. evaluated

Study	Sample size	Genotypes	SVR	Treatment protocol
Ajlan [81]	36	4	91.6%	SOF+RBV+PEG-INF for 12 weeks or SOF+RBV for 24 weeks
Dabbous [82]	39	4	76%	SOF+RBV 24 weeks
Forns [95]	104	1, 2, 3, 4	59%	SOF+RBV for 24–48 weeks
Abaalkhail [93]	50	4	86%	LDV-SOF+/-RBV 12-24 weeks
Mann [94]	227	1,4 (n=27)	92.5%	SOF+LDV+RBV 12-24 weeks
Dumortier [108]	125	All(11 G4)	92%	SOF/DCV+/-RBV 12-24 weeks
Coilly [107]	137	All (12 G 4)	96%	SOF+DAC
Leroy [102]	23 (all with FCH)	All (3 G4)	96%	SOF+DCV for 24 weeks
Reau [128]	100	All (3 G4)	100% for G4	Glecaprevir/Pibrentasvir for 12 weeks
Agarwal [131]	79	1,4 (n=4)	100% for G4	SOF/VEL

SVR = sustained virological response, SOF = sofosbuvir, RBV = ribavirin, LDV = ledipsavir, DCV = daclatasvir, SIM = simeprevir, FCH = fibrosing cholestatic hepatitis, Peg-INF = pegylated interferon.

Table 2.
Prospective studies that included HCV-G4 patients following liver transplantation.

12 weeks of combination therapy with LDV and SOV for patients with chronic HCV-G4 infections. 20 (95%) of 21 patients completed 12 weeks of treatment and achieved SVR (95% CI 76-100), including seven patients with cirrhosis. One patient was non-adherent to study drugs and withdrew from the study, but was included in the intention-to-treat analysis. No patients discontinued treatment because of adverse events [88]. Crespo et al. investigated the effectiveness and safety of DAAs in patients with HCV-G4 infection in routine practice. 130 patients with HCV-G4 were treated with LDV/SOV, SVR was achieved in 93. 2% of cirrhotic patients [89]. Abergel et al. also evaluated the efficacy and safety of therapy with LDV and SOF in patients with HCV-G4. Forty-four patients (22 treatments naïve and 22 treatment experienced) received a fixed-dose combination tablet of 90 mg LDV and 400 mg SOV orally once daily for 12 weeks. Ten patients (23%) had compensated cirrhosis. The SVR rate was 93% and was similar in treatment-naïve (95%, 21/22) and treatment-experienced (91%, 20/22) patients. Treatment was well tolerated with no serious adverse events [90]. Sanai et al. assessed real-world safety and efficacy of LDV/SOF with or without RBV in HCV-G4 infected patients with compensated and decompensated cirrhosis. This observational cohort (n = 213) included HCV-G4 treatment-naïve (59.6%) and -experienced (40.4%) patients with advanced fibrosis (F3, Metavir; n = 30), compensated (F4, n = 135) and decompensated cirrhosis (n = 48) treated for 12 (n = 202) or 24 weeks (n = 11) with LDV/SOF. RBV was dosed by physician discretion between 600 and 1200 mg daily. Patients with prior DAA failure were excluded from the analysis. Overall, 197 (92.5%) of the patients achieved SVR [91]. The SVR rate was as high as 98% for genotype 4 when using this combination to treat treatment-niave cirrhotic patients for 12 weeks [92]. Abaalkhail et al. evaluated prospectively the safety and efficacy of LDV-SOF for 12 to 24 weeks with or without RBV in treating HCV-4 infected patients with cirrhosis (cohort A) or post-liver transplantation (cohort B). A total of 111 patients (61 cirrhotic; 50 postliver transplants) with HCV genotype 4 were included. SVR was achieved in 91.8% and 86% of cohorts A and B, respectively. There were no treatment-related mortality or significant side effects [93].

Cohort B of the SOLAR-1 study enrolled patients who had undergone liver transplantation and included patients with post-transplant liver cirrhosis. Patients were randomly assigned to receive a fixed-dose combination tablet containing LDV and SOF plus RBV for 12 or 24 weeks. The cohort included 108 post-transplant patients. SVR was achieved in 96–98% of patients without cirrhosis or with compensated cirrhosis, in 85%–88% of patients with moderate hepatic impairment, in 60%–75% of patients with severe hepatic impairment, and in all six patients with FCH [87]. Similarly, an open-label study at 34 sites in Europe, Canada, Australia, and New Zealand evaluated treatment outcome in the pre and post-transplant settings. Cohort A included patient with cirrhosis who had not undergone liver transplantation. Cohort B included post-transplantation patients who had either no cirrhosis; CTP-A, CTP-B, or CTP-C cirrhosis; or fibrosing cholestatic hepatitis. Patients in each group were randomly assigned to receive 12 or 24 weeks of LDV (90 mg) and SOF (400 mg) once daily, plus RBV (600–1200 mg daily). The majority of patients were infected with HCV genotype 1 and only 37 were infected with genotype 4. Among all patients with genotype 4 HCV, SVR was achieved by 14 of 18 (78%) patients (12 weeks' treatment) and 16 of 17 (94%) patients (24 weeks' treatment) [94]. SOF/LDV combination was also evaluated in the post-transplant setting in a recently published German study that included both genotypes 1, 4. An overall SVR was achieved in 97% of patients [95].

The safety profile of LVD/SOF with RBV was evaluated in a pooled analysis of SOLAR-1 and -2 studies. These two studies included cirrhotic or post–liver transplantation patients infected with genotypes 1 and 4 and were randomized to 12 or 24 weeks of treatment. Treatment in the two trials was well tolerated and safe. RBV-associated anemia was the most common adverse effect, representing over 50% of reported drug-related adverse events [96].

4.3 Sofosbuvir/daclatasvir (DCV)

DCV is a pangenotypic NS5A inhibitor with a very low potential for drug interaction and a favorable safety profile. EL-khayat et al. investigated the efficacy and safety of SOF/DCV for treatment of patients with HCV-G4 induced cirrhosis. This was a multicenter study involving 551 patients with HCV-G4 related cirrhosis; 432 naïve patients and 119 treatment-experienced patients. All patients received SOF/DCV/RBV for 12 weeks and when RBV is contraindicated the treatment duration was extended to 24 weeks. SVR rate was 92% in naïve cirrhotic patients and 87% in previous treated patients [97]. In a French study, 176 HCV-G4 patients were treated with SOF and DCV. All the patients enrolled had advanced stages of liver fibrosis. The overall SVR rate was 90%, with the highest rate (97%) reached in cirrhotic patients treated with RBV, a the lowest (88%) in those treated without RBV [98]. In another recently published study involving only HCV-G4 patients, SVR was achieved in 100% of patients who received SOF/DCV with or without RBV. This study included patients with advanced fibrosis and cirrhosis. Adverse events occurred in 32% of patients, but none discontinued treatment [99]. The Phase II, open-label, nonrandomized IMPACT study assessed the efficacy of three DAAs (simeprevir, sofosbuvir, and daclatasvir) in HCV genotype 1/ 4-infected cirrhotic patients with portal hypertension or decompensated liver disease. All patients received simeprevir (SIM) 150 mg, DCV 60 mg, and SOF 400 mg once-daily for 12 weeks. All 40 patients included in the study achieved SVR and the combination was well tolerated [100]. The outcome of SOF/DCV/RBV in non-responders to prior sofosbuvir-based therapy was evaluated in a large Egyptian study that included 1014 patients in which 47% were cirrhotic. Overall SVR was 90.6% with no major side effects [101].

Multiple other studies showed high SVR rates among genotype 4 infected patients [102–106].

Data on the use of DCV in the post-transplant setting for HCV-G4-infected patients are limited.

In a multicenter prospective study 137 patients with post-transplant HCV recurrence received SOF and DCV. This cohort included 12 patients infected with HCV-G4. The SVR rate after completing treatment was 96% under the intention-to treat analysis. No clinically relevant drug–drug interactions were noted, but 52% of patients required a change to the dosage of immunosuppressive drugs [107]. A recent prospective multicenter study evaluating SOF based therapy in the post liver transplant setting was conducted and included all genotpes. The main combination regimen was SOF/DCV (73.6%). SVR was 92.8% (on an intent-to-treat basis) [108]. Leroy *et al*. analyzed data from 23 patients with FCH who participated in a prospective cohort study in France and Belgium to assess the effects of antiviral agents in patients with recurrence of HCV infection after liver transplantation. Three patients with G4 infection were included in this study and all 3 achieved SVR [109].

4.4 Sofosbuvir/Simeprevir (SIM)

SIM is a NS3/4A protease inhibitor with antiviral activity against G1, G2, G4, G5, and G6.

An open-label, multicentre, phase IIa study evaluated the outcome of SIM plus SOF for eight or 12 weeks in HCV-G4 infected patients. This study included 23 cirrhotic patients who received a 12 week course of therapy. Treatment comprised SIM 150 mg and SOF 400 mg daily. All cirrhotic patients achieved SVR and the treatment was well tolerated [110]. In a phase III, open-label, single-arm study the efficacy and safety of 12 weeks of SIM plus SOF in treatment-naïve and experienced HCV-G4 infection, including cirrhotic patients was conducted. All patients achieved SVR including the cirrhotic patients. No serious adverse events were reported and no patients discontinued study treatment [111]. The combination of SIM/SOF in a recently published Egyptian study involving genotype 4 infected patients resulted in a SVR rate of 92% in 100 treated patients [112]. The Phase II IMPACT study was conducted in HCV genotype 1- or 4-infected cirrhotic patients with portal hypertension or decompensated liver disease and assessed the combination of the three direct-acting antivirals SIM, DCV and SOF. All 40 patients achieved SVR [113]. Multiple other studies that included cirrhotic and treatment experienced patients treated with SIM and SOF revealed high SVR rates [114–116].

The efficacy and safety of SOF-based regimens in the real world among a cohort of Egyptian patients with recurrent HCV post LDLT was evaluated in HCV-G4 infected patients. 190 patients were included. Out of 190, 119 received SOF/RBV, 38 SOF/SIM, 22 SOF/DCV)/ ± RBV, and 11 received SOF/LDV/ ± RBV. SVR rates were as follow: 84.9% in SOF/RBV group, 94.7% in SOF/SIM, 100% in SOF/DCV, and 100% in SOF/LDV. Treatment was well tolerated with no significant drug–drug interactions [117]. The outcome of the combination SIM + SOF ± RBV in a group of liver transplant patients with HCV genotype 4 infection in Spain was evaluated in a real life study. This was a multicenter retrospective study, including 28 HCV genotype 4 patients from 11 liver transplant centers. The SVR was 95.23% including patients with advanced fibrosis and cirrhosis [118].

4.5 Ombitasvir, ritonavir and paritaprevir

The combination of ombitasvir, ritonavir and paritaprevir was evaluated in multiple studies involving compensated cirrhotic HCV-G4 patients and revealed high SVR rates reaching 100% in some studies [119–124]. In a recent meta-analyses, 20 cohorts across 12 countries were identified, totaling 5158 patients infected with

G1 and 4. The overall SVR rates were 98.9% for HCV-G4 infected patients [125]. The regimen is contraindicated in Child Pugh classes B and C cirrhosis, therefor its use in the pre transplant setting is limited.

4.6 Glecaprevir/Pibrentasvir

The EXPEDITION-1 trial enrolled 146 patients with compensated cirrhosis, 16 (11%) patients were infected with HCV-G4. Patients in this trial received a fixed dose of glecaprevir (300 mg)/pibrentasvir (120 mg) for 12 weeks. SVR was 100% for patients infected with HCV-G4 [126].

EXPEDITION-8 is a randomized trial that enrolled 343 patients with HCV Genotypes 1–6 and compensated cirrhosis. All patients received an 8-week course of Glecaprevir/Pibrentasvir. Of 343 patients, 13 had HCV-G4. The SVR12 rate in HCV-G4 was 100% [127].

On the other hand, MAGELLAN-2 trial was a phase 3, open-label trial for patients at least 3 months post transplantation. The study enrolled 100 patients of HCV. Three patients with genotype 4 underwent LT. After a 12-week course, all HCV-G4 infected patients achieved SVR 12 [128].

Immunosuppressive therapy should be monitored closely due to the possibility of drug–drug interaction when used with protease inhibitors.

4.7 Sofosbuvir/Velpatasvir (VEL)

In 2015, ASTRAL-1 evaluated the efficacy and safety of 12-week course of VEL and SOF. Of the 624 patients, 116 (19%) had genotype 4. One fourth of genotype 4 patients had cirrhosis. After a 12-week course of SOV/VEL, all patients (100%) with HCV-G4 achieved SVR [129].

ASTRAL-4 trial enrolled 267 patients with decompensated cirrhosis, CPT B. The study was open label with 3 arms that included: SOF/VEL for 12 weeks, SOF/VEL in addition to RBV for 12 weeks, or SOF/VEL for 24 weeks. In this trial, 8 (3%) patients had genotype 4. Regardless of the assigned arm, all genotype 4 patients (100%) achieved SVR. In this study, 81% of patients with MELD score above 15 had improvement after completion of treatment. This study was one of the earliest trials to evaluate SOV/VEL for decompensated cirrhotic patients [130].

In a recent trial 79 post liver transplant patients with HCV-G 1 and 4 received SOF/VEL daily for 12 weeks. In this trial, 4 patients were infected with HCV-G4. All patients with genotype 4 achieved SVR. There were no deaths or rejection episodes during the study period [131].

4.8 Sofosbuvir/Velpatasvir/Voxilaprevir (VOX)

POLARIS-1 trial assessed the safety and efficacy of SOF/VEL/VOX taken for 12 weeks vs. placebo. Patients with cirrhosis represented 46% of the study population. All patients with genotype 4 (22) were in the active treatment arm. By the end of the study period, 20 patients (91%) achieved SVR. One cirrhotic patient developed NS5A Y93H resistance-associated substitution and the other one did not receive treatment.

In the POLARIS-4 trial, patients were assigned to either SOF/VEL/VOX or SOF/VEL once daily for 12 weeks. All genotype 4 patients received SOF/VEL/VOX. The SVR rate was 100% for HCV-G4 infected patients [132].

The use of combined SOF/VEL/VOX is not recommended in patients with advanced liver disease CPT C. There are no currently strong data to support SOF/VEL/VOX use post liver transplantation. Case reports showed favorable outcome in the post-transplant setting [133].

4.9 Elbasvir/Grazoprevir (EBR/GZR)

A randomized controlled open label trial assessed the effectiveness of EBR/GZR with or without RBV for 12 or 16 weeks. The study population was 420 patients out of whom 36 had HCV-G4. The SVR for HCV-G4 patients was 89% which improved with a longer duration of treatment [134].

Jacobson et al. published the integrated analysis of 6 clinical trials. The analysis included 402 patients who received EBR/GZR once daily +/− RBV, for 12-18 weeks. Twenty-three patients with HCV-G4 were included in the analysis. Six patients were treatment naïve and they all achieved SVR. In the treatment experienced group, 4 patients (100%) achieved SVR after 16-18 week of treatment. However, the success rate was lower in treatment experienced patients with a 12-week course without RBV (66.7%) or with RBV (80%) [135].

Data for this combination in the post-transplant setting is limited.

4.10 DAA treatment failures

Despite the high SVR rate associated with DAA in HCV-G4 infected patients, a small percentage of patients do not respond to treatment. In the early era of DAA the most common approach was to add RBV or in some studies PEG-IFN and extend the treatment duration. However, with the emergence of new DAA choices, changing to another DAA became the most common approach. Yousif et al. conducted a prospective cohort study to assess the safety and efficacy of 12 weeks' retreatment with either combination of SOF/DCV/SMV/RBV (45 patients) or SOF/OBV/PTV/r/RBV (163 patients) in patients who had previously failed NS5A inhibitors-based regimens. The overall SVR rates in the two groups were 98. 1% [136]. In another study, patients who failed SOF/DCV were retreated successfully with other DAAs [137]. In a recently published study quadruple regimen of (sofosbuvir, daclatasvir, and simeprevir with a weight-based ribavirin) in chronic HCV-G4 DAAs-experienced patients was successful in eradicating the virus [138]. Multiple other studies revealed similar results [139, 140].

5. Timing of treatment for patients on the transplant list

The management of hepatitis C virus (HCV) infection in patients with decompensated cirrhosis has evolved dramatically. DAAs have shown to be safe and effective in patients with decompensated cirrhosis with high SVR rates. However, it is still debatable on when to initiate treatment in patients with advanced liver disease. Krassenburg et al. evaluated the impact of SVR in a large international multicenter cohort study, including a large number of patients with HCV-related cirrhosis treated with DAAs. Achievement of SVR was independently associated with a 2. 5-fold lower risk of cirrhosis-related complications or death in patients with compensated cirrhosis. On the other hand, no clinical benefit was apparent with HCV eradication in patients with decompensated liver disease. Among patients with CP-B/C cirrhosis, the event-free survival and LT-free survival did not differ between those with SVR and those without SVR. Furthermore, MELD score improvement did not translate to a beneficial clinical outcome in these subset of patients. Thus, DAA therapy may lower prioritization for LT through MELD score reduction, which is likely to primarily affect those with a more urgent need liver transplantation [141]. Other recently published studies assessed the impact of DAAs on patients awaiting liver transplant. They evaluated whether patients can be first inactivated due to clinically improvement and subsequently delisted in a real life setting. Treated patient had a significant improvement in the median MELD and Child Pugh score. They concluded that all oral DAAs were able to reverse liver dysfunction and may result in delisting of about 20-30% of patients. Patients with lower MELD scores had higher chances to be delisted. However, the longer term benefits of therapy need to be ascertained [142, 143]. Similarly, Afdahl et al. evaluated the outcome of DAA in compensated and decompensated cirrhotic patients. They also measured the hepatic venous pressure gradient before and after treatment in fifty patients with Child-Pugh-Turcotte (CPT) A and B cirrhosis and portal hypertension. They observed a clinically meaningful improvement in portal hypertension in addition to improvements in liver biochemistry, Child–Pugh score and Model for End-Stage Liver Disease scores [144]. The potential benefits of treating patients on the waiting list include potential improvements in overall clinical status that may salvage these patients from liver transplantation; reducing post-transplant recurrence; and avoiding possible post-transplant drug–drug interactions. One concern is that treating these patients may lower their MELD scores and drive them down the transplant list, thus delaying transplantation despite persistent portal hypertensive complications.

Author details

Saad Alghamdi[1] and Waleed Al-hamoudi[1,2]*

1 Department of Liver Transplantation and Hepatobiliary Surgery, King Faisal Specialist Hospital and Research Center, Riyadh, Saudi Arabia

2 Gastroenterology Unit, Department of Medicine, College of Medicine, King Saud University, Riyadh, Saudi Arabia

*Address all correspondence to: walhamoudi@ksu.edu.sa; walhamoudi@gmail.com

References

[1] Kim WR. The burden of hepatitis C in the United States. Hepatology 2002; 36: S30-S34.

[2] Wiesner RH, Sorrell M, Villamil F. Report of the first International Liver Transplantation Society expert panel consensus conference on liver transplantation and hepatitis C. Liver Transpl 2003; 9: S1-S9.

[3] Garcia-Retortillo M, Forns X, Feliu A, Moitinho E, Costa J, Navasa M, et al. Hepatitis C virus kinetics during and immediately after liver transplantation. Hepatology 2002; 35: 680-687.

[4] Vinaixa C, Rubín A, Aguilera V, Berenguer M. Recurrence of hepatitis C after liver transplantation. Ann Gastroenterol 2013; 26:304-313.

[5] Fehily SR, Papaluca T, Thompson AJ. Long-Term Impact of Direct-Acting Antiviral Agent Therapy in HCV Cirrhosis: Critical Review. Semin Liver Dis. 2019 Jul;39(3):341-353.

[6] Messina JP, Humphreys I, Flaxman A, Brown A, Cooke GS, Pybus OG, et al. Global distribution and prevalence of hepatitis C virus genotypes. Hepatology 2015;61:77-87.

[7] Abdel-Aziz F, Habib M, Mohamed MK, Abdel-Hamid M, Gamil F, Madkour S, et al. Hepatitis C virus (HCV) infection in a community in the Nile Delta: Population description and HCV prevalence. Hepatology 2000;32:111-115.

[8] Al Traif I, Al Balwi MA, Abdulkarim I, Handoo FA, Alqhamdi HS, Alotaibi M, et al. HCV genotypes among 1013 Saudi nationals: A multicenter study. Ann Saudi Med 2013;33:10-12.

[9] Xu LZ, Larzul D, Delaporte E, Bréchot C, Kremsdorf D. Hepatitis C virus genotype 4 is highly prevalent in central Africa (Gabon). J Gen Virol 1994;75:2393-2398.

[10] Yosry A, Esmat G, El-Serafy M, Omar A, Doss W, Said M, et al. Outcome of living donor liver transplantation for Egyptian patients with hepatitis c (genotype 4)-related cirrhosis. Transplant Proc 2008;40:1481-1484.

[11] Al-Sebayel M, Khalaf H, Al-Sofayan M, Al-Saghier M, Abdo A, Al-Bahili H, et al. Experience with 122 consecutive liver transplant procedures at King Faisal Specialist Hospital and Research Center. Ann Saudi Med 2007;27:333-338.

[12] Rustgi VK. The epidemiology of hepatitis C infection in the United States. J Gastroenterol 2007;42:513-21.

[13] Roche B, Samuel D. Risk factors for hepatitis C recurrence after liver transplantation. J Viral Hepat 2007;14(Suppl 1):89-96.

[14] Katsoulidou A, Sypsa V, Tassopoulos NC, Boletis J, Karafoulidou A, Ketikoglou I, et al. Molecular epidemiology of hepatitis C virus (HCV) in Greece: Temporal trends in HCV genotype-specific incidence and molecular characterization of genotype 4 isolates. J Viral Hepat 2006;13:19-27.

[15] Ansaldi F, Bruzzone B, Salamaso S, Rota MC, Durando P, Gasparini R, et al. Different seroprelavence and molecular epidemiology pattern of hepatitis C virus infection in Italy. J Med Virol 2005;76:327-332.

[16] Fernández-Arcás N, López-Siles J, Trapero S, Ferraro A, Ibá-ez A, Orihuela F, et al. High prevalence of hepatitis C virus subtypes 4c and 4d in Malaga (Spain): Phylogenetic and epidemiological analyses. J Med Virol 2006;78:1429-1435.

[17] Nicot F, Legrand-Abravanel F, Sandres-Saune K, Boulestin A, Dubois M, Alric L, et al. Heterogeneity of hepatitis C virus genotype 4 strains circulating in south-western France. J Gen Virol 2005;86:107-114.

[18] Dahlan Y, Ather HM, Al-ahmadi M, Batwa F, Al-hamoudi W. Sustained virological response in a predominantly hepatitis C virus genotype 4 infected population. World J Gastroenterol 2009;15:4429-4433.

[19] Al Ashgar H, Helmy A, Khan MQ, Al Kahtani K, Al Quaiz M, Rezeig M, et al. Predictors of sustained virological response to a 48-week course of pegylated interferon alfa-2a and ribavirin in patients infected with hepatitis C virus genotype 4. Ann Saudi Med 2009;29:4-14.

[20] Derbala MF, El Dweik NZ, Al Kaabi SR, Al-Marri AD, Pasic F, Bener AB, et al. Viral kinetic of HCV genotype-4 during pegylated interferon alpha 2a: Ribavirin therapy. J Viral Hepat 2008;15:591-599.

[21] El Khayat HR, Fouad YM, El Amin H, Rizk A. A randomized trial of 24 versus 48 weeks of peginterferon alpha-2a plus ribavirin in Egyptian patients with hepatitis C virus genotype 4 and rapid viral response. Trop Gastroenterol 2012;33:112-7.

[22] Kamal SM, El Kamary SS, Shardell MD, Hashem M, Ahmed IN, Muhammadi M, et al. Pegylated interferon alpha-2b plus ribavirin in patients with genotype 4 chronic hepatitis C: The role of rapid and early virologic response. Hepatology 2007;46:1732-1740.

[23] Kamal SM. Hepatitis C genotype 4 therapy: Increasing options and improving outcomes. Liver Int 2009;29(Suppl 1):39-48.

[24] Kamal SM, Fouly AE, Kamel RR, Hockenjos B, Al Tawil A, Khalifa KE, et al. Peginterferon alfa-2b therapy in acute hepatitis C: Impact of onset of therapy on sustained virologic response. Gastroenterology 2006;130:632-638.

[25] Kamal SM, Moustafa KN, Chen J, Fehr J, Abdel Moneim A, Khalifa KE, et al. Duration of peginterferon therapy in acute hepatitis C: A randomized trial. Hepatology 2006;43:923-931.

[26] Kamal S, Nasser I. Hepatitis C genotype 4: What we know and what we don't yet know. Hepatology 2008;47:1371-1383.

[27] AlQaraawi AM, Sanai FM, Al-Husseini H, Albenmousa A, AlSheikh A, Ahmed LR, et al. Prevalence and impact of hepatic steatosis on the response to antiviral therapy in Saudi patients with genotypes 1 and 4 chronic hepatitis C. Dig Dis Sci 2011;56:1222-1228.

[28] Antonini TM, Furlan V, Teicher E, Haim-Boukobza S, Sebagh M, Coilly A, Bonhomme-Faivre L, et al. Therapy with boceprevir or telaprevir in HIV/hepatitis C virus co-infected patients to treat recurrence of hepatitis C virus infection after liver transplantation. AIDS 2015 Jan 2;29(1):53-8.

[29] Gane EJ, Stedman CA, Hyland RH, Ding X, Svarovskaia E, Symonds WT, Hindes RG, et al. Nucleotide polymerase inhibitor sofosbuvir plus ribavirin for hepatitis C. N Engl J Med 2013;368:34-44.

[30] Kowdley KV, Lawitz E, Crespo I, Hassanein T, Davis MN, DeMicco M, Bernstein DE, et al. Sofosbuvir with pegylated interferon alfa-2a and ribavirin for treatment-naive patients with hepatitis C genotype-1 infection (ATOMIC): an open-label, randomised, multicentre phase 2 trial. Lancet 2013;381:2100-2107.

[31] Lawitz E, Lalezari JP, Hassanein T, Kowdley KV, Poordad FF, Sheikh AM, et al. Sofosbuvir in combination with

peginterferon alfa-2a and ribavirin for non-cirrhotic, treatment-naive patients with genotypes 1, 2, and 3 hepatitis C infection: a randomised, double-blind, phase 2 trial. Lancet Infect Dis 2013;13:401-408.

[32] Lalezari JP ND, Hyland RH. Once daily sofosbuvir plus ribavirin for 12 and 24 weeks in treatment-naïve patients with HCV infection: the QUANTUM study. J Hepatol 2013;58:S236.

[33] Lawitz E, Mangia A, Wyles D, Rodriguez-Torres M, Hassanein T, Gordon SC, Schultz M, et al. Sofosbuvir for previously untreated chronic hepatitis C infection. N Engl J Med 2013;368:1878-1887.

[34] Jacobson IM, Gordon SC, Kowdley KV, Yoshida EM, Rodriguez-Torres M, Sulkowski MS, et al. Sofosbuvir for hepatitis C genotype 2 or 3 in patients without treatment options. N Engl J Med 2013;368:1867-1877.

[35] Osinusi A, Meissner EG, Lee YJ, Bon D, Heytens L, Nelson A, Sneller M, et al. Sofosbuvir and ribavirin for hepatitis C genotype 1 in patients with unfavorable treatment characteristics: a randomized clinical trial. Jama 2013;310:804-811.

[36] AASLD/IDSA HCV Guidance Panel. Hepatitis C guidance: AASLD-IDSA recommendations for testing, managing, and treating adults infected with hepatitis C virus. Hepatology. 2015 Sep;62(3):932-954.

[37] van der Meer AJ, Veldt BJ, Feld JJ, Wedemeyer H, Dufour JF, Lammert F, Duarte-Rojo A, et al. Association between sustained virological response and all-cause mortality among patients with chronic hepatitis C and advanced hepatic fibrosis. JAMA. 2012 Dec 26;308(24):2584-2593.

[38] Flemming JA, Kim WR, Brosgart CL, Terrault NA. Reduction in liver transplant wait-listing in the era of direct-acting antiviral therapy. Hepatology. 2017;65(3):804-812.

[39] Belli LS, Perricone G, Adam R, Cortesi PA, Strazzabosco M, Facchetti R, et al. Impact of DAAs on liver transplantation: major effects on the evolution of indications and results. An ELITA study based on the ELTR registry. J Hepatol. 2018;69(4):810-817.

[40] Crespo G, Trota N, Londoño M-C, Mauro E, Baliellas C, Castells L, et al. The efficacy of direct anti-HCV drugs improves early post-liver transplant survival and induces significant changes in waiting list composition. J Hepatol. 2018;69(1):11-17.

[41] Murag S, Dennis BB, Kim D, Ahmed A, Cholankeril G. Recent advances in liver transplantation with HCV seropositive donors. F1000Res. 2019 Dec 30;8:F1000 Faculty Rev-2151.

[42] Berenguer M, Prieto M, Rayón JM, Mora J, Pastor M, Ortiz V, et al. Natural history of clinically compensated hepatitis C virus-related graft cirrhosis after liver transplantation. Hepatology 2000;32:852-858.

[43] Zekry A, Whiting P, Crawford DH, Angus PW, Jeffrey GP, Padbury RT, et al.; Australian and New Zealand Liver Transplant Clinical Study Group. Liver transplantation for HCV-associated liver cirrhosis: Predictors of outcomes in a population with significant genotype 3 and 4 distribution. Liver Transpl 2003;9:339-347.

[44] Gane EJ, Portmann BC, Naoumov NV, Smith HM, Underhill JA, Donaldson PT, et al. Long-term outcome of hepatitis C infection after liver transplantation. N Engl J Med 1996;334:815-820.

[45] Wali MH, Heydtmann M, Harrison RF, Gunson BK, Mutimer DJ. Outcome of liver transplantation

for patients infected by hepatitis C, including those infected by genotype 4. Liver Transpl 2003;9:796-804.

[46] Wali M, Harrison RF, Gow PJ, Mutimer D. Advancing donor liver age and rapid fibrosis progression following transplantation for hepatitis C. Gut 2002;51:248-252.

[47] Burak KW, Kremers WK, Batts KP, Wiesner RH, Rosen CB, Razonable RR, et al. Impact of cytomegalovirus infection, year of transplantation, and donor age on outcomes after liver transplan-tation for hepatitis C. Liver Transpl 2002;8:362-369.

[48] Berenguer M, Prieto M, San Juan F, Rayon JM, Martinez F, Carrasco D, et al. Contribution of donor age to the recentdecrease in patient survival among HCV-infected liver transplant recipients. Hepatology 20021;36:202-210.

[49] Al-Sebayel M. Survival after liver transplantation: Experience with 89 cases. Ann Saudi Med 1999;19:216-8.

[50] Kizilisik TA, al-Sebayel M, Hammad A, al-Traif I, Ramirez CG, Abdulla A. Hepatitis C recurrence in liver transplant recipients. Transplant Proc 1997;29:2875-2877.

[51] Al Sebayel M, Kizilisik AT, Ramirez C, Altraif I, Hammad AQ, Littlejohn W, et al. Liver transplantation: Experience at King Fahad National Guard Hospital, Riyadh, Saudi Arabia. Transplant Proc 1997;29:2870-2871.

[52] al Sebayel M. Liver transplantation: Five-year experience in Saudi Arabia. Transplant Proc 1999;31:3157.

[53] Al Sebayel MS, Ramirez CB, Abou Ella K. The first 100 liver transplants in Saudi Arabia. Transplant Proc 2001;33:2709.

[54] Mudawi H, Helmy A, Kamel Y, Al Saghier M, Al Sofayan M, Al Sebayel M, et al. Recurrence of hepatitis C virus genotype-4 infection following liver transplantation: Natural history and predictors of outcome. Ann Saudi Med 2009;29:91-7.

[55] Yosry A, Abdel-Rahman M, Esmat G, El-Serafy M, Omar A, Doss W, et al. Recurrence of hepatitis c virus (genotype 4) infection after living-donor liver transplant in Egyptian patients. Exp Clin Transplant 2009;7:157-163.

[56] Allam N, Al Saghier M, El Sheikh Y, Al Sofayan M, Khalaf H, Al Sebayel M, et al. Clinical outcomes for Saudi and Egyptian patients receiving deceased donor liver transplantation in China. Am J Transplant 2010;10:1834-1841.

[57] Zhou S, Terrault NA, Ferrell L, Hahn JA, Lau JY, Simmonds P, et al. Severity of liver disease in liver transplantation recipients with hepatitis C virus infection: Relationship to genotype and level of viremia. Hepatology 1996;24:1041-1046.

[58] Alfaleh FZ, Hadad Q, Khuroo MS, Aljumah A, Algamedi A, Alashgar H, et al. Peginterferon alpha-2b plus ribavirin compared with interferon alpha-2b plus ribavirin for initial treatment of chronic hepatitis C in Saudi patients commonly infected with genotype 4. Liver Int 2004;24:568-574.

[59] Khuroo MS, Khuroo MS, Dahab ST. Meta-analysis: A randomized trial of peginterferon plus ribavirin for the initial treatment of chronic hepatitis C genotype 4. Aliment Pharmacol Ther 2004;20:931-8.

[60] Kamal SM, El Tawil AA, Nakano T, He Q, Rasenack J, Hakam SA, et al. Peginterferon {alpha}-2b and ribavirin therapy in chronic hepatitis C genotype 4: Impact of treatment duration and viral kinetics on sustained virological response. Gut 2005;54:858-866.

[61] Roulot D, Bourcier V, Grando V, Deny P, Baazia Y, Fontaine H, et al.; Observational VHC4 Study Group. Epidemiological characteristics and response to peginterferon plus ribavirin treatment of hepatitis C virus genotype 4 infection. J Viral Hepat 2007;14:460-467.

[62] Fortune BE, Martinez-Camacho A, Kreidler S, Gralla J, Everson GT. Post-transplant survival is improved for hepatitis C recipients who are RNA negative at time of liver transplantation. Transpl Int 2015;28:980-989.

[63] Everson GT. Treatment of hepatitis C in the patient with decompensated cirrhosis. Clin Gastroenterol Hepatol 2005;3(Suppl 2):S106-S112.

[64] Everson GT, Trotter J, Forman L, Kugelmas M, Halprin A, Fey B, et al. Treatment of advanced hepatitis C with a low accelerating dosage regimen of antiviral therapy. Hepatology 2005;42:255-262.

[65] Crippin JS, McCashland T, Terrault N, Sheiner P, Charlton MR. A pilot study of the tolerability and efficacy of antiviral therapy in hepatitis C virus-infected patients awaiting liver transplantation. Liver Transpl 2002;8:350-355.

[66] Everson GT, Terrault NA, Lok AS, Rodrigo del R, Brown RS Jr, Saab S, et al.; Adult-to-Adult Living Donor Liver Transplantation Cohort Study. A randomized controlled trial of pretransplant antiviral therapy to prevent recurrence of hepatitis C after liver transplantation. Hepatology 2013;57:1752-1762.

[67] Dabbous HM, Elmeteini MS, Sakr MA, Montasser IF, Bahaa M, Abdelaal A, et al. Optimizing outcome of recurrent hepatitis C virus genotype 4 after living donor liver transplantation: Moving forward by looking back. Transplant Proc 2014;46:822-827.

[68] Ponziani FR, Milani A, Gasbarrini A, Zaccaria R, Viganò R, Donato MF, et al. Treatment of recurrent genotype 4 hepatitis C after liver transplantation: Early virological response is predictive of sustained virological response. An AISF RECOLT-C group study. Ann Hepatol 2012;11:338-342.

[69] Al-hamoudi W, Mohamed H, Abaalkhail F, Kamel Y, Al-Masri N, Allam N, et al. Treatment of genotype 4 hepatitis C recurring after liver transplantation using a combination of pegylated interferon alfa-2a and ribavirin. Dig Dis Sci 2011;56:1848-52.

[70] Poordad F, Dieterich D. Treating hepatitis C: current standard of care and emerging direct-acting antiviral agents. J Viral Hepat. 2012 Jul;19(7):449-464.

[71] Pawlotsky JM. Treatment of chronic hepatitis C: Current and future. Curr Top Microbiol Immunol 2013;369:321-42. doi.org/10.1007/978-3-642-27340-7_13

[72] Gane EJ, Stedman CA, Hyland RH, Ding X, Svarovskaia E, Symonds WT, et al. Nucleotide polymerase inhibitor sofosbuvir plus ribavirin for hepatitis C. N Engl J Med 2013;368:34-44. doi.org/10.1056/NEJMoa1208953

[73] Kowdley KV, Lawitz E, Crespo I, Hassanein T, Davis MN, DeMicco M, et al. Sofosbuvir with pegylated interferon alfa-2a and ribavirin for treatment-naive patients with hepatitis C genotype-1 infection (ATOMIC): An open-label, randomised, multicentre phase 2 trial. Lancet 2013;381:2100-2107. doi.org/10.1016/S0140-6736(13)60247-0

[74] Lawitz E, Lalezari JP, Hassanein T, Kowdley KV, Poordad FF, Sheikh AM, et al. Sofosbuvir in combination with peginterferon alfa-2a and ribavirin for non-cirrhotic, treatment-naive patients with genotypes 1, 2, and 3 hepatitis

C infection: A randomised, double-blind, phase 2 trial. Lancet Infect Dis 2013;13:401-8. doi.org/10.1016/S1473-3099(13)70033-1

[75] Lawitz E, Mangia A, Wyles D, Rodriguez-Torres M, Hassanein T, Gordon SC, et al. Sofosbuvir for previously untreated chronic hepatitis C infection. N Engl J Med 2013;368:1878-87. doi.org/10.1056/NEJMoa1214853.

[76] Curry MP, Forns X, Chung RT, Terrault NA, Brown R Jr, Fenkel JM, et al. Sofosbuvir and ribavirin prevent recurrence of HCV infection after liver transplantation: An open-label study. Gastroenterology 2015;148:100-7.e1. doi.org/10.1053/j.gastro.2014.09.023.

[77] Ruane PJ, Ain D, Stryker R, Meshrekey R, Soliman M, Wolfe PR, et al. Sofosbuvir plus ribavirin for the treatment of chronic genotype 4 hepatitis C virus infection in patients of Egyptian ancestry. J Hepatol. 2015;62(5):1040.

[78] 78Doss W, Shiha G, Hassany M, Soliman R, Fouad R, Khairy M, et al. Sofosbuvir plus ribavirin for treating Egyptian patients with hepatitis c genotype 4. J Hepatol 2015. doi.org/10.1016/j.jhep.2015.04.023.

[79] Abd-Elsalam S, Sharaf-Eldin M, Soliman S, Elfert A, Badawi R, Ahmad YK. Efficacy and safety of sofosbuvir plus ribavirin for treatment of cirrhotic patients with genotype 4 hepatitis C virus in real-life clinical practice. Arch Virol. 2018 Jan;163(1):51-56.

[80] Elsharkawy A, Fouad R, El Akel W, El Raziky M, Hassany M, Shiha G, et al. Sofosbuvir-based treatment regimens: real life results of 14 409 chronic HCV genotype 4 patients in Egypt. Aliment Pharmacol Ther. 2017 Mar;45(5):681-687.

[81] Ajlan A, Al-Jedai A, Elsiesy H, Alkortas D, Al-Hamoudi W, Alarieh R, et al, Clinical Study Sofosbuvir-Based Therapy for Genotype 4 HCV Recurrence Post-Liver Transplant Treatment-Experienced Patients. Can J Gastroenterol Hepatol. 2016;2016:2872371.

[82] Dabbous HM, Montasser IF, Sakr MA, Refai R, Sayam M, Abdelmonem A, Sayed H, et al. Safety, Efficacy, and Tolerability of Sofosbuvir and Ribavirin in Management of Recurrent Hepatitis C Virus Genotype 4 After Living Donor Liver Transplant in Egypt: What Have We Learned so far? Hepat Mon. 2016 Apr 30;16(5):e35339.

[83] Charlton M, Gane E, Manns MP, Brown RS Jr, Curry MP, Kwo PY, et al. Sofosbuvir and ribavirin for treatment of compensated recurrent hepatitis C virus infection after liver transplantation. Gastroenterology 2015;148:108-117.

[84] Forns X, Charlton M, Denning J, McHutchison JG, Symonds WT, Brainard D, et al. Sofosbuvir compassionate use program for patients with severe recurrent hepatitis C after liver transplantation. Hepatology 2015;61:1485-1494.

[85] Colombo M, Aghemo A, Liu H, Zhang J, Dvory-Sobol H, Hyland R, et al. Treatment With Ledipasvir-Sofosbuvir for 12 or 24 Weeks in Kidney Transplant Recipients With Chronic Hepatitis C Virus Genotype 1 or 4 Infection: A Randomized Trial. Ann Intern Med. 2017 Jan 17;166(2):109-117.

[86] Ioannou GN, Beste LA, Chang MF, Green PK, Lowy E, Tsui JI, et al. Effectiveness of Sofosbuvir, Ledipasvir/Sofosbuvir, or Paritaprevir/Ritonavir/Ombitasvir and Dasabuvir Regimens for Treatment of Patients with Hepatitis C in the Veterans Affairs National Health Care System. Gastroenterology. 2016 Sep;151(3):457-471.e5.

[87] Charlton M, Everson GT, Flamm SL, Kumar P, Landis C, Brown

RS Jr, et al. Ledipasvir and sofosbuvir plus ribavirin for treatment of HCV infection in patients with advanced liver disease. Gastroenterology 2015 Sep; 149(3):649-659.

[88] Kohli A, Kapoor R, Sims Z, Nelson A, Sidharthan S, Lam B, et al. Ledipasvir and sofosbuvir for hepatitis C genotype 4: a proof-of-concept, single-centre, open-label phase 2a cohort study. Lancet Infect Dis. 2015;15(9):1049.

[89] Crespo J, Calleja JL, Fernández I, Sacristan B, Ruiz-Antorán B, Ampuero J, et al; Spanish Group for the Study of the Use of Direct-acting Drugs Hepatitis C Collaborating Group. Real-World Effectiveness and Safety of Oral Combination Antiviral Therapy for Hepatitis C Virus Genotype 4 Infection. Clin Gastroenterol Hepatol. 2017 Jun;15(6):945-949.e1.

[90] Abergel A, Metivier S, Samuel D, Jiang D, Kersey K, Pang PS, et al. Ledipasvir plus sofosbuvir for 12 weeks in patients with hepatitis C genotype 4 infection. Hepatology. 2016 Oct;64(4):1049-1056.

[91] Sanai FM, Altraif IH, Alswat K, AlZanbagi A, Babatin MA, AlMousa A, et al. Real life efficacy of ledipasvir/sofosbuvir in hepatitis C genotype 4-infected patients with advanced liver fibrosis and decompensated cirrhosis. J Infect. 2018 Jun;76(6):536-542.

[92] Shiha G, Esmat G, Hassany M, Soliman R, Elbasiony M, Fouad R, et al. Ledipasvir/sofosbuvir with or without ribavirin for 8 or 12 weeks for the treatment of HCV genotype 4 infection: results from a randomised phase III study in Egypt. Gut. 2019 Apr;68(4):721-728.

[93] Abaalkhail F, Elsiesy H, Elbeshbeshy H, Shawkat M, Yousif S, Ullah W, et al. Treatment of Patients With Hepatitis C Virus Infection With Ledipasvir-Sofosbuvir in the Liver Transplant Setting. Transplantation. 2017 Nov;101(11):2739-2745.

[94] Manns M, Forns X, Samuel D, Denning J, Arterburn S, Brandt-Sarif T, et al. Ledipasvir/sofosbuvir with ribavirin is safe and efficacious in decompensated and post-liver transplantation patients with HCV infection: Preliminary results of the SOLAR-2 trial. J Hepatol 2015;62:S187.

[95] Ciesek S, Proske V, Otto B, Pischke S, Costa R, Lüthgehetmann M, et al. Efficacy and safety of sofosbuvir/ledipasvir for the treatment of patients with hepatitis C virus re-infection after liver transplantation. Transpl Infect Dis. 2016 Jun;18(3):326-332.

[96] Samuel D, Manns M, Forns X, Flamm SL, Reddy KR, Denning J, et al. Ledipasvir/sofosbuvir with ribavirin is safe in >600 decompensated and post-liver transplantation patients with HCV infection: An integrated safety analysis of the SOLAR-1 and SOLAR-2 trials. Lancet Infect Dis. 2016 Jun;16(6):685-697.

[97] El-Khayat H, Fouad Y, Mohamed HI, El-Amin H, Kamal EM, Maher M, et al. Sofosbuvir plus daclatasvir with or without ribavirin in 551 patients with hepatitis C-related cirrhosis, genotype 4. Aliment Pharmacol Ther. 2018 Mar;47(5):674-679.

[98] Hezode C, Abergel A, Chas J, et al. Sustanined virologic response to daclatasvir and sofosbuvir with or without ribavirin, among patients in the French daclatasvir ATU programme infected with HCV genotypes 4,5,6. J Hepatol. 2016;64:S133–S142.

[99] Babatin MA, Alghamdi AS, Albenmousa A, Alaseeri A, Aljarodi M, Albiladi H, et al. Efficacy and Safety of Simeprevir or Daclatasvir in Combination with Sofosbuvir for the

Treatment of Hepatitis C Genotype 4 Infection. J Clin Gastroenterol. 2018 May/Jun;52(5):452-457.

[100] Lawitz E, Poordad F, Gutierrez JA, Beumont M, Beets G, Vandevoorde A, et al. Simeprevir, daclatasvir, and sofosbuvir for hepatitis C virus-infected patients: Long-term follow-up results from the open-label, Phase II IMPACT study. Health Sci Rep. 2020 Feb 22;3(2):e145.

[101] Darweesh SK, Elsaeed K, Omar H, El Raziky M, Elakel W, Elserafy M, et al. High SVR rate following retreatment of non-sustained virological responders to sofosbuvir based anti-HCV therapies regardless of RAS testing: A real-life multicenter study. Expert Rev Gastroenterol Hepatol. 2019 Sep;13(9):907-914.

[102] Lashen SA, Shamseya MM, Madkour MA, Aboufarrag GA. Tolerability and effectiveness of generic direct-acting antiviral drugs in eradication of hepatitis C genotype 4 among Egyptian patients. Liver Int. 2019 May;39(5):835-843.

[103] El-Nahaas SM, Fouad R, Elsharkawy A, Khairy M, Elhossary W, Anwar I, et al. High sustained virologic response rate using generic directly acting antivirals in the treatment of chronic hepatitis C virus Egyptian patients: single-center experience. Eur J Gastroenterol Hepatol. 2018 Oct;30(10):1194-1199.

[104] Abdel-Moneim A, Aboud A, Abdel-Gabaar M, Zanaty MI, Ramadan M. Efficacy and safety of sofosbuvir plus daclatasvir with or without ribavirin: large real-life results of patients with chronic hepatitis C genotype 4. Hepatol Int. 2018 Jul;12(4):348-355.

[105] Ahmed OA, Elsebaey MA, Fouad MHA, Elashry H, Elshafie AI, Elhadidy AA, et al. Outcomes and predictors of treatment response with sofosbuvir plus daclatasvir with or without ribavirin in Egyptian patients with genotype 4 hepatitis C virus infection. Infect Drug Resist. 2018 Mar 28;11:441-445.

[106] Omar H, El Akel W, Elbaz T, El Kassas M, Elsaeed K, El Shazly H, et al. Generic daclatasvir plus sofosbuvir, with or without ribavirin, in treatment of chronic hepatitis C: real-world results from 18 378 patients in Egypt. Aliment Pharmacol Ther. 2018 Feb;47(3):421-431.

[107] Coilly A, Fougerou-Leurent C, de Ledinghen V, Houssel-Debry P, Duvoux C, Di Martino V, et al. Multicentre experience using daclatasvir and sofosbuvir to treat hepatitis C recurrence after liver transplantation - The CO23 ANRS CUPILT study. J Hepatol. 2016 Jun 1. pii: S0168-8278(16)30253-7.

[108] Dumortier J, Leroy V, Duvoux C, de Ledinghen V, Francoz C, Houssel-Debry P, et al. Sofosbuvir-based treatment of hepatitis C with severe fibrosis (METAVIR F3/F4) after liver transplantation. Liver Transpl. 2016 Oct;22(10):1367-1378.

[109] Leroy V, Dumortier J, Coilly A, Sebagh M, Fougerou-Leurent C, Radenne S, et al. Efficacy of sofosbuvir and daclatasvir in patients with fibrosing cholestatic hepatitis C after liver transplantation. Clin Gastroenterol Hepatol 2015 Nov; 13(11):1993-2001. doi: 10.1016/j.cgh.2015.05.030.

[110] El Raziky M, Gamil M, Ashour MK, Sameea EA, Doss W, Hamada Y, et al. Simeprevir plus sofosbuvir for eight or 12 weeks in treatment-naïve and treatment-experienced hepatitis C virus genotype 4 patients with or without cirrhosis. J Viral Hepat. 2017 Feb;24(2):102-110.

[111] Buti M, Calleja JL, Lens S, Diago M, Ortega E, Crespo J, et al.

Simeprevir in combination with sofosbuvir in treatment-naïve and -experienced patients with hepatitis C virus genotype 4 infection: a Phase III, open-label, single-arm study (PLUTO). Aliment Pharmacol Ther. 2017 Feb;45(3):468-475.

[112] Abdel-Moneim A, Aboud A, Abdel-Gabbar M, Zanaty MI, Elbary AAA, Ramadan M. Sofosbuvir in combination with ribavirin or simeprevir: real-life study of patients with hepatitis C genotype 4. Ann Gastroenterol. 2019 Jan-Feb;32(1):93-98.

[113] Lawitz E, Poordad F, Gutierrez JA, Kakuda TN, Picchio G, Beets G, et al. Simeprevir, daclatasvir and sofosbuvir for hepatitis C virus-infected patients with decompensated liver disease. J Viral Hepat. 2017 Apr;24(4):287-294.

[114] Ahmed OA, Elsebaey MA, Fouad MHA, Elkadeem M, Badawi R, Khayyal A, et al. Outcomes of Treatment and Predictors of Response to Sofosbuvir Plus Simeprevir in Hepatitis C Virus with Genotype-4 Infection. Infect Disord Drug Targets. 2020;20(3):389-395.

[115] Eletreby R, Elakel W, Said M, El Kassas M, Seif S, Elbaz T, et al. Real life Egyptian experience of efficacy and safety of Simeprevir/Sofosbuvir therapy in 6211 chronic HCV genotype IV infected patients. Liver Int. 2017 Apr;37(4):534-541.

[116] Wang BQ, Wang YL, Shi KQ. Real life Egyptian experience of efficacy and safety of Simeprevir/Sofosbuvir therapy in HCV genotype IV infected patients. Liver Int. 2017 May;37(5):765.

[117] Yosry A, Gamal Eldeen H, Medhat E, Mehrez M, Zayed N, Elakel W, et al. Efficacy and safety of sofosbuvir-based therapy in hepatitis C virus recurrence post living donor liver transplant: A real life egyptian experience. J Med Virol. 2019 Apr;91(4):668-676.

[118] Sanchez Antolin G, Testillano M, Pascasio JM, Narvaez Rodriguez I, Prieto M, et al; Spanish Society of Liver Transplantation Study Group Collaborating Group. Efficacy and Safety of Therapy with Simeprevir and Sofosbuvir in Liver Transplant Recipients Infected by Hepatitis C Virus Genotype 4: Cohort Spanish Society of Liver Transplantation Cohort. Transplant Proc. 2016 Nov;48(9):3013-3016.

[119] Ferenci P, Bourgeois S, Buggisch P, Norris S, Curescu M, Larrey D, et al. Real-world safety and effectiveness of ombitasvir/paritaprevir/ritonavir ± dasabuvir ± ribavirin in hepatitis C virus genotype 1- and 4-infected patients with diverse comorbidities and comedications: A pooled analysis of post-marketing observational studies from 13 countries. J Viral Hepat. 2019 Jun;26(6):685-696.

[120] Waked I, Shiha G, Qaqish RB, Esmat G, Yosry A, Hassany M, et al. Ombitasvir, paritaprevir, and ritonavir plus ribavirin for chronic hepatitis C virus genotype 4 infection in Egyptian patients with or without compensated cirrhosis (AGATE-II): a multicentre, phase 3, partly randomised open-label trial. Lancet Gastroenterol Hepatol. 2016 Sep;1(1):36-44.

[121] Asselah T, Hézode C, Qaqish RB, ElKhashab M, Hassanein T, Papatheodoridis G, et al. Ombitasvir, paritaprevir, and ritonavir plus ribavirin in adults with hepatitis C virus genotype 4 infection and cirrhosis (AGATE-I): a multicentre, phase 3, randomised open-label trial. Lancet Gastroenterol Hepatol. 2016 Sep;1(1):25-35.

[122] Aygen B, Demirtürk N, Yıldız O, Çelen MK, Çelik İ, Barut Ş, et al. Real-world efficacy, safety, and clinical outcomes of ombitasvir/paritaprevir/ritonavir ± dasabuvir ± ribavirin combination therapy in patients with hepatitis C virus genotype 1 or

4 infection: The Turkey experience experience. Turk J Gastroenterol. 2020 Apr;31(4):305-317.

[123] Petta S, Marzioni M, Russo P, Aghemo A, Alberti A, Ascione A, et al; ABACUS study group; AIFA team. Ombitasvir, paritaprevir, and ritonavir, with or without dasabuvir, plus ribavirin for patients with hepatitis C virus genotype 1 or 4 infection with cirrhosis (ABACUS): a prospective observational study. Lancet Gastroenterol Hepatol. 2017 Jun;2(6):427-434.

[124] Perelló C, Carrión JA, Ruiz-Antorán B, Crespo J, Turnes J, Llaneras J, et al. Spanish Collaborative Group for the Study of the Use of Hepatitis C Direct-Acting Drugs. Effectiveness and safety of ombitasvir, paritaprevir, ritonavir ± dasabuvir ± ribavirin: An early access programme for Spanish patients with genotype 1-4 chronic hepatitis C virus infection. J Viral Hepat. 2017;24:226-237.

[125] Wedemeyer H, Craxí A, Zuckerman E, Dieterich D, Flisiak R, Roberts SK, et al. Real-world effectiveness of ombitasvir/paritaprevir/ritonavir±dasabuvir±ribavirin in patients with hepatitis C virus genotype 1 or 4 infection: A meta-analysis. J Viral Hepat. 2017 Nov;24(11):936-943.

[126] Forns X, Lee SS, Valdes J, Lens S, Ghalib R, Aguilar H, et al. Glecaprevir plus pibrentasvir for chronic hepatitis C virus genotype 1, 2, 4, 5, or 6 infection in adults with compensated cirrhosis (EXPEDITION-1): a single-arm, open-label, multicentre phase 3 trial. Lancet Infect Dis. 2017 Oct;17(10):1062-1068.

[127] Brown RS Jr, Buti M, Rodrigues L, Chulanov V, Chuang WL, Aguilar H, et al. Glecaprevir/pibrentasvir for 8 weeks in treatment-naïve patients with chronic HCV genotypes 1-6 and compensated cirrhosis: The EXPEDITION-8 trial. J Hepatol. 2020 Mar;72(3):441-449.

[128] Reau N, Kwo PY, Rhee S, Brown RS Jr, Agarwal K, Angus P, et al. Glecaprevir/Pibrentasvir Treatment in Liver or Kidney Transplant Patients with Hepatitis C Virus Infection. Hepatology. 2018 Oct;68(4):1298-1307.

[129] Feld JJ, Jacobson IM, Hézode C, Asselah T, Ruane PJ, Gruener N, et al. Sofosbuvir and Velpatasvir for HCV Genotype 1, 2, 4, 5, and 6 Infection. N Engl J Med. 2015 Dec 31;373(27):2599-2607.

[130] Curry MP, O'Leary JG, Bzowej N, Muir AJ, Korenblat KM, Fenkel JM, et al; ASTRAL-4 Investigators. Sofosbuvir and Velpatasvir for HCV in Patients with Decompensated Cirrhosis. N Engl J Med. 2015 Dec 31;373(27):2618-2628.

[131] Agarwal K, Castells L, Müllhaupt B, Rosenberg WMC, McNabb B, Arterburn S, et al. Sofosbuvir/velpatasvir for 12 weeks in genotype 1-4 HCV-infected liver transplant recipients. J Hepatol. 2018 Sep;69(3):603-607.

[132] Bourlière M, Gordon SC, Flamm SL, Cooper CL, Ramji A, Tong M, et al; POLARIS-1 and POLARIS-4 Investigators. Sofosbuvir, Velpatasvir, and Voxilaprevir for Previously Treated HCV Infection. N Engl J Med. 2017 Jun 1;376(22):2134-2146.

[133] Cardona-Gonzalez MG, Goldman JD, Narayan L, Brainard DM, Kowdley KV. Sofosbuvir, Velpatasvir, and Voxilaprevir for Treatment of Recurrent Hepatitis C Virus Infection After Liver Transplantation. Hepatol Commun. 2018 Nov 14;2(12):1446-1450.

[134] Asselah T, Reesink H, Gerstoft J, de Ledinghen V, Pockros PJ, Robertson M, et al. Efficacy of elbasvir and grazoprevir in participants with hepatitis C virus genotype 4 infection: A pooled analysis. Liver Int. 2018 Sep;38(9):1583-1591.

[135] Jacobson IM, Lawitz E, Kwo PY, Hézode C, Peng CY, Howe AYM, et al Safety and Efficacy of Elbasvir/Grazoprevir in Patients with Hepatitis C Virus Infection and Compensated Cirrhosis: An Integrated Analysis. Gastroenterology. 2017 May;152(6):1372-1382.e2.

[136] Yousif MM, Ahmed H, Elsadek HM, Shendi AM, Gouda TM, Elsayed IA, et al. Real-world safety and effectiveness of retreatment of Egyptian chronic hepatitis C patients not responding to NS5A inhibitor-based therapies. J Viral Hepat. 2020 Nov;27(11):1190-1201.

[137] Said EM, Abdulaziz BA, El Kassas M, El Attar IH, Emadeldeen M, Abd-Elsalam SM. High success rates for the use of sofosbuvir/ombitasvir/paritaprevir/ritonavir + ribavirin and sofosbuvir/simeprevir/daclatasvir + ribavirin in retreatment of chronic hepatitis C infection after unsuccessful sofosbuvir/daclatasvir therapy: a real-life experience. Arch Virol. 2020 Jul;165(7):1633-1639.

[138] Abo-Amer YE, Badawi R, El-Abgeegy M, Elsergany HF, Mohamed AA, Mostafa SM, et al. Quadruple Therapy Offers High SVR Rates in Patients with HCV Genotype 4 with Previous Treatment Failure. Adv Virol. 2020 Jul 24;2020:9075905.

[139] de Lédinghen V, Laforest C, Hézode C, Pol S, Renault A, Alric L, et al. Retreatment With Sofosbuvir Plus Grazoprevir/Elbasvir Plus Ribavirin of Patients With Hepatitis C Virus Genotype 1 or 4 Who Previously Failed an NS5A- or NS3-Containing Regimen: The ANRS HC34 REVENGE Study. Clin Infect Dis. 2018 Mar 19;66(7):1013-1018.

[140] Kondili LA, Gaeta GB, Brunetto MR, Di Leo A, Iannone A, Santantonio TA, et al. Incidence of DAA failure and the clinical impact of retreatment in real-life patients treated in the advanced stage of liver disease: Interim evaluations from the PITER network. PLoS One. 2017 Oct 4;12(10):e0185728.

[141] Krassenburg LAP, Maan R, Ramji A, Manns MP, Cornberg M, Wedemeyer H, et al. Clinical outcomes following DAA therapy in patients with HCV-related cirrhosis depend on disease severity. J Hepatol. 2020 Nov 23:S0168-8278(20)33805-8.

[142] Belli LS, Berenguer M, Cortesi PA, Strazzabosco M, Rockenschaub SR, Martini S, et al. Delisting of liver transplant candidates with chronic hepatitis C after viral eradication: A European study. J Hepatol. 2016 May 17. pii: S0168-8278(16)30196-9.

[143] Perricone G, Duvoux C, Berenguer M, Cortesi PA, Vinaixa C, Facchetti R, et al; European Liver and Intestine Transplant Association (ELITA). Delisting HCV-infected liver transplant candidates who improved after viral eradication: Outcome 2 years after delisting. Liver Int. 2018 Dec;38(12):2170-2177.

[144] Afdhal N, Everson GT, Calleja JL, McCaughan G, Bosch J, Denning J, et al. Effect of long term viral suppression with sofosbuvir + ribavirin on hepatic venous pressure gradient in HCV-infected patients with cirrhosis and portal hypertension. J Hepatol 2015;62(Suppl 2):S269–S270.

Section 6

Hepatocellular Carcinoma and Antiviral Therapies

Chapter 7

Hepatocellular Carcinoma and Antiviral Therapies in HCV Chronic Infection

Laura Iliescu

Abstract

The development of direct-acting antiviral (DAA) therapies in chronic HCV infection has been associated with increased expectations regarding the prognosis of this infection in the medical community, as the possibility of HCV eradication is now in sight. While the cure of the HVC infection has been associated with a dramatic decrease in its systemic complications, the impact on the progression of the liver disease, especially in patients with cirrhosis, is still controversial. Furthermore, the risk of developing hepatocellular carcinoma (HCC) after direct-acting antiviral therapy is debatable, with studies presenting an increased prevalence of HCC early after the introduction of these therapies, as well as newer contradicting studies. This chapter aims to examine the current literature data available regarding the impact of new HCV therapies in the incidence and prognosis of hepatocellular carcinoma.

Keywords: hepatocellular carcinoma, hepatitis C virus, direct-acting antiviral agents

1. Introduction

Hepatitis C virus (HCV) chronic infection is one of the leading causes of morbidity and mortality, with over 71 million people infected worldwide. [1] Its natural evolution comprises liver cirrhosis and its complications, including hepatocellular carcinoma (HCC). HCV infection is the leading factor associated with HCC in Western European countries and USA, with an increased risk of up to 20 times greater than the general population. [2] The association between HCC and HCV occurs in cirrhotic patients; an estimated 20% of patients with HCV chronic infection develop cirrhosis within 20–30 years of infection, and, of those, 1–4% develop HCC each year. [3] The risk of developing HCC in the course of HCV infection is related not only to the presence of the virus, but also to viral genotype, concurrent liver disease or metabolic syndrome (diabetes mellitus, obesity) and lifestyle factors. [4]

HCV genotypes 3 and 6 are associated with higher HCC risks [5, 6]. Furthermore, co-infection with hepatitis B virus (HBV) or human immunodeficiency virus (HIV) doubles the risk of developing HCC in younger HCV infected patients. [7] Smoking and alcohol abuse are associated with an increased risk of HCC in HCV infected patients as follows: a relative risk of HCC of 23 in smoking patients, as opposed to 7.7 in non-smokers [8] and a 2 fold increase in the risk of HCC in patients with an alcohol intake over 60 g daily. [9] On the other hand, coffee-drinking has beneficial effects on both the progression of liver disease and the HCC development. [10]

Diabetes mellitus is an important cofactor in the development of HCC associated with the HCV infection. On the one hand, the presence of HCV is an important risk factor for the development of type 2 diabetes. [11] HCV has a direct action against beta-pancreatic cells [12] and also a systemic pro-inflammatory action, inducing the expression of TNF-α and IL-6 which promote insulin-resistance. [13] On the other hand, the development of diabetes is associated with an increased risk of HCC of up to 3 fold, due to insulin resistance, increased inflammation, inhibition of apoptosis and the generation of pro-oncogenic mutations. [14] Obesity is also a risk factor for the development of HCC, due to increased production of pro-inflammatory cytokines and insulin resistance which mediate carcinogenesis.

2. Relationship between HCV and HCC

There are two main mechanisms of carcinogenesis in HCV chronic infection: the carcinogenetic hepatic environment produced by the HCV infection per se and the direct carcinogenetic effect of several HCV proteins, both structural (core, E1, E2) and non-structural (p7, NS2, NS3, NS4A, NS4B, NS5A, and NS5B). [15]

Experimental studies have revealed the impact of the viral protein expressions on cellular proliferation. For example, over-expression of core proteins, NS3, NS5A promotes cellular proliferation and tumor transformation in mice, via oncogenic molecular pathways. [16, 17] The core protein also inhibits tumor suppressor genes (TP53 TP73) and negative regulation factors of the cell cycle. [18] Aggressive phenotypes of HCC are associated with the activation of cellular proliferative pathways (RAF/MAPK/ERK kinase) by the HCV core protein as well as by NS5A and NS5B. [19] Furthermore, HCV core protein stimulates the production of oxygen reactive species, with an important role in the pathogenesis of HCC, and also inhibits the tumor suppression activity of TGF- beta. [20, 21] NS5A protein inhibits caspase-3 enzyme (thus stimulating evasion from apoptosis) and prevents nuclear translocation of Smad proteins, inhibiting TGF beta signaling with the final outcome of down-regulating tumor suppressor cyclin-dependent kinase inhibitor 1. [22, 23] NS5A also induces chromosomal instability and mitotic dysregulation as well as apoptosis mediated by TNF-alpha. [24, 25]

Alterations of the host genomic DNA are described in HCV infection (oncogenic mutations, deletion of tumor suppressor genes), with an important impact on HCC carcinogenesis. The core protein inhibits mitotic spindle checkpoint function, increases chromosomal polyploidy, while the chronic oxidative stress induces mitochondrial and chromosomal DNA alterations. [20, 26]. HCV induces endoplasmic reticulum perturbations and prolonged stress, which leads to accumulation of DNA mutations and a predisposition to carcinogenesis. [27]

Chronic inflammation also plays a part in HCC development. In support of the inflammatory model of carcinogenesis, it has been shown that inhibition of cyclooxygenase 2 prevents HCC in experimental models. [28] The core protein of HCV inhibits immune responses mediated by the nuclear factor kappa-B (NF- kB), involved in the progression of initiated tumor clones. [29] Extracellular core protein may inhibit antigen-presenting cells via the IL-6 pathway. [30] NS5A interacts with TNF receptor-associated factor 2 and activates the JNK pathway (c-Jun N terminal kinase) generating an inflammatory environment in the liver that is the basis for HCC carcinogenesis. [31] Other viral proteins also affect immune mechanisms and promote carcinogenesis; for instance, NS3 has an immune suppressive effect by cleavage of mitochondrial antiviral signaling proteins and E2 viral protein contributes to immune evasion by inhibiting natural killer cells. [32, 33]

HCV is an important factor in the dysregulation of normal liver metabolism and a promoter of steatosis. [34] It has been shown, in experimental animal models, that the expression of HCV core protein is associated with progressive steatosis and HCC, as well as insulin resistance and suppression of the assembly and secretion of very low density lipoproteins. [35–37] HCV core protein modulates cell differentiation and proliferation, accentuates steatosis and oxidative stress via peroxisome activated receptor alpha. [38]

Normal hepatocellular senescence is also impaired in HCV infected patients. In the stage of cirrhosis, after regeneration cycles, cellular senescence is stimulated by telomere shortening, which decreases hepatocyte proliferation and prevents carcinogenesis. [39] In the HCV infection, hepatocyte senescence is inhibited and somatic mutations of the telomerase reverse-transcriptase promoter stimulate carcinogenesis. [40]

Fibrosis is the most important background in the development of hepatocellular carcinoma, as it stimulates genetic aberrations. [41] There is a direct correlation between the degree of liver fibrosis and the increased risk of HCV associated HCC in some patients, which may persist despite obtaining sustained virologic response by antiviral treatments, as there is still progression of liver fibrosis and its associated HCC risk. [42, 43] HCV core and other non- structural proteins stimulate profibrogenic, mitogenic and pro-inflammatory cytokines (TGF-beta, platelet-derived growth factor, IL-8, Il-32). [15] In addition, HCV infected apoptotic cells may amplify fibrogenic signals. [44] Portal hypertension secondary to liver cirrhosis increases gut mucosa permeability and bacterial translocation, resulting in increased circulatory bacterial lipopolysaccharides, an important stimuli of fibrogenesis and carcinogenesis. [45] The interaction between the HCV protein E2 and CD81 (pertaining to the complex responsible for HCV internalization) stimulates an inflammatory response resulting in liver damage. [46] Experimental studies have suggested the role of renin-angiotensin system in carcinogenesis, as administration of angiotensin-converting enzymes inhibitors inhibits angiogenic factors and decreases insulin-resistance related carcinogenesis. [47]

Different host-specific mechanisms have been incriminated in the development of HCV associated HCC. For example, is has been demonstrated that the epidermal growth factor (EGF) pathway is activated in hepatic stellate cells, stimulating cellular growth, proliferation, differentiation and carcinogenesis, and its inhibition via EGF receptor inhibitor, erlotinib, diminishes fibrosis and reduces the risk of HCC. [48] In other trials, erlotinib has proven effective in preventing HCV infection, by inhibiting HCV cellular entry. [49] In addition, gefitinib (another EGF inhibitor) has proven effective in experimental animal models in suppressing HCC growth in subjects with established HCC lesions. [50] Sorafenib, a multi-kinase inhibitor, inhibits angiogenesis and has beneficial roles in portal hypertension as well as HCC by blocking the response to vascular endothelial growth factor. [51] Host related factors predicting response to antiviral therapy appear to play a role in HCV associated HCC risk. Il28B variants CT or TT, used to predict virologic response to interferon therapy, also increases the risk of developing HCC. [52] Molecules pertaining to the major histocompatibility complex class I are involved in fibrogenesis and carcinogenesis by inflammatory mechanisms. [53] Metabolic disturbances, such as those involved in the iron metabolism leading to hepatic iron overload, stimulate steatosis, mitochondrial alterations and carcinogenesis, especially in HCV-based models. [54] The presence of HCV infection dysregulates the activity of microRNAs in a distinct pattern. [55]

3. Hepatocellular carcinoma in the setting of DAA treatments

Currently, the most important international panels recommend using direct acting antiviral (DAA) therapies for all degrees of liver fibrosis, customized for all HCV genotypes, with significant advantages: very high response rates (over 90%), short treatment duration and few adverse effects [56–58] These options are summarized in **Table 1**.

Not only do all guidelines recommend antiviral treatment in chronic HCV infection regardless of degree of liver fibrosis or other comorbidities, but they also indicate that the presence of HCV associated comorbidities is a strong argument in favor of antiviral therapy. The use of DAA in patients with HCC is still under debate. The European guidelines recommend that HCV treatment in patients with HCC should be administered after curative (ablation, resection) or palliative procedures (transarterial chemoembolisation). [59] The reasoning behind this recommendation is that patients with HCC have lower response rates to DAA. [60] A recent meta-analysis on over 5500 patients with HCC revealed a SVR rate of 88%, with higher rates reported in patients who received curative HCC treatment compared to those with non-curative therapies or not treated. [61] Furthermore, patients with HCC awaiting liver transplantation who received DAA had a lower risk of dropout caused by tumor progression or death. [62] Strong recommendations are made in favor of treating HCV associated HCC patients after liver transplantation. [63] In HCV patients with treated HCC, without indication for liver transplantation, the indication of DAA treatment is uncertain. Large cohort studies show that obtaining SVR is associated with lower risks of de novo HCC and liver-related mortality in the mid and long term. [64, 65] On the other hand, a large study has shown that the high HCC risks persist up to 10 years after SVR in patients with advanced fibrosis. [66] There is no clear conclusion regarding the impact of DAA treatment on the risk of HCC recurrence following curative procedures, as shown by a review and meta-analysis on 13000 patients. [67] Another retrospective cohort study on 797 patients with HCV infection and a history of HCC with complete response to ablation, resection, transarterial chemo- or radio-embolisation concluded that DAA therapy decreases the incidence of overall deaths. [68] A recent expert literature review states that DAA treatment decreases the risk of de novo HCC in patients with and without cirrhosis, while the presence of active HCC significantly decreases SVR rates. [69] There was no association between antiviral therapy and the baseline risk, aggressiveness, time of progression of HCC.

	Genotype 1a	Genotype 1b	Genotype 2	Genotype 3	Genotype 4	Genotype 5	Genotype 6
SOF/VEL							
GLE/PIB							
SOF/VEL/ VOX							
SOF/LDV							
GZR/ EBRGZR/ EBR							
OBV/ PTV/r + DSV							

SOF sofosbuvir; VEL velpatasvir, GLE glecaprevir, PIB pibrentasvir VOX voxilaprevir, LDV ledipasvir, GZR grazoprevir, ERB elbasvir, OBV ombitasvir, PTV paritaprevir, r ritonavir, DSV dasabuvir.

Table 1.
Direct acting antiviral agents currently in use (regimens marked with orange are not indicated in the respective genotypes.

The guidelines presented by the American Association for the Study of Liver Diseases in 2019 recommend screening for HCC in patients with advanced fibrosis before any antiviral therapy and elaborate simple treatment strategies for non-cirrhotic patients including diagnosis, pre-therapeutic evaluation and follow-up so as to be accessible to a broad range of health care professionals. [57] In patients with decompensated cirrhosis or cirrhosis complications, a case-based decision is required. [70] An interesting study presented in the APASL consensus statements and recommendations on treatment of hepatitis C shows that, in patients with compensate cirrhosis and HCC, DAA treatment (sofosbuvir and ribavirin) administered at least 4 weeks prior to liver transplantation reduced the risk of allograft recurrence by 50%. [71]

4. SOF/VEL

SOF/VEL is a pan-genotypic all oral treatment regimen, consisting of a NS5B polymerase inhibitor (sofosbuvir) and a NS5A inhibitor (velpatasvir). [72] In a real life study of over 2800 HCV infected patients, this regimen showed an efficacy of 94.6% in the general population, with an SVR rate of 88,6% in cirrhotic patients. Notably the number of cirrhotic patients included was significantly low. [73] In a trial on 102 Japanese patients with decompensated cirrhosis, HCC was diagnosed in 3 patients after the completion of antiviral therapy with SOF/VEL (in days 1, 70 and 124 respectively). Four other patients had a history of HCC resolved for more than 2 years prior to therapy and did not experience recurrence. [74] Another prospective multicenter trial studied the efficacy of SOF/VEL in 71 patients with decompensated cirrhosis; among those, 22 patients (31%) had a history of treated HCC (by resection, ablation, transarterial chemoembolization, chemotherapy, heavy ion therapy, proton therapy), during a timeframe ranging from 2 months to 13 years prior to DAA treatment. None of the patients had evidence of active HCC at the initiation of DAA therapy; however, the maximum level of alpha-fetoprotein noted at initiation was over 2000 ng/ml. 90.9% of patients with a history of HCC obtained SVR (compared to 94.4% in the entire study population); 4 patients presented HCC recurrence; no de novo HCC cases were reported. [75] 16 patients in a large trial involving 729 Chinese patients infected with genotype 2 HCV were given SOF/VEL, among which one had a history of HCC; all the patients obtained SVR and there was no recurrence in the HCC patient.

5. SOF/VEL/VOX

This is a pan-genotypic regimen, containing a NS5B polymerase inhibitor (sofosbuvir), a NS5A inhibitor (velpatasvir) and a NS3/4A protease inhibitor (voxilaprevir), with over 90% SVR rates in treatment naïve patients but especially in DAA- experienced patients and hard-to-treat categories, for which this regimen is currently reserved. [76, 77] One adverse reactions report has been filed regarding a treatment experienced patient developing HCC after treatment with SOF/VEL/VOX. [78] Another case report considers the undiagnosed presence of HCC as the cause of non-response to antiviral therapy re-treatment in a patient with HCV genotype 1b. [79] A large multicenter clinical trial reports HCC (alongside the presence of cirrhosis) as the only cause of treatment resistance in 179 patients with various degrees of fibrosis. [80]

6. GLE/PIB

The combination between Glecaprevir (a NS3/4A protease inhibitor) and Pibrentasvir (a NS5A inhibitor) is another pan-genotypic antiviral option in patients without cirrhosis or with compensated cirrhosis. [81] It has shown response rates of up to 100% and a rate of discontinuation due to severe adverse events of 0.7% in clinical trials (SURVEYOR-I and SURVEYOR-II, comprising 449 patients). [82] Furthermore, newer trials reveal excellent response rates with a lower duration of therapy (8 weeks instead of 12 weeks) even in patients with compensated cirrhosis, without the identification of post-baseline cases of HCC. [83] An interesting study performed in Japan (a country with one of the highest rates of HCV infection and HCC incidence) evaluates the cost-effectiveness of GLE/PIB compared to other DAAs. [84] This study revealed a lower lifetime risk of HCC in patients treated with GLE/PIB or SOF/LDV (3.66%) compared to EBV/GRZ (4.99%). However, in a study evaluating safety and efficacy of GLE/PIB in DAA experienced patients, which enrolled 177 subjects (17 with a history of HCC but no active disease 6 month prior to treatment initiation) one death from HCC was reported, occurring after the end of the treatment but before the SVR12 evaluation. This was a non- cirrhotic patient, without history or proof of HCC at baseline, diagnosed with advanced HCC shortly before the end of treatment. Virologic failure occurred in 17.7% of patients with a history of HCC. [85] A large real-life cohort study evaluated the efficacy of several antiviral regimens in patients with and without HCC in Taiwan. [86]. Among the 1237 patients, 193 received GLE/PIB; 9 of them had a history of HCC and one had active disease. The study notes no differences regarding SVR in patients with or without HCC. The same conclusion was drawn in regard to OBV/PVT/r + DVS (5 patients with active HCC), SOF/LDV and ELB/GZR (each with one patient with active HCC).

7. SOF/LDV

This is one of the first used all oral regimens, combining the well-known sofosbuvir (NS5B polymerase inhibitor) with an NS5A inhibitor (ledipasvir). It is one of the few therapeutic regimens suited for patients with decompensated cirrhosis. [87] In a real life observational trial, SOV/LDV demonstrated a rate of SVR of 86%, in patients with cirrhosis Child A, B or C and transplant recipients, with a significant improvement in MELD score. Out of 200 patients, only one HCC was newly diagnosed, while out of 35 patients with a history of HCC, 17 developed recurrence, depending on the previous (curative or non-curative therapies). [88] A retrospective analysis evaluating 62,354 patients treated for HCV chronic infection, either by interferon, DAA (including SOV/LDV) or both, revealed that achievement of SVR is associated with a 61% reduction in the risk of HCC. A higher incidence of HCC was noted after DAA only therapy (compared to interferon alone or interferon and DAA) but, after evaluating risk factors for HCC, analysis showed that the presence of cirrhosis, impaired liver function and diabetes (more prevalent in the DAA subgroup) were responsible for the differences. [89] Another trial comparing the HCC risk after DAA with the risk after interferon-based therapy (819 patients treated with DAA, 380 treated with SOV/LDV), found that 9/380 patients developed new HCCs. The patients were older and had Child A or Child B cirrhosis; most of them were interferon-experienced. [90] Notably, in the same cohort, out of 120 patients treated with OBV/ PTV/r + DSV, 3 patients developed HCC. Failure to achieve SVR was the strongest risk factor associated with de novo HCC. In contrast, in the historical cohort of patients treated with interferon 19/283 patients developed HCC;

11 patients had no signs of cirrhosis at the time of therapy. A prospective multicenter trial studied the risk of de novo HCC after DAA therapies, including 158 cirrhotic patients and 31 patients with advanced fibrosis receiving SOF/LDV. Newly diagnosed HCC was reported in 35/985 patients after 48 weeks of surveillance. [91] Risk factors for HCC included male gander, failure to obtain SVR, presence of cirrhosis and hepatocytolytic syndrome; DAA therapy was not associated with an increased risk of HCC. In another retrospective trial, 1082 HCV patients receiving DAA or interferon-based therapies were monitored for de novo HCC; during follow-up 33% developed HCC. The patients received different antiviral therapies, among them: SOF/LVD 41 patients, GLE/PIB 49 patients, GZR/EBR 44 patients and OBV/PTV/r + DSV 41 patients. None of the antiviral therapies represented risk factors for HCC. [92]

8. GZR/EBR

This treatment regimen contains an NS3/4A protease inhibitor (grazoprevir) and an NS5A inhibitor (elbasvir) and can only be used in patients with genotypes 1 and 4 HCV infection, with SVR rates of 92–99% in patients with chronic hepatitis and compensated cirrhosis. [93] In a real life retrospective study, out of 149 patients, 27 of with had a history of HCC, no new or recurrent cases of HCC were reported. [94] According to a recent model, in patients with chronic HCV infection and renal disease, the estimated incidence of HCC was 1,2% in the GZR/ EBR group, 21,64% in the no-treatment group and 8,9% in the interferon group. [95] Furthermore, in a prospective report on 40 hemodialysis patients with genotype 1b infection, there was one documented case of HCC at week 4 of therapy. [96] A trial of 349 patients treated with DAA, including 45 patients with a history of HCC, found 15 cases of HCC recurrence and 3 cases of de novo HCC, after a median surveillance of 22 months after DAA (for recurrent HCC) and 16 months (for de novo HCC). 2 cases of recurrence occurred in the 19 patients treated with GZR/EBR. The most important risk factor for recurrence was the previous HCC management. [97]

9. OBV/PTV/r + DSV

This is a genotype 1 specific DAA combination including an NS5A inhibitor (ombitasvir) an NS3/4A protease inhibitor (paritaprevir) and an NS5B polymerase inhibitor (dasabuvir), while ritonavir acts as a pharmacokinetic enhancer. [56] A prospective analysis on 24 patients with HCV associated compensated cirrhosis and history of HCC revealed a decrease in HCC recurrence rate, as well as survival without recurrence, when compared to a control group. Patients had been previously managed with resection, radiofrequency ablation, and trans-arterial chemoembolization, had a history of 6 month of disease free survival and were monitored by CT scan or MRI every 6 months. The SVR rate in the study group was 87% (lower than that recorded in patients without HCC). [98] Another prospective study on 278 patients with HCV related advanced fibrosis (F3-F4), without HCC history, revealed 11 cases on newly diagnosed HCC (5 during antiviral therapy, 2 at the end of therpy and 4 at 3 months after the end of therapy). The overall incidence of HCC did not surpass the general incidence. Notably, patients presented an infiltrative type HCC, difficult to observe on abdominal ultrasonography or even CT scan, requiring MRI. [99] In a multicenter trial in Brazil, out of 222 patients with advanced fibrosis, one patient was diagnosed with HCC at the end of therapy, despite initial screening, was not evaluated for SVR and subsequently died. [100]

A large real world cohort study of 941 patients including 131 patients with concomitant HCC (79 without viable tumors and 52 with viable tumors) evaluated safety and efficacy of OBV/PTV/r + DSV. There were no differences in SVR between patients with and without HCC; risk factors for no response were Child Pugh A 6 and low serum albumin. One patient died during treatment due to HCC rupture. [101] On the other hand, one of the first studies of HCC recurrence in the setting of DAA therapy which was performed in 4 Spanish hospitals, revealed a recurrence rate of 27.6% (16/58 patients); notably, initial evaluations showed no active disease for more than 6 months prior to DAA therapy. One of the 15 patients treated with OBV/PTV/r + DSV developed "non-characterized" nodules on liver imaging. [102]

10. Conclusion

The benefits of DAA therapy in patients with HCC have been proven by a propensity-matched trial on 1239 patients, with HCC managed by curative options or palliation. The results showed a decrease in 5-years all- cause mortality and liver related mortality in both groups. [103] However, the current opinion is that the risk of HCC may persist up to 10 years after obtaining SVR; the HCV infection appears to leave behind an epigenetic scar, inducing carcinogenesis. [104] Therefore, the international consensus is that HCC surveillance should continue after antiviral therapy, and its duration and periodicity should be based on the general risk of HCC of the patient, even deciding on a case to case basis. [105] Besides, the reduction of HCC risk in patients with decompensated cirrhosis is also controversial, thus stimulating further debate regarding the best timing for liver transplantation in these patients. [106]

Author details

Laura Iliescu[1,2]

1 Department of Internal Medicine, Fundeni Clinical Institute, Bucharest, Romania

2 "Carol Davila" University of Medicine and Pharmacy, Bucharest, Romania

*Address all correspondence to: laura_ate@yahoo.com

References

[1] https://www.who.int/news-room/fact-sheets/detail/hepatitis-c

[2] de Martel C, Maucort-Boulch D, Plummer M, Franceschi S. World-wide relative contribution of hepatitis B and C viruses in hepatocellular carcinoma. Hepatology. 2015;62:1190-1200. doi: 10.1002/hep.27969

[3] Omland LH, Krarup H, Jepsen P, Georgsen J, Harritshøj LH, Riisom K, et al. Mortality in patients with chronic and cleared hepatitis C viral infection: a nationwide cohort study. J Hepatol. 2010;53:36-42. doi: 10.1016/j.jhep.2010.01.033

[4] Axley P, Ahmed Z, Ravi S, Singal AK. Hepatitis C Virus and Hepatocellular Carcinoma: A Narrative Review. J Clin Transl Hepatol. 2018;6(1):79-84. doi:10.14218/JCTH.2017.00067

[5] Kanwal F, Kramer JR, Ilyas J, Duan Z, El-Serag HB. HCV genotype 3 is associated with an increased risk of cirrhosis and hepatocellular cancer in a national sample of U.S. Veterans with HCV. Hepatology. 2014;60:98-105. doi: 10.1002/hep.27095

[6] Lee MH, Hsiao TI, Subramaniam SR, Le AK, Vu VD, Trinh HN, et al. HCV genotype 6 increased the risk for hepatocellular carcinoma among asian patients with liver cirrhosis. Am J Gastroenterol. 2017;112:1111-1119. doi: 10.1038/ajg.2017.123

[7] Kruse RL, Kramer JR, Tyson GL, Duan Z, Chen L, El-Serag HB, et al. Clinical outcomes of hepatitis B virus coinfection in a United States cohort of hepatitis C virus-infected patients. Hepatology. 2014;60:1871-1878. doi: 10.1002/hep.27337

[8] Chuang SC, Lee YC, Hashibe M, Dai M, Zheng T, Boffetta P. Interaction between cigarette smoking and hepatitis B and C virus infection on the risk of liver cancer: a meta-analysis. Cancer Epidemiol Biomarkers Prev. 2010;19:1261-1268. doi: 10.1158/1055-9965.EPI-09-1297

[9] Donato F, Tagger A, Gelatti U, Parrinello G, Boffetta P, Albertini A, et al. Alcohol and hepatocellular carcinoma: the effect of lifetime intake and hepatitis virus infections in men and women. Am J Epidemiol. 2002;155:323-331. doi: 10.1093/aje/155.4.323

[10] Saab S, Mallam D, Cox GA, 2nd, Tong MJ. Impact of coffee on liver diseases: a systematic review. Liver Int. 2014;34:495-504. doi: 10.1111/liv.12304

[11] Lecube A, Hernández C, Genescà J, Esteban JI, Jardí R, Simó R: High prevalence of glucose abnormalities in patients with hepatitis C virus infection: a multivariate analysis considering the liver injury. Diabetes Care 27 : 1171-1175,2004

[12] Masini M, Campani D, Boggi U, Menicagli M, Funel N, Pollera M, Lupi R, Del Guerra S, Bugliani M, Torri S, Del Prato S, Mosca F, Filipponi F, Marchetti P: Hepatitis C virus infection and human pancreatic β-cell dysfunction (Brief Report). Diabetes Care 28 : 940-941,2005

[13] Albert Lecube, Cristina Hernández, Joan Genescà, Rafael Simó. Glucose Abnormalities in Patients with Hepatitis C Virus Infection. Diabetes Care May 2006, 29 (5) 1140-1149; DOI: 10.2337/dc05-1995

[14] Li X, Xu H, Gao Y, Pan M, Wang L, Gao P. Diabetes mellitus increases the risk of hepatocellular carcinoma in treatment-naïve chronic hepatitis C patients in China. Medicine (Baltimore) 2017;96:e6508. doi: 10.1097/MD.0000000000006508

[15] Hoshida Y, Fuchs BC, Bardeesy N, Baumert TF, Chung RT. Pathogenesis and prevention of hepatitis C virus-induced hepatocellular carcinoma, Journal of Hepatology 2014 vol. 61 j S79–S90

[16] Fukutomi T, Zhou Y, Kawai S, Eguchi H, Wands JR, Li J. Hepatitis C virus core protein stimulates hepatocyte growth: correlation with upregulation of wnt-1 expression. Hepatology 2005;41:1096-1105

[17] Arima N, Kao CY, Licht T, Padmanabhan R, Sasaguri Y. Modulation of cell growth by the hepatitis C virus nonstructural protein NS5A. J Biol Chem 2001;276:12675-12684

[18] Alisi A, Giambartolomei S, Cupelli F, Merlo P, Fontemaggi G, Spaziani A, et al. Physical and functional interaction between HCV core protein and the different p73 isoforms. Oncogene 2003;22:2573-2580

[19] Zhao LJ, Wang L, Ren H, Cao J, Li L, Ke JS, et al. Hepatitis C virus E2 protein promotes human hepatoma cell proliferation through the MAPK/ERK signalling pathway via cellular receptors. Exp Cell Res 2005;305: 23-32

[20] Koike K. Hepatitis C virus contributes to hepatocarcinogenesis by modulating metabolic and intracellular signalling pathways. J Gastroenterol Hepatol 2007;22:S108–S111

[21] Pavio N, Battaglia S, Boucreux D, Arnulf B, Sobesky R, Hermine O, et al. Hepatitis C virus core variants isolated from liver tumor but not from adjacent non-tumor tissue interact with Smad3 and inhibit the TGF-beta pathway. Oncogene 2005;24(40):6119-6132

[22] Street A, Macdonald A, McCormick C, Harris M. Hepatitis C virus NS5Amediated activation of phosphoinositide 3-kinase results in stabilization of cellular beta-catenin and stimulation of beta-catenin-responsive transcription. J Virol 2005;79:5006-5016

[23] Choi SH, Hwang SB. Modulation of the transforming growth factor-beta signal transduction pathway by hepatitis C virus nonstructural 5A protein. J Biol Chem 2006;281:7468-7478

[24] Wu SC, Chang SC, Wu HY, Liao PJ, Chang MF. Hepatitis C virus NS5A protein down-regulates the expression of spindle gene Aspm through PKR-p38 signalling pathway. J Biol Chem 2008;283:29396-29404

[25] Ghosh AK, Majumder M, Steele R, Meyer K, Ray R, Ray RB. Hepatitis C virus NS5A protein protects against TNF-alpha mediated apoptotic cell death. Virus Res 2000;67:173-178

[26] Machida K, Liu JC, McNamara G, Levine A, Duan L, Lai MM. Hepatitis C virus causes uncoupling of mitotic checkpoint and chromosomal polyploidy through the Rb pathway. J Virol 2009;83:12590-12600

[27] Tardif KD, Mori K, Siddiqui A. Hepatitis C virus subgenomic replicons induce endoplasmic reticulum stress activating an intracellular signalling pathway. J Virol 2002;76:7453-7459

[28] Nagahara T, Okano J, Fujise Y, Abe R, Murawaki Y. Preventive effect of JTE522, a selective cyclooxygenase-2 inhibitor, on DEN-induced hepatocarcinogenesis in rats. Biomed Pharmacother 2010;64:319-326

[29] Joo M, Hahn YS, Kwon M, Sadikot RT, Blackwell TS, Christman JW. Hepatitis C virus core protein suppresses NF-jB activation and cyclooxygenase-2 expression by direct interaction with IkappaB kinase beta. J Virol 2005;79:7648-7657

[30] Tacke RS, Tosello-Trampont A, Nguyen V, Mullins DW, Hahn YS. Extracellular hepatitis C virus core

protein activates STAT3 in human monocytes/ macrophages/dendritic cells via an IL-6 autocrine pathway. J Biol Chem 2011;286:10847-10855

[31] Hui L, Zatloukal K, Scheuch H, Stepniak E, Wagner EF. Proliferation of human HCC cells and chemically induced mouse liver cancers requires JNK1-dependent p21 downregulation. J Clin Invest 2008;118:3943-3953

[32] Li XD, Sun L, Seth RB, Pineda G, Chen ZJ. Hepatitis C virus protease NS3/ 4A cleaves mitochondrial antiviral signaling protein off the mitochondria to evade innate immunity. Proc Natl Acad Sci U S A 2005;102: 17717-17722

[33] Tseng CT, Klimpel GR. Binding of the hepatitis C virus envelope protein E2 to CD81 inhibits natural killer cell functions. J Exp Med 2002;195: 43-49

[34] Hwang SJ, Lee SD. Hepatic steatosis and hepatitis C: still unhappy bedfellows? J Gastroenterol Hepatol 2011;26:96-101

[35] Moriya K, Fujie H, Shintani Y, Yotsuyanagi H, Tsutsumi T, Ishibashi K, et al. The core protein of hepatitis C virus induces hepatocellular carcinoma in transgenic mice. Nat Med 1998;4:1065-1067

[36] Koike K, Moriya K. Metabolic aspects of hepatitis C viral infection: steatohepatitis resembling but distinct from NASH. J Gastroenterol 2005;40:329-336

[37] Perlemuter G, Sabile A, Letteron P, Vona G, Topilco A, Chretien Y, et al. Hepatitis C virus core protein inhibits microsomal triglyceride transfer protein activity and very low density lipoprotein secretion: a model of viral-related steatosis. FASEB J 2002;16:185-194

[38] Koike K. Steatosis, liver injury, and hepatocarcinogenesis in hepatitis C viral infection. J Gastroenterol 2009;44:82-88

[39] Herbig U, Jobling WA, Chen BP, Chen DJ, Sedivy JM. Telomere shortening triggers senescence of human cells through a pathway involving ATM, p53, and p21(CIP1), but not p16(INK4a). Mol Cell 2004;14:501-513

[40] Lim JS, Park SH, Jang KL. Hepatitis C virus core protein overcomes stressinduced premature senescence by down-regulating p16 expression via DNA methylation. Cancer Lett 2012;321:154-161

[41] Aihara T, Noguchi S, Sasaki Y, Nakano H, Imaoka S. Clonal analysis of regenerative nodules in hepatitis C virus-induced liver cirrhosis. Gastroenterology 1994;107:1805-1811

[42] Fattovich G, Stroffolini T, Zagni I, Donato F. Hepatocellular carcinoma in cirrhosis: incidence and risk factors. Gastroenterology 2004;127:S35–S50

[43] Hernandez-Gea V, Toffanin S, Friedman SL, Llovet JM. Role of the microenvironment in the pathogenesis and treatment of hepatocellular carcinoma. Gastroenterology 2013;144:512-527

[44] Gieseler RK, Marquitan G, Schlattjan M, Sowa JP, Bechmann LP, Timm J, et al. Hepatocyte apoptotic bodies encasing nonstructural HCV proteins amplify hepatic stellate cell activation: implications for chronic hepatitis C. J Viral Hepat 2011;18:760-767

[45] Dapito DH, Mencin A, Gwak GY, Pradere JP, Jang MK, Mederacke I, et al. Promotion of hepatocellular carcinoma by the intestinal microbiota and TLR4. Cancer Cell 2012;21:504-516

[46] Mazzocca A, Sciammetta SC, Carloni V, Cosmi L, Annunziato F, Harada T, et al. Binding of hepatitis C virus envelope protein E2 to CD81 up-regulates matrix metalloproteinase-2

in human hepatic stellate cells. J Biol Chem 2005;280:11329-11339

[47] Yoshiji H, Noguchi R, Kaji K, Ikenaka Y, Shirai Y, Namisaki T, et al. Attenuation of insulin-resistance-based hepatocarcinogenesis and angiogenesis by combined treatment with branched-chain amino acids and angiotensin-converting enzyme inhibitor in obese diabetic rats. J Gastroenterol 2010;45:443-450

[48] Fuchs BC, Hoshida Y, Fujii T, Wei L, Yamada S, Lauwers GY, et al. Epidermal growth factor receptor inhibition attenuates liver fibrosis and development of hepatocellular carcinoma. Hepatology 2014;59:1577-1590

[49] Zona L, Lupberger J, Sidahmed-Adrar N, Thumann C, Harris HJ, Barnes A, et al. HRas signal transduction promotes hepatitis C virus cell entry by triggering assembly of the host tetraspanin receptor complex. Cell Host Microbe 2013;13:302-313

[50] Schiffer E, Housset C, Cacheux W, Wendum D, Desbois-Mouthon C, Rey C, et al. Gefitinib, an EGFR inhibitor, prevents hepatocellular carcinoma development in the rat liver with cirrhosis. Hepatology 2005;41:307-314

[51] Horwitz E, Stein I, Andreozzi M, Nemeth J, Shoham A, Pappo O, et al. Human and mouse VEGFA-amplified hepatocellular carcinomas are highly sensitive to sorafenib treatment. Cancer Discov 2014;4(6):730-743

[52] Fabris C, Falleti E, Cussigh A, Bitetto D, Fontanini E, Bignulin S, et al. IL-28B rs12979860 C/T allele distribution in patients with liver cirrhosis: role in the course of chronic viral hepatitis and the development of HCC. J Hepatol 2011;54:716-722

[53] Hoshida Y, Fuchs BC, Tanabe KK. Genomic risk of hepatitis C-related hepatocellular carcinoma. J Hepatol 2012;56:729-730

[54] Furutani T, Hino K, Okuda M, Gondo T, Nishina S, Kitase A, et al. Hepatic iron overload induces hepatocellular carcinoma in transgenic mice expressing the hepatitis C virus polyprotein. Gastroenterology 2006;130: 2087-2098

[55] Ura S, Honda M, Yamashita T, Ueda T, Takatori H, Nishino R, et al. Differential microRNA expression between hepatitis B and hepatitis C leading disease progression to hepatocellular carcinoma. Hepatology 2009;49:1098-1112

[56] EASL recommendations on treatment of hepatitis C: Final update of the seriesq European Association for the Study of the Liver*, Journal of Hepatology 2020 vol. 73 j 1170-1218

[57] Ghany, M.G., Morgan, T.R. and (2020), Hepatitis C Guidance 2019 Update: American Association for the Study of Liver Diseases–Infectious Diseases Society of America Recommendations for Testing, Managing, and Treating Hepatitis C Virus Infection. Hepatology, 71: 686-721

[58] Omata M, Kanda T, Wei L, Yu ML, Chuang WL, Ibrahim A, Lesmana CR, Sollano J, Kumar M, Jindal A, Sharma BC, Hamid SS, Dokmeci AK, Mamun-Al-Mahtab, McCaughan GW, Wasim J, Crawford DH, Kao JH, Yokosuka O, Lau GK, Sarin SK. APASL consensus statements and recommendation on treatment of hepatitis C. Hepatol Int. 2016 Sep;10(5):702-726. doi: 10.1007/s12072-016-9717-6

[59] EASL recommendations on treatment of hepatitis C: Final update of the series. European Association for the Study of the Liver*, Journal of Hepatology 2020 vol. 73 j 1170-1218

[60] Beste LA, Green PK, Berry K, Kogut MJ, Allison SK, Ioannou GN. Effectiveness of hepatitis C antiviral treatment in a USA cohort of veteran patients with hepatocellular carcinoma. J Hepatol 2017;67:32-39

[61] He S, Lockart I, Alavi M, Danta M, Hajarizadeh B, Dore GJ. Systematic review with meta-analysis: effectiveness of direct-acting antiviral treatment for hepatitis C in patients with hepatocellular carcinoma. Aliment Pharmacol Ther 2020;51:34-52

[62] Huang AC, Mehta N, Dodge JL, Yao FY, Terrault NA. Direct-acting antivirals do not increase the risk of hepatocellular carcinoma recurrence after local-regional therapy or liver transplant waitlist dropout. Hepatology 2018;68:449-461

[63] Cortesi PA, Belli LS, Facchetti R, Mazzarelli C, Perricone G, De Nicola S, et al. The optimal timing of hepatitis C therapy in liver transplanteligible patients: cost-effectiveness analysis of new opportunities. J Viral Hepat 2018;25:791-801

[64] Ioannou GN, Green PK, Berry K. HCV eradication induced by directacting antiviral agents reduces the risk of hepatocellular carcinoma. J Hepatol 2018;68:25-32

[65] Nahon P, Bourcier V, Layese R, Audureau E, Cagnot C, Marcellin P, et al. Eradication of hepatitis C virus infection in patients with cirrhosis reduces risk of liver and non-liver complications. Gastroenterology 2017;152:142-156

[66] Ioannou GN, Beste LA, Green PK, Singal AG, Tapper EB, Waljee AK, et al. Increased risk for hepatocellular carcinoma persists up to 10 years after HCV eradication in patients with baseline cirrhosis or high FIB-4 scores. Gastroenterology 2019;157:1264-1278

[67] Waziry R, Hajarizadeh B, Grebely J, Amin J, Law M, Danta M, et al. Hepatocellular carcinoma risk following direct-acting antiviral HCV therapy: a systematic review, meta-analyses, and meta-regression. J Hepatol 2017;67:1204-1212

[68] Singal AG, Rich NE, Mehta N, Branch AD, Pillai A, Hoteit M, et al. Directacting antiviral therapy for hepatitis C virus infection is associated with increased survival in patients with a history of hepatocellular carcinoma. Gastroenterology 2019;157:1253-1263

[69] Singal AG, Lim JK, Kanwal F. AGA clinical practice update on interaction between oral direct-acting antivirals for chronic hepatitis C infection and hepatocellular carcinoma: expert review. Gastroenterology 2019;156:2149-2157

[70] HCV Guidance: Recommendations for Testing, Managing, and Treating Hepatitis C Last Updated: August 27, 2020 www.hcvguidelines.org

[71] Curry MP, Forns X, Chung RT, Terrault NA, Brown R, Jr, Fenkel JM, et al. Sofosbuvir and ribavirin prevent recurrence of HCV infection after liver transplantation: an open-label study. Gastroenterology. 2015;148:100-107. doi: 10.1053/j.gastro.2014.09.023

[72] Greig SL. Sofosbuvir/Velpatasvir: A Review in Chronic Hepatitis C. Drugs. 2016 Oct;76(16):1567-1578. doi: 10.1007/s40265-016-0648-2

[73] Wilton J, Wong S, Yu A, Ramji A, Cook D, Butt ZA et al, for the BC Hepatitis Testers Cohort Team, Real-world Effectiveness of Sofosbuvir/Velpatasvir for Treatment of Chronic Hepatitis C in British Columbia, Canada: A Population-Based Cohort Study, Open Forum Infectious Diseases, Volume 7, Issue 3, March 2020

[74] Takehara T, Sakamoto N, Nishiguchi S, et al. Efficacy and safety

of sofosbuvir-velpatasvir with or without ribavirin in HCV-infected Japanese patients with decompensated cirrhosis: an open-label phase 3 trial. J Gastroenterol. 2019;54(1):87-95. doi:10.1007/s00535-018-1503-x

[75] Atsukawa, M., Tsubota, A., Kondo, C. et al. Real-World Clinical Application of 12-Week Sofosbuvir/Velpatasvir Treatment for Decompensated Cirrhotic Patients with Genotype 1 and 2: A Prospective, Multicenter Study. Infect Dis Ther 9, 851-866 (2020)

[76] Bourlière M, Gordon SC, Flamm SL, Cooper CL, Ramji A, Tong M, et al. POLARIS-1 and POLARIS-4 Investigators Sofosbuvir, velpatasvir and voxilaprevir for previously treated HCV infection. N Engl J Med 2017;376:2134-2146. 10.1056/NEJMoa1613512

[77] Childs-Kean LM, Brumwell NA, Lodl EF. Profile of sofosbuvir/velpatasvir/voxilaprevir in the treatment of hepatitis C. Infect Drug Resist. 2019;12:2259-2268. Published 2019 Jul 23. doi:10.2147/IDR.S171338

[78] Food and Drug Administration. FDA adverse event reporting system (FAERS) public dashboard. Available from: https://www.fda.gov/drugs/fda-adverse-event-reporting-system-faers/fda-adverse-event-reporting-system-faers-public-dashboard. Accessed March22, 2019

[79] Tandy A, Shiva V, Alexander L, A Rare Case of Sofosbuvir/Velpatasvir/Voxilaprevir Failure in a Patient With Hepatitis C Virus Infection and Previously Undiagnosed Hepatocellular Carcinoma, The American Journal of Gastroenterology: October 2019 - Volume 114 - Issue - p S1375 doi: 10.14309/01.ajg.0000599536.00418.14

[80] Degasperi E, Spinetti A, Lombardi A, Landonio S, Rossi MC, Pasulo L, et al.NAVIGATORE-Lombardia and Veneto Study Groups. Real-life effectiveness and safety of sofosbuvir/velpatasvir/voxilaprevir in hepatitis C patients with previous DAA failure J Hepatol, 71 (2019), pp. 1106-1115

[81] Lamb YN. Glecaprevir/Pibrentasvir: First Global Approval. Drugs. 2017 Oct;77(16):1797-1804. doi: 10.1007/s40265-017-0817-y

[82] Kwo PY, Poordad F, Asatryan A, Wang S, Wyles DL, Hassanein T, et al. Glecaprevir and pibrentasvir yield high response rates in patients with HCV genotype 1-6 without cirrhosis. J Hepatol. 2017 Aug;67(2):263-271. doi: 10.1016/j.jhep.2017.03.039

[83] Brown RS Jr, Buti M, Rodrigues L, Chulanov V, Chuang WL, Aguilar H, et al. Glecaprevir/pibrentasvir for 8 weeks in treatment-naïve patients with chronic HCV genotypes 1-6 and compensated cirrhosis: The EXPEDITION-8 trial. J Hepatol. 2020 Mar;72(3):441-449. doi: 10.1016/j.jhep.2019.10.020

[84] Kawaguchi, I., Chayama, K., Gonzalez, Y.S. et al. A Cost-Effectiveness Analysis of Glecaprevir/Pibrentasvir Versus Existing Direct-Acting Antivirals to Treat Chronic Hepatitis C in Japan. Adv Ther 37, 457-476 (2020). https://doi.org/10.1007/s12325-019-01166-3

[85] Lok AS, Sulkowski MS, Kort JJ, Willner I, Reddy KR, Shiffman ML, et al. Efficacy of Glecaprevir and Pibrentasvir in Patients With Genotype 1 Hepatitis C Virus Infection With Treatment Failure After NS5A Inhibitor Plus Sofosbuvir Therapy. Gastroenterology. 2019 Dec;157(6):1506-1517.e1. doi: 10.1053/j.gastro.2019.08.008

[86] Dai CY, Huang CF, Hsieh MH, Huang CI, Yeh ML, Tsai PC, Lin CC, Lee MS, Yang JF, Hsu PY, Wei YJ, Hsu CT, Liang PC, Lin YH, Huang JF, Chuang WL, Yu ML. Treatment efficacy

for patients with chronic hepatitis C and preexisting hepatocellular carcinoma by directly acting antivirals. Hepatoma Res 2020;6:16

[87] Keating GM. Ledipasvir/Sofosbuvir: a review of its use in chronic hepatitis C. Drugs. 2015 Apr;75(6):675-685

[88] Idilman, R, Demir, M, Aladag, M, et al.; Early Access Program Study Group. Low recurrence rate of hepatocellular carcinoma following ledipasvir and sofosbuvir treatment in a real-world chronic hepatitis C patients cohort. J Viral Hepat. 2019; 26: 666-674

[89] Ioannou GN, Green PK, Berry K. HCV eradication induced by direct-acting antiviral agents reduces the risk of hepatocellular carcinoma [published online ahead of print, 2017 Sep 5]. J Hepatol. 2017;S0168-8278(17)32273-0. doi:10.1016/j.jhep.2017.08.030

[90] Finkelmeier F, Dultz G, Peiffer K, –H, Kronenberger B, Krauss F, Zeuzem S, Sarrazin C, Vermehren J, Waidmann O: Risk of de novo Hepatocellular Carcinoma after HCV Treatment with Direct-Acting Antivirals. Liver Cancer 2018;7:190-204

[91] Rinaldi, L., Perrella, A., Guarino, M. et al. Incidence and risk factors of early HCC occurrence in HCV patients treated with direct acting antivirals: a prospective multicentre study. J Transl Med 17, 292 (2019)

[92] Lee HW, Han DH, Shin HJ, Lee JS, Kim SU, Park JY, Kim DY, Ahn SH, Kim BK. Hepatocellular Carcinoma Risk According to Regimens for Eradication of Hepatitis C Virus; Interferon or Direct Acting Antivirals. Cancers. 2020; 12(11):3414

[93] Morikawa K, Nakamura A, Shimazaki T, Sakamoto N. Safety and efficacy of elbasvir/grazoprevir for the treatment of chronic hepatitis C: current evidence. Drug Des Devel Ther. 2018;12:2749-2756. Published 2018 Sep 5. doi:10.2147/DDDT.S133697

[94] Tsai TC, Deng ST, Hsu CW. The efficacy and safety of elbasvir/grazoprevir treatment in HCV genotype 1 patients in Taiwan [published correction appears in J Med Virol. 2020 Aug;92(8):1369]. J Med Virol. 2020;92(2):219-226. doi:10.1002/jmv.25605

[95] Chizoba Nwankwo, Shelby L. Corman, Elamin H. Elbasha, Projected impact of elbasvir/grazoprevir in patients with hepatitis C virus genotype 1 and chronic kidney disease in Vietnam,Journal of Infection and Public Health, Volume 12, Issue 4, 2019, Pages 502-508

[96] Liu, CH., Peng, CY., Fang, YJ. et al. Elbasvir/grazoprevir for hepatitis C virus genotype 1b East-Asian patients receiving hemodialysis. Sci Rep 10, 9180 (2020)

[97] Kogiso T, Sagawa T, Kodama K, et al. Hepatocellular carcinoma after direct-acting antiviral drug treatment in patients with hepatitis C virus. JGH Open. 2018;3(1):52-60. Published 2018 Nov 9. doi:10.1002/jgh3.12105

[98] Preda CM, Baicus C, Sandra I, Oproiu A, Manuc T, Constantinescu I, Gavrila D, Diculescu M, Dumitru R, Vasilescu C, Tieranu C, Istratescu D, Voiosu T, Manuc M. Recurrence rate of hepatocellular carcinoma in patients with treated hepatocellular carcinoma and hepatitis C virus-associated cirrhosis after ombitasvir/paritaprevir/ritonavir+dasabuvir+ribavirin therapy. United European Gastroenterol J. 2019 Jun;7(5):699-708

[99] Iliescu EL, Mercan-Stanciu A, Toma L, Ioanitescu ES, Dumitru R, Rusie D. Hepatocellular carcinoma in the setting of interferon-free treatment for chronic HCV hepatitis - experience

of a single center. Hepatoma Res 2018;4:3

[100] Pessoa MG, Ramalho-Madruga JV, Alves K, Nunes EP, Cheinquer H, Brandão-Mello CE, et al. Efficacy and Safety of Ombitasvir/Paritaprevir/ Ritonavir and Dasabuvir ± Ribavirin for HCV in Brazilian Adults with Advanced Fibrosis. Ann Hepatol. 2018 Oct 16;17(6):959-968

[101] Chen, CH., Chen, CH., Lin, CL. et al. Real-world safety and efficacy of paritaprevir/ritonavir/ombitasvir plus dasabuvir ± ribavirin in patients with hepatitis C virus genotype 1 and advanced hepatic fibrosis or compensated cirrhosis: a multicenter pooled analysis. Sci Rep 9, 7086 (2019)

[102] Reig M, Mariño Z, Perelló C, Iñarrairaegui M, Ribeiro A, Lens S, Díaz A, Vilana R, Darnell A, Varela M, Sangro B, Calleja JL, Forns X, Bruix J. Unexpected high rate of early tumor recurrence in patients with HCV-related HCC undergoing interferon-free therapy. J Hepatol. 2016 Oct;65(4):719-726

[103] Dang H, Yeo YH, Yasuda S, Huang CF, Iio E, Landis C, et al. Cure with interferon free DAA is associated with increased survival in patients with HCV related HCC from both East and West. Hepatoology 2019 Oct 14;[Epub ahead of print]

[104] Ioannou GN, Beste LA, Green PK, Singal AG, Tapper EB, Waljee AK, et al. Increased risk for hepatocellular carcinoma persists up to 10 years after HCV eradication in patients with baseline cirrhosis or high FIB-4 scores. Gastroenterology 2019;157:1264-1278 e4

[105] Na SK, Song BC. Development and surveillance of hepatocellular carcinoma in patients with sustained virologic response after antiviral therapy for chronic hepatitis C. Clin Mol Hepatol 2019;25:234-244

[106] Calvaruso V, Cabibbo G, Cacciola I, Petta S, Madonia S, Bellia A, et al. Incidence of hepatocellular carcinoma in patients with HCV-associated cirrhosis treated with direct-acting antiviral agents. Gastroenterology 2018;155:411-421 e4

Section 7

Non-alcoholic Fatty Liver Disease

Chapter 8

Diagnosis of Nonalcoholic Steatohepatitis

Eira Cerda-Reyes, Alicia Sarahi Ojeda-Yuren, Julián Torres-Vazquez, María del Rosario Herrero Maceda, Martín Uriel Vázquez-Medina, Perla Denice Flores-Rangel, Yailin Fabiola Velásquez Palacios, Saraid Cerda-Reyes and Graciela Elia Castro-Narro

Abstract

The prevalence of non-alcoholic fatty liver disease (NAFLD) has increased in the last years up to 25% in the adult population. This disease includes a large spectrum of disorders, from simple fatty liver disease to cirrhosis and Hepatocellular Carcinoma (HCC), and they are related to chronic metabolic conditions. NAFLD is characterized by the presence of at least 5% of hepatic steatosis without evidence of hepatocellular injury. The diagnosis of this disease should be of exclusion and focused on its progression, treatment, and identification of the prognosis. The European Association for the Study of the Liver (EASL), the National Institute for Health and Care Excellence (NICE), the Italian Association for the Study of the Liver (AISF), and the American Association for the Study of the Liver (AASLD), published their Clinical Guidelines that have identified the criteria for the diagnosis of NAFLD, several, using imaging or histological diagnostic methods, although they imply a different approach and screening. The Fatty Liver Index and the NAFLD Liver Fat Score are used by 3 out of 5 Guidelines and they are easily calculated using blood tests and clinical information. Other non-invasive scales for NAFLD are the NAFLD fibrosis score (NFS), Fib-4, AST/ALT ratio index; also the ELF panel, Fibrometer, Fibrotest, Hepascore; and some imaging techniques that include transient elastography, magnetic resonance elastography (MRE), and shear wave elastography. Finally, proteomic's and glycomic's technologic biomarkers are currently under investigation and recent use, such as Cytokeratin 18 and Sirtuin 1. Still, liver biopsy remains the gold standard to distinguish between steatohepatitis and simple steatosis, using the histological classification and staging scoring systems of NAFLD Activity Score (NAS) and the Steatosis Activity Fibrosis (SAF), to evaluate the disease's activity.

Keywords: non alcoholic liver disease, no invasive diagnosis, diagnosis

1. Introduction

In the last years, the prevalence of non-alcoholic fatty liver disease (NAFLD) has raised at a worldwide level, affecting up to 25% of the adult population [1].

The prevalence of type 2 diabetes, cardiovascular diseases, cancer associated with obesity, and advanced hepatic diseases (liver cirrhosis and liver cancer), have increased together with the growth of the prevalence of NAFLD [1–4].

The broad spectrum of disorders that involve NAFLD range from simple fatty liver to nonalcoholic steatohepatitis, and the increasing of fibrosis that concludes in cirrhosis [5, 6]. Among the most relevant metabolic conditions related to this disease, are obesity, insulin resistance, dyslipidemia, and type 2 diabetes [5–7].

Furthermore, the European Association for the Study of the Liver (EASL) and the Asia-Pacific Guidelines point out the relation between Hepatocellular Carcinoma (HCC) and NAFLD, since it can occur in patients with NAFLD but without cirrhosis [8, 9].

2. Definition

Nonalcoholic fatty liver is characterized by the presence of at least 5% of hepatic steatosis without evidence of hepatocellular injury (ballooning). On the other hand, the definition of NASH (non-alcoholic steatohepatitis) is the appearance of at least 5% of hepatic steatosis and inflammation, hepatocytic injury (eg. ballooning) with or without fibrosis [10].

3. Diagnosis

The diagnosis' approach should focus on the non-invasive evaluation to first identify NAFLD in patients with metabolic risk factors, and then, monitor the progression of the disease, the treatment, and the response, in order to identify early patients with a worse prognosis [6, 11].

The risk with NAFLD is that it is a silent entity that is diagnosed incidentally, because abnormal liver enzymes are reported in liver biochemistry or through images, such as in ultrasound with steatosis reported. NAFLD is a diagnosis of exclusion, therefore once it is suspected, the diagnosis should be confirmed by ruling out other possible causes of steatosis; for example, alcoholic hepatitis and NASH are clinically indistinguishable. For this exclusion, it is necessary to evaluate if there is a significant consumption of alcohol, which is generally considered of more than 20 g per day [12]; also, it is important to carry out a good clinical record to identify risk factors for liver disease, such as the use of medications or a family history of liver disease. Several Clinical Guidelines have identified criteria for the diagnosis of NAFLD (**Table 1**).

All of these considerations imply a different approach to NAFLD detection by Scientific Societies. Only the recommendations of the Asia-Pacific Associations, EASL and NICE (National Institute for Health and Care Excellence) [13] recommend screening, in particular, of high-risk groups (**Table 2**). In contrast, the AASLD (American Association for the Study of the Liver) recommends a concept of surveillance in the metabolic risk factor populations since there is no cost-effectiveness evidence to support a test to determine NAFLD in adults [6, 14].

3.1 Liver biochemistry

The liver biochemistry of NAFLD usually presents within normal parameters, although a slight increase in aspartate aminotransferase (AST) or alanine aminotransferase (ALT) or gamma-glutamyl transpeptidase (γGT) can occur. However, since liver enzymes are not a sensitive screening test, all the recommendations agree that their normal values may not exclude NAFLD [13]. Besides, liver enzyme

	EASL	NICE	Asia-Pacific	AISF	AASLD
Criteria	Steatosis in>5% of hepatocytes by imaging or histology. There are no other causes of steatosis. Insulin resistance	Excessive fat in the liver. There are no other causes of steatosis. No significant alcohol consumption.	Hepatic steatosis by imaging or histology. There are no other causes of steatosis. No significant alcohol consumption.	Hepatic steatosis in images or histology. There are no other causes of steatosis. No significant alcohol consumption.	Evidence of hepatic steatosis by imaging or histology. There are no other causes of steatosis. No significant alcohol consumption. Non-coexisting chronic liver disease.
Alcohol consumption limit (males)	30 g/d	30 g/d	2 standard drinks / day 140 g / week	30 g/d	21 standard drink / week 294 g / week
Alcohol consumption limit (females)	20 g/d	20 g/d	1 standard drink / day 70 g / week	20 g/d	14 standard drinks / week 196 g / week

Translated from Leoni S. World J Gastroenterol. 2018 Aug 14;24(30):3361–3373. EASL: European Association for the Study of the Liver, NICE: National Institute for Health and Care Excellence, AISF: Italian Association for the Study of the Liver, AASLD: American Association for the Study of the Liver.

Table 1.
Diagnostic criteria for NAFLD according to various clinical guidelines.

	EASL	NICE	Asia-Pacific	AISF	AASLD
Generalized screening	No	No	No	No	No
Screening in high-risk groups Screening type	Yes Obesity Metabolic syndrome Altered liver enzymes Yes, hepatic enzymes	Yes Obesity Type 2 diabetes No, hepatic enzymes. Yes, ultrasound.	Yes Obesity Type 2 diabetes No, hepatic enzymes Yes, ultrasound If transient elastography	Not mentioned	No (active surveillance)

Translated from Leoni S. World J Gastroenterol. 2018 Aug 14;24(30):3361–3373. EASL: European Association for the Study of the Liver, NICE: National Institute for Health and Care Excellence, AISF: Italian Association for the Study of the Liver, AASLD: American Association for the Study of the Liver.

Table 2.
Comparisons of recommendations for screening of NAFLD.

abnormalities can mask another cause of liver disease, in which steatosis is a coexisting condition. Also, abnormalities in laboratory tests (such as ferritin or autoantibodies) do not always diagnose the presence of another liver disease but could be an epiphenomenon of NAFLD with no other clinical consequence. In particular, according to the AASLD guidelines, elevated serum ferritin and low autoimmune antibody titers (especially antinuclear and smooth muscle antibodies) are frequent features in patients with NAFLD and may not demonstrate hemochromatosis or autoimmune liver disease [6, 15, 16].

3.2 Non-invasive techniques

Currently, the absence of highly specific and sensitive non-invasive markers that can predict inflammation and fibrosis has increased the efforts in the identification of new markers of the disease's progression and the development of clinical scores of disease's severity. To evaluate steatosis, the Fatty Liver Index (FLI) and the NAFLD Liver Fat Score are used by the EASL, the Asia Pacific Association, and the Italian guidelines. These scores can be calculated easily by using common blood tests and simple clinical information. For instance, FLI is calculated from triglyceride levels, body mass index, waist circumference, and gamma-glutamyltransferase, while NAFLD liver fat score is determined by evaluating the presence/absence of the metabolic syndrome and type 2 diabetes, fasting serum insulin, and aminotransferases. Both of them have been validated in a cohort of severely obese patients and in the general population, which can predict the presence of steatosis, but not its severity [6, 17–19].

Respectively, there has been an increase in the investigation of different tools in this regard, that include non-invasive scales (NAFLD fibrosis score (NFS), FIB-4, AST/ALT ratio index), serum biomarkers (ELF panel, Fibrometer, Fibrotest, Hepascore), and techniques of imaging, such as transient elastography, magnetic resonance elastography (MRE), and shear wave elastography. According to the NICE guideline, the best cost–benefit ratio in identifying patients with advanced fibrosis stages was demonstrated by the liver fibrosis (ELF) blood test, and therefore, these tests should be offered to all patients with an incidental diagnosis of NAFLD. On the contrary, the EASL and Italian guidelines suggest the use of the NAFLD fibrosis score (NFS) and the FIB-4 as non-invasive scores to identify patients with different risks of advanced fibrosis. Both scores predict liver-related mortality and cardiovascular disease since they have been validated in several ethnically NAFLD patients. Furthermore, in a recent study of the AASLD is highlighted that both NFS and FIB-4 present the best predictive value for advanced fibrosis in NAFLD patients with histological diagnosis (**Table 3**) [20–22].

3.3 Proteomics, glycomics and microRNA

The new technology in proteomics, glycomics, and microRNA (miRNA) can tell us about the pathophysiology of NAFLD/NASH [23].

Sirtuin 1 (Sirt 1) is a heat shock protein that is related to toxic immune reactions, antimicrobial activity, and mitophagy. Mitophagy is very important in NAFLD along with other diseases, therefore there is an increasing interest in maintaining the regulation and homeostasis of the mitochondria, due that it is necessary for the survival of many tissues [24]. The nuclear receptor of Sirt 1 is a nicotinamide adenine dinucleotide (NAD+) dependent class III histone deacetylase (HDAC) that modifies the gene expression to the metabolic activity of transcription factors, such as p53, and deacetylation of nuclear receptors. Its functions involve the metabolism of cholesterol, fatty acids, glucose, and xenobiotics, as well as the expression of p450 in the hepatic metabolism [25]. This is why the regulation of the nuclear receptor Sirt 1 is crucial to prevent NAFLD and other metabolic diseases. The proteome blood clinical analysis for the proteomic biomarkers, especially Sirt 1, with its measurement in plasma, cytoplasm, and nucleus, is the key to detect, evaluate and determine mitochondrial apoptosis and the progression of the disease [24, 25].

The most studied biomarker is cytokeratin 18 that is used to evaluate the presence of inflammation. There is a lot of research about its circulating levels as a signal of hepatocellular apoptotic activity and as a specific feature of NASH [6, 26].

Panel	Study	Biomarkers	Sensitivity (%)	Specificity (%)
Validated diagnostic panels to predict hepatic steatosis				
SteatoTest	Poynard et.at, 2005	α-MG, Haptoglobin, Apolipoprotein A1, Total Bilirubin, GGT, Glucose, Triglycerides, Cholesterol, ALT, Age, Gender, and BMI	90	70
FLI	Bedogni et al. 2006	Triglycerides, BMI, GGT, waist circumference	87	86
NAFLD-LFS	Kotronen et al. 2009	Mets, DT2, AST, ALT, insulin	95	95
LAP	Bedogni et al. 2010	Waist circumference, triglycerides	NA	NA
Diagnostic dashboards to predict NASH				
NASH Test	Poynard et al. 2006	NASH panels Undisclosed formula, α-MG, Haptoglobulin, Apoliprotein A1, Total Bilirubin, GGT, AST, Triglycerides, Cholesterol, ALT, Age, Gender, Weight and Height	33	94
Nash Diagnosis	Younossi et al. 2008	Undisclosed formula, CK18-M30, CK 18-M65, adiponectin and resistin	72	91
Apoptosis Panel	Tamimi et.al 2011	Cytokeratin 18 fragments, Fas ligand, soluble Fas	88	89
Diagnostic panels to predict fibrosis in NASH				
NAFLD fibrosis score	Angulo et al.2007	Age, glucose, BMI, platelets, albumin, AST / ALT	82	98
Fibrotest	Ratziu et al. 2006	Age,,α2-macroglobuline, Total bilirubin, GGT and apolipoprotein A1	77	98
BARD	Harrison et al. 2008	BMI ≥ 28 Kg/m^2, AST/ALT≥0.8, DT2	NA	NA
FibroMeter	Cales et al. 2009	Glucose, AST, ferritin, platelets, ALT, weight, age	79	96
FIB-A	McPherson et al. 2011	Age, AST / platelets, ALT	85	65

α-MG: alpha 2 macroglobulin, FLI: liver fat index, LAP. Lipid accumulation product, NA: not applicable. Translated from Machado MV, Cortez-Pinto H. Non-invasive diagnosis of non-alcoholic fatty liver disease. A critical appraisal. J Hepatol 2013;58(5):1007–1019.

Table 3.
Different scores and models to predict steatosis, NASH, and fibrosis.

The Asia Pacific Association guidelines recommend that elevated levels of cytokeratin18 have a good predictive value for NAFLD in comparison to healthy livers, but it makes no difference between NASH versus simple steatosis. However, the EASL recommendations highlight that serum levels of cytokeratin 18 has an inverse relation with the histological improvement, although its predictive value is no better than ALT in identifying histological responders [6, 27–29].

3.4 Liver ultrasound and imaging techniques

The first line of diagnosis of hepatic steatosis is liver ultrasound because it is inexpensive, non-invasive, and widely accessible. Also, it is used currently in clinical practice and is quite accurate with an overall sensitivity of 85% and a specificity of 94% [30]. On the ultrasound can be observed that there is usually a visual decrease in the vascular margins, a loss of definition of the diaphragm, hepatomegaly, and hyperechogenicity of the liver parenchyma, as well as focal fat deposition in the hyperechoic area. If hepatocyte steatosis is not inferior to 31%, the transabdominal ultrasound is very effective [31].

There is a consensus for the use of abdominal ultrasound (USA). On the other hand, it can miss the diagnosis when the fat hepatic content is <20% because the sensitivity of USA among patients with morbid obesity (BMI > 40 kg/m2) is low [6, 32, 33].

Transient elastography has been recently approved by the United States (US) Food and Drug Administration (FDA) as a diagnostic tool for adult and pediatric patients with liver disease. Its cut-off value for advanced fibrosis in adults with NAFLD has been established at 9.9 KpA with a sensitivity of 95% and a specificity of 77%. Particularly, for clinically significant fibrosis, the elastography score has been shown to have good diagnostic accuracy with an AUROC of 0.93 (95% CI: 0.890.096) for advanced fibrosis (F3) and cirrhosis, and a negative predictive value of 90% in ruling out cirrhosis when a cutoff of 7.9 kPa is used. Although, it has a weaker capacity to make a difference between F2 and F3. Due to this high rate of false positive results, the EASL and the Asia Pacific recommendations mention that its low specificity limits its use in daily practice in the diagnosis of the advanced degree of fibrosis and cirrhosis, as well as a high failure rate. Moreover, the EASL highlights that it should not be used only as a first-line screening tool to identify advanced fibrosis or cirrhosis because of the unreliable results among patients with high BMI and thoracic fold thickness. However, by using M or XLprobe, the performance can improve and increase the success rate. For the identification of different degrees in fibrosis in NAFLD patients, especially in the intermediate stage, the US guidelines recommend magnetic resonance elastography (MRE), since it has a better performance than transient elastography in this regard, but shows the same predictive value for advanced stages of fibrosis. As a result, the AASLD concludes that ERM and transient elastography are useful tools to identify NAFLD patients with advanced liver fibrosis. Although, like transient elastography, shear wave elastography seems to be inadequate to distinguish between intermediate stages of fibrosis and to provide reliable results in 73% of patients with a BMI of 30 kg/m^2 [34–37].

Nevertheless, the gold standard for evaluating and quantifying hepatic steatosis and detecting the amount of liver fat as low as 5%–10% is magnetic resonance imaging (MRI), either by proton density fat fraction (1H-MRS) or by spectroscopy, although it is not commonly used in the clinical practice. This MRI is not recommended in the daily clinical setting despite its accurate precision, because of its limited availability, high costs, and long execution time [6, 38].

Another imaging technique used to quantify the fat content in the liver is transient ultrasound-based ultrasound (TE) using the continuous attenuation parameter (CAP). Due to that it simultaneously measures liver stiffness and evaluates the severity of NAFLD in the same setting, it has become a promising tool with good sensitivity [39]. However, despite its low cost and speed of implementation, its role in clinical practice has not yet been defined. In fact, according to the EASL, it has never been compared to hepatic steatosis as measured by 1H-MRS and there is limited data on its ability to discriminate different histological patterns.

On the other hand, the Asia Pacific Association proposes the CAP as a useful screening tool for the diagnosis of NAFLD, as well as to demonstrate an improvement in hepatic steatosis after the intervention in lifestyle and the reduction of the bodyweight [6].

The stiffness of the liver measured by the M probe is not always successful in obese patients. The XL probe, an improved FibroScan probe, has been demostrated to achieve better diagnostic accuracy. The cutoff values, compared to the M probe values, are approximately 1.5 to 2 kPa lower. In conclusion, in the diagnosis of fibrosis and cirrhosis, a strong alternative to liver biopsy can be ET in patients with NAFLD [23].

The optimal strategy for stratifying patients with NAFLD and monitoring disease progression has yet to be established. The EASL and the Italian guidelines mention that the combination of noninvasive scores (NFS and FIB4) and transient elastography should be used to identify patients at low risk for advanced liver disease and clinical decision making. Also, in combination, they can identify patients who must undergo a liver biopsy to confirm advanced fibrosis, and in whom a more intensive approach is needed.

3.5 Liver biopsy

The gold standard remains the liver biopsy, although it may not always be required to diagnose NAFLD, because it can distinguish steatohepatitis from simple steatosis, provide an evaluation of the degree of necroinflammatory activity, visualize fibrosis, and architectural alterations. The most widely used histological classification and staging system for NAFLD [23, 40] is the NAFLD Activity Score (NAS) and the Steatosis Activity Fibrosis (SAF) scoring systems to assess disease activity [6].

The SAF score simplified the identification of a subset of NAFLD, which includes the assessment of steatosis (S), activity (A), and fibrosis (F): NASH. The histopathologic features of NAFLD include lobular and portal inflammation, steatosis, hepatocellular ballooning, glycogenated nuclei, apoptotic hepatocytes (acidophilic bodies), deposition, megamitochondria, Mallory-Denk bodies, and fibrosis, with the characteristic pattern centered on the perisinusoidal/pericellular area. This fibrotic pattern typically originated in the adult zone, is known as chicken wire fibrosis [6, 41].

A score of ≥5 with steatosis and ballooning of hepatocytes is generally considered diagnostic of NASH, although patients may have NASH with lower NAS scores if there is the presence of steatosis and ballooning of hepatocytes [6, 40].

4. Conclusions

The incidence and prevalence of NAFLD are increasing. Clinical guidelines agree that noninvasive tests are currently not available to detect NAFLD and distinguish it from simple steatosis. Identifying people at risk of disease progression to NASH, fibrosis, and cirrhosis is extremely important because most patients are asymptomatic.

The current gold standard for the diagnosis of NAFLD / NASH is liver biopsy. Noninvasive tests such as proteomic biomarkers, transient elastography, and elastoMR to evaluate NAFLD/NASH are promising.

The most validated diagnostic panels include the NAFLD fibrosis score, FIB-4, and FibroMeter. Transient elastography is very useful in the evaluation of advanced fibrosis and cirrhosis.

Author details

Eira Cerda-Reyes[1]*, Alicia Sarahi Ojeda-Yuren[2], Julián Torres-Vazquez[3], María del Rosario Herrero Maceda[4], Martín Uriel Vázquez-Medina[5], Perla Denice Flores-Rangel[6], Yailin Fabiola Velásquez Palacios[7], Saraid Cerda-Reyes[8] and Graciela Elia Castro-Narro[9]

1 Head of Academic Coordination, Central Military Hospital, Mexico

2 Anahuac University, Mexico

3 Chief Resident of Internal Medicine, Central Military Hospital, Mexico

4 Appointed Physician at the Gastroenterology Section, Central Military Hospital, Mexico

5 National Polytechnic Institute, Mexico

6 Gastroenterology Resident, Central Military Hospital, Mexico

7 Internal Medicine Resident, Central Military Hospital, Mexico

8 Allergology Service, Medical Specialties Unit, Mexico

9 Head of Transplant Service, Medica Sur Hospital, Mexico

*Address all correspondence to: arieirace@yahoo.com.mx

References

[1] Younossi ZM, Koenig AB, Abdelatif D, Fazel Y, Henry L, Wymer M. Global epidemiology of nonalcoholic fatty liver disease meta-analytic assessment of prevalence, incidence, and outcomes. Hepatology 2016; 64: 73-84.

[2] GBD 2016 Disease and Injury Incidence and Prevalence Collaborators. Global, regional, and national incidence, prevalence, and years lived with disability for 328 diseases and injuries for 195 countries, 1990-2016: a systematic analysis for the Global Burden of Disease Study 2016. Lancet 2017; 390: 1211-59.

[3] GBD 2016 Risk Factors Collaborators. Global, regional, and national comparative risk assessment of 84 behavioural, environmental and occupational, and metabolic risks or clusters of risks, 1990-2016: a systematic analysis for the Global Burden of Disease Study 2016. Lancet 2017; 390: 1345-422.

[4] Pearson-Stuttard J, Zhou B, Kontis V, Bentham J, Gunter MJ, Ezzati M. Worldwide burden of cancer attributable to diabetes and high body-mass index: a comparative risk assessment. Lancet Diabetes Endocrinol 2018; 6: e6-15. 7

[5] De Minicis S, Day C, Svegliati-Baroni G. From NAFLD to NASH and HCC: pathogenetic mechanisms and therapeutic insights. Curr Pharm Des 2013; 19: 5239-5249

[6] Leoni S, Tovoli F, Napoli L, Serio I, Ferri S, Bolondi L. Current guidelines for the management of non-alcoholic fatty liver disease: A systematic review with comparative analysis World J Gastroenterol. 2018 Aug 14;24(30):3361-3373

[7] Schwimmer JB, Deutsch R, Kahen T, Lavine JE, Stanley C, Behling C. Prevalence of fatty liver in children and adolescents. Pediatrics 2006; 118: 1388-1393

[8] Paradis V, Zalinski S, Chelbi E, Guedj N, Degos F, Vilgrain V, Bedossa P, Belghiti J. Hepatocellular carcinomas in patients with metabolic syndrome often develop without significant liver fibrosis: a pathological analysis. *Hepatology* 2009; 49: 851-859

[9] Piscaglia F, Svegliati-Baroni G, Barchetti A, Pecorelli A, Marinelli S, Tiribelli C, Bellentani S; HCC-NAFLD Italian Study Group. Clinical patterns of hepatocellular carcinoma in nonalcoholic fatty liver disease: A multicenter prospective study. *Hepatology* 2016; 63: 827-838

[10] Naga Chalasani N, Younossi Z, Lavine, JE, Charlton M, Cusi K, Rinella M, Harrison SA, Brunt EM, and Sanyal AJ. Practice Guidance. The Diagnosis and Management of Nonalcoholic Fatty Liver Disease: Practice Guidance From the American Association for the Study of Liver Diseases. Hepatology 2018;67: 328-357

[11] European Association for the Study of the Liver (EASL). European Association for the Study of Diabetes (EASD); European Association for the Study of Obesity (EASO). EASL-EASD-EASO Clinical Practice Guidelines for the management of non-alcoholic fatty liver disease. J Hepatol 2016; 64: 1388-1402

[12] Angulo P, Keach JC, Batts KP, et al. Independent predictors of liver fibrosis in patients with nonalcoholic steatohepatitis. Hepatology 1999; 30: 1356-1362.

[13] Cheah MC, McCullough AJ, Goh GB. Current Modalities of Fibrosis Assessment in Non-alcoholic Fatty Liver Disease. *J Clin Transl Hepatol* 2017; 5: 261-271

[14] Chalasani N, Younossi Z, Lavine JE, Charlton M, Cusi K, Rinella M, Harrison SA, Brunt EM, Sanyal AJ. The diagnosis and management of nonalcoholic fatty liver disease: Practice guidance from the American Association for the Study of Liver Diseases. *Hepatology* 2018; 67: 328-357

[15] Valenti L, Fracanzani AL, Bugianesi E, Dongiovanni P, Galmozzi E, Vanni E, Canavesi E, Lattuada E, Roviaro G, Marchesini G, Fargion S. HFE genotype, parenchymal iron accumulation, and liver fibrosis in patients with nonalcoholic fatty liver disease. *Gastroenterology* 2010; 138: 905-912

[16] Vuppalanchi R, Gould RJ, Wilson LA, Unalp-Arida A, Cummings OW, Chalasani N, Kowdley KV; Nonalcoholic Steatohepatitis Clinical Research Network (NASH CRN). Clinical significance of serum autoantibodies in patients with NAFLD: results from the nonalcoholic steatohepatitis clinical research network. *Hepatol Int* 2012; 6: 379-385

[17] Bedogni G, Bellentani S, Miglioli L, Masutti F, Passalacqua M, Castiglione A, Tiribelli C. The Fatty Liver Index: a simple and accurate predictor of hepatic steatosis in the general population. *BMC Gastroenterol* 2006; 6: 33 [PMID: 17081293 DOI: 10.1186/1471-230X-6-33]

[18] Kotronen A, Peltonen M, Hakkarainen A, Sevastianova K, Bergholm R, Johansson LM, Lundbom N, Rissanen A, Ridderstråle M, Groop L, Orho-Melander M, Yki-Järvinen H. Prediction of non- alcoholic fatty liver disease and liver fat using metabolic and genetic factors. *Gastroenterology* 2009; 137: 865-872

[19] Fedchuk L, Nascimbeni F, Pais R, Charlotte F, Housset C, Ratziu V; LIDO Study Group. Performance and limitations of steatosis biomarkers in patients with nonalcoholic fatty liver disease. *Aliment Pharmacol Ther* 2014; 40: 1209-1222

[20] Kaswala DH, Lai M, Afdhal NH. Fibrosis Assessment in Nonalcoholic Fatty Liver Disease (NAFLD) in 2016. *Dig Dis Sci* 2016; 61: 1356-1364 [PMID: 27017224 DOI: 10.1007/s10620-016-4079-4]

[21] Fagan KJ, Pretorius CJ, Horsfall LU, Irvine KM, Wilgen U, Choi K, Fletcher LM, Tate J, Melino M, Nusrat S, Miller GC, Clouston AD, Ballard E, O'Rourke P, Lampe G, Ungerer JP, Powell EE. ELF score □9.8 indicates advanced hepatic fibrosis and is influenced by age, steatosis and histological activity. *Liver Int* 2015; 35: 1673-1681

[22] Guha IN, Parkes J, Roderick P, Chattopadhyay D, Cross R, Harris S, Kaye P, Burt AD, Ryder SD, Aithal GP, Day CP, Rosenberg WM. Noninvasive markers of fibrosis in nonalcoholic fatty liver disease: Validating the European Liver Fibrosis Panel and exploring simple markers. *Hepatology* 2008; 47: 455-460

[23] Tsai E, Lee T-P. Diagnosis and Evaluation of Nonalcoholic Fatty Liver Disease/Nonalcoholic Steatohepatitis, Including Noninvasive Biomarkers and Transient Elastography. Clin Liver Dis 22 (2018) 73-92

[24] Martins IJ. Evaluation of diagnostic tests in human health and disease. J Clin Path Lab Med. 2018;2(1):13-15.

[25] Martins IJ. "Sirtuin 1, a Diagnostic Protein Marker and its Relevance to Chronic Disease and Therapeutic Drug Interventions". EC Pharmacology and Toxicology 6.4. 2018: 209-215

[26] Feldstein AE, Wieckowska A, Lopez AR, Liu YC, Zein NN, McCullough AJ. Cytokeratin-18

fragment levels as noninvasive biomarkers for nonalcoholic steatohepatitis: a multicenter validation study. *Hepatology* 2009; 50: 1072-1078

[27] Chan WK, Sthaneshwar P, Nik Mustapha NR, Mahadeva S. Limited utility of plasma M30 in discriminating non-alcoholic steatohepatitis from steatosis--a comparison with routine biochemical markers. PLoS One 2014; 9: e105903

[28] Shen J, Chan HL, Wong GL, Chan AW, Choi PC, Chan HY, Chim AM, Yeung DK, Yu J, Chu WC, Wong VW. Assessment of non-alcoholic fatty liver disease using serum total cell death and apoptosis markers. Aliment Pharmacol Ther 2012; 36: 1057-1066 [PMID: 23066946 DOI: 10.1111/apt.12091]

[29] Vuppalanchi R, Jain AK, Deppe R, Yates K, Comerford M, Masuoka HC, Neuschwander-Tetri BA, Loomba R, Brunt EM, Kleiner DE, Molleston JP, Schwimmer JB, Lavine JE, Tonascia J, Chalasani N. Relationship between changes in serum levels of keratin 18 and changes in liver histology in children and adults with nonalcoholic fatty liver disease. Clin Gastroenterol Hepatol 2014; 12: 2121-2130. e1-2

[30] Bril F, Cusi K. Management of nonalcoholic fatty liver disease in patients with type 2 diabetes: a call to action. Diabetes Care 2017; 40: 419-30

[31] Lucas C, Lucas G, Lucas N, Krzowska-Firych J, Tomasiewicz K. A systematic review of the present and future of non-alcoholic fatty liver disease. Clin Exp Hepatol 2018; 4, 3: 165-174

[32] Saadeh S, Younossi ZM, Remer EM, Gramlich T, Ong JP, Hurley M, Mullen KD, Cooper JN, Sheridan MJ. The utility of radiological imaging in nonalcoholic fatty liver disease. Gastroenterology 2002; 123: 745-750

[33] Ryan CK, Johnson LA, Germin BI, Marcos A. One hundred consecutive hepatic biopsies in the workup of living donors for right lobe liver transplantation. Liver Transpl 2002; 8: 1114-1122

[34] Tapper EB, Challies T, Nasser I, Afdhal NH, Lai M. The Performance of Vibration Controlled Transient Elastography in a US Cohort of Patients With Nonalcoholic Fatty Liver Disease. Am J Gastroenterol 2016; 111: 677-684

[35] Wong VW, Vergniol J, Wong GL, Foucher J, Chan AW, Chermak F, Choi PC, Merrouche W, Chu SH, Pesque S, Chan HL, de Lédinghen V. Liver stiffness measurement using XL probe in patients with nonalcoholic fatty liver disease. Am J Gastroenterol 2012; 107: 1862-1871

[36] Wong VW, Vergniol J, Wong GL, Foucher J, Chan HL, Le Bail B, Choi PC, Kowo M, Chan AW, Merrouche W, Sung JJ, de Lédinghen V. Diagnosis of fibrosis and cirrhosis using liver stiffness measurement in nonalcoholic fatty liver disease. Hepatology 2010; 51: 454-462

[37] Imajo K, Kessoku T, Honda Y, Tomeno W, Ogawa Y, Mawatari H, Fujita K, Yoneda M, Taguri M, Hyogo H, Sumida Y, Ono M, Eguchi Y, Inoue T, Yamanaka T, Wada K, Saito S, Nakajima A. Magnetic Resonance Imaging More Accurately Classifies Steatosis and Fibrosis in Patients With Nonalcoholic Fatty Liver Disease Than Transient Elastography. Gastroenterology 2016; 150: 626-637.e7

[38] Szczepaniak LS, Nurenberg P, Leonard D, Browning JD, Reingold JS, Grundy S, Hobbs HH, Dobbins RL. Magnetic resonance spectroscopy to measure hepatic triglyceride content: prevalence of hepatic steatosis in the general population. Am J Physiol Endocrinol Metab 2005; 288: E462-E468

[39] Kwok R, Choi KC, Wong GL, Zhang Y, Chan HL, Luk AO, Shu SS, Chan AW, Yeung MW, Chan JC, Kong AP, Wong VW. Screening diabetic patients for non-alcoholic fatty liver disease with controlled attenuation parameter and liver stiffness measurements: a prospective cohort study. Gut 2016; 65: 1359-1368

[40] Kleiner DE, Brunt EM, Van Natta M, et al. Design and validation of a histological scoring system for nonalcoholic fatty liver disease. Hepatology 2005; 41: 1313-1321.

[41] Valenti L, Fracanzani AL, Bugianesi E, et al. HFE genotype, parenchymal iron accumulation, and liver fibrosis in patients with nonalcoholic fatty liver disease. Gastroenterology 2010; 138: 905-912.

Chapter 9

Treatment of Nonalcoholic Fatty Liver Disease through Changes in Gut Microbiome and Intestinal Epithelial Barrier

Hassan M. Heshmati

Abstract

Nonalcoholic fatty liver disease (NAFLD) is a leading liver disease worldwide with a prevalence of approximately 25% among adult population. The highest prevalence is observed in Middle East and the lowest prevalence in Africa. NAFLD is a spectrum of liver disorders ranging from simple steatosis to nonalcoholic steatohepatitis (NASH). Pro-inflammatory diet, overweight/obesity, inflammation, insulin resistance, prediabetes, type 2 diabetes, dyslipidemia, disrupted gut microbiome, and impaired intestinal barrier function are important risk factors associated with and/or contributing to NAFLD. Gut microbiome is a complex and diverse microbial ecosystem essential for the maintenance of human health. It is influenced by several factors including diet and medications. Gut microbiome can be disrupted in NAFLD. Intestinal epithelial barrier is the largest and most important barrier against the external environment and plays an important role in health and disease. Several factors including diet and gut microbiome impact intestinal barrier function. NAFLD can be associated with impaired intestinal barrier function (increased intestinal permeability). There are no specific drugs that directly treat NAFLD. The first-line therapy of NAFLD is currently lifestyle intervention. Weight loss is an important component in the treatment of NAFLD subjects who have excess body weight. Gut microbiome and intestinal epithelial barrier are becoming promising targets for the treatment of several diseases including NAFLD. In the absence of approved pharmacotherapy for the treatment of NAFLD/NASH, in addition to lifestyle intervention and weight loss (in case of excess body weight), focus should also be on correcting gut microbiome and intestinal permeability (directly and/or through gut microbiome modulation) using diet (e.g., low-fat diet, high-fiber diet, and Mediterranean diet), prebiotics (nondigestible food ingredients), probiotics (nonpathogenic living microorganisms), synbiotics (combination of prebiotics and probiotics), and fecal microbiota transplantation (transfer of healthy stool).

Keywords: nonalcoholic fatty liver disease, gut microbiome, intestinal epithelial barrier, targeted treatment

1. Introduction

NAFLD is a leading liver disease worldwide with a prevalence of approximately 25% among adult population. It is the most common cause of chronic liver disease in Western countries. NAFLD is a spectrum of liver disorders ranging from simple steatosis to NASH [1–9].

Pro-inflammatory diet, overweight/obesity, inflammation, insulin resistance, prediabetes, type 2 diabetes, dyslipidemia, disrupted gut microbiome, and impaired intestinal barrier function are important risk factors associated with and/or contributing to NAFLD [2, 4–27].

In the absence of approved drugs for the treatment of NAFLD/NASH, management relies mainly on lifestyle intervention and weight loss (in case of excess body weight) [1, 2, 8, 28–30].

Gut microbiome and intestinal epithelial barrier are becoming promising targets for the treatment of several diseases including NAFLD [4, 17, 18, 20–22, 24, 25, 31–43].

2. Physiology

2.1 Liver

The liver is the largest visceral organ. It weighs approximately 1.5 kg. Macroscopically, the liver is divided into four lobes. The basic functional unit of the liver is the liver lobule which includes the hepatocytes. Approximately 30% of the liver volume is made up by blood (**Figure 1**) [44].

The liver is a vital organ. It has numerous important roles including secretion of bile (700–1,200 mL/day), metabolism of bilirubin, metabolism of nutrients (e.g., glucose homeostasis, fat synthesis, and albumin synthesis), endocrine function (e.g., production of angiotensinogen and activation of vitamin D), storage of minerals and vitamins (e.g., iron, copper, vitamin A, vitamin B12, and vitamin D), hematologic and vascular functions (e.g., hemostatic function and capacity to store/release large volume of blood), immunologic and protective functions, and metabolic inactivation and detoxification (e.g., catabolism or alteration of hormones, toxins, and drugs) [44].

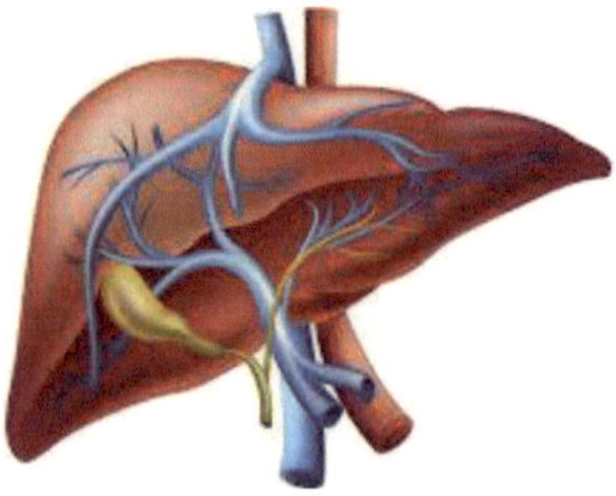

Figure 1.
Normal liver.

2.2 Gut microbiome

Gut microbiome is a complex and diverse microbial ecosystem living in the digestive tract, mainly in the colon. It is established within the few first years of life and contains up to 100 trillion microbes, mainly bacteria (more than 1,000 species) but also fungi, protozoa, archaea, and viruses (**Figure 2**) [45–51].

Gut microbiome is involved in multiple physiological functions and is essential for the maintenance of human health [50–57]. It is influenced by several factors including diet and medications [31, 32, 50, 53, 58–69].

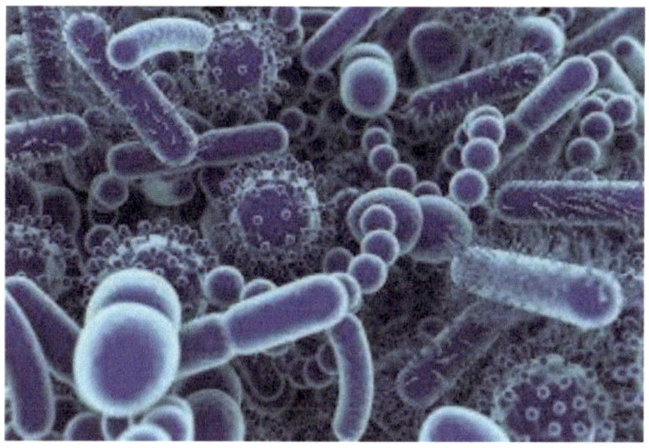

Figure 2.
Gut microbiome.

2.3 Intestinal epithelial barrier

The intestine is lined by layer of epithelial cells that are connected by cell–cell junctions (tight junction, adherens junction, desmosome). These junctions are responsible for maintenance of tissue integrity, creation of a barrier, and signaling. The barrier, which is important for tissue homeostasis, controls the passage of water, ions, molecules, cells, and pathogens across the epithelial layer. Intestinal epithelial barrier is the largest and most important barrier against the external environment (barrier between luminal contents and the underlying immune system). It covers a surface of approximately 400 m^2 and requires approximately 40% of the body energy expenditure (**Figure 3**) [23, 41–43, 70, 71].

Intestinal epithelial barrier is constantly challenged by gut microbiome. It plays an important role in health and disease [23, 41–43, 70, 71]. Several factors including diet and gut microbiome impact intestinal barrier function [20, 41–43]. A high-fiber diet has a beneficial effect while a high-fructose diet and a high-fat diet have a deleterious effect on intestinal barrier function.

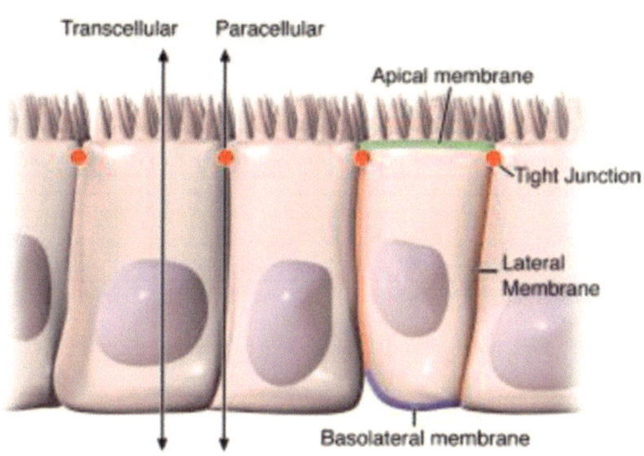

Figure 3.
Intestinal epithelial barrier.

3. NAFLD

3.1 Definition

NAFLD is a liver disease characterized by hepatic steatosis (≥ 5% fat deposit) on either imaging or histology, with no excessive alcohol consumption (< 30 g/day for men and < 20 g/day for women), in the absence of other causes of steatosis (e.g., viral hepatitis and medications). It is a spectrum of liver disorders ranging from simple steatosis to NASH. Up to 30% of NAFLD subjects develop NASH. NASH is the aggressive form of NAFLD that can progress to fibrosis, cirrhosis, and hepatocellular cancer. The presence of fibrosis is the strongest predictor of mortality (**Figure 4**) [1–9].

Recently, a consensus of international experts proposed to change the acronym NAFLD to MAFLD (metabolic dysfunction-associated fatty liver disease) [72].

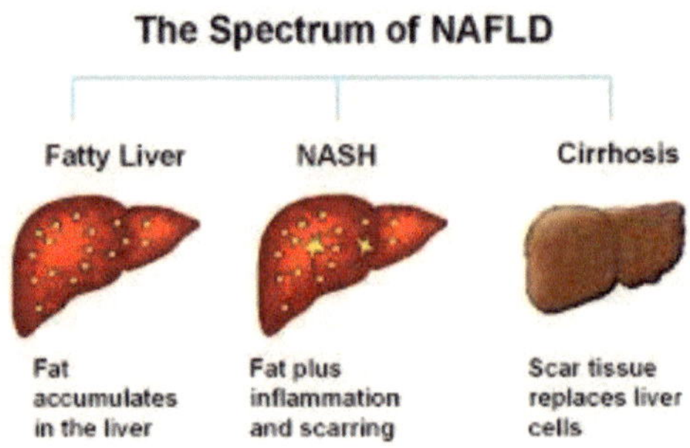

Figure 4.
Spectrum of NAFLD.

3.2 Prevalence

NAFLD is a pandemic with a prevalence of approximately 25% among adult population worldwide. The highest prevalence is observed in Middle East and the lowest prevalence in Africa. More than 1 billion people are affected by NAFLD worldwide (**Table 1**) [3, 8]. The differences in prevalence can be explained, at least partially, by genetic background and lifestyle. NAFLD prevalence continues to rise in all age groups, including in the adolescent population, especially in the setting of the obesity pandemic.

NAFLD is a sexual dimorphic disease. The prevalence of NAFLD is higher in men than in women (protective role of estrogen) [73, 74].

Region	NAFLD Prevalence
World	**25%**
Middle East	32%
South America	30%
Asia	27%
North America	24%
Europe	24%
Africa	13%

Table 1.
Prevalence of NAFLD in adult population by region.

3.3 Pathophysiology

The pathophysiology underlying NAFLD is complex with both non-genetic and genetic components [2, 4–27, 75–79].

Pro-inflammatory diet, overweight/obesity, inflammation, insulin resistance, prediabetes, type 2 diabetes, dyslipidemia, disrupted gut microbiome, and impaired intestinal barrier function are important risk factors associated with and/or contributing to NAFLD [2, 4–27]. In addition, some miscellaneous endocrine disorders including growth hormone (GH) deficiency, hypothyroidism, polycystic ovary syndrome, and hypogonadism and deficiency in epigenetic regulators such as sirtuin 1 have been reported as possible contributing factors to NAFLD [75–79].

There are several genetic forms of NAFLD including variations in patatin-like phospholipase domain-containing protein 3 (*PNPLA3*), transmembrane 6 superfamily 2 (*TM6SF2*), membrane-bound O-acyltransferase domain-containing protein 7 (*MBOAT7*), and glucokinase regulatory protein (*GCKR*) genes [5, 6].

Excessive fat deposition in the liver (hepatocytes) leading to NAFLD can result from one or several combined mechanisms including increased delivery of lipids to the liver from diet or adipose tissue, increased *de novo* synthesis of lipids in the liver, decreased hepatic oxidation of fatty acids, and decreased export of triglycerides from the liver [7–9].

3.3.1 Pro-inflammatory diet

Various common food components have pro-inflammatory potential and by contributing to chronic inflammation, can promote the development of NAFLD [10]. They can either directly alter liver metabolism or act through disruption of gut microbiome. The Western diet which is a diet rich in saturated fat, red meat, fructose, alcohol, and salt is associated with an increased risk of NAFLD.

3.3.2 Overweight/obesity, inflammation

Excess body weight (overweight and obesity) is considered as the main cause of several abnormalities that are contributing to the pathogenesis of NAFLD (e.g., inflammation and insulin resistance). NAFLD is commonly associated with overweight/obesity [74]. It is independently associated with both subcutaneous and visceral obesity. The adipose tissue inflammation observed in overweight/obesity and characterized by increased cytokine production leads to systemic inflammation which is responsible for insulin resistance [10, 11, 80]. Clinical studies have shown that cellular and molecular adipose tissue inflammation correlate with the degree of liver inflammation and the importance of liver disease.

Based on body mass index (BMI), up to approximately 19% of NAFLD subjects do not have excess body weight (lean NAFLD) [74, 81, 82].

The prevalence of NAFLD by BMI in a Chinese population of Shanghai is reported in **Table 2** [74].

BMI	NAFLD Prevalence
< 18.5 (n = 445)	0.4%
18.5 to < 24.0 (n = 4,899)	12.7%
24.0 to < 28.0 (n = 2,801)	49.2%
≥ 28.0 (672)	82.4%

Table 2.
Prevalence of NAFLD by BMI in a Chinese population of Shanghai (n = 8,817).

3.3.3 Insulin resistance, prediabetes, type 2 diabetes

Insulin resistance plays an important role in the in the development of NAFLD. Overweight/obesity and systemic inflammation are responsible for insulin resistance which in its turn is an important contributing factor to the pathogenesis of prediabetes, type 2 diabetes, and NAFLD [2, 10, 80]. NAFLD is highly correlated with prediabetes and type 2 diabetes. There is a reciprocal association between prediabetes/type 2 diabetes and NAFLD [13]. The global prevalence of NAFLD in subjects with prediabetes and type 2 diabetes is around 48% and more than 55%, respectively (**Figure 5**) [5, 10, 12, 15].

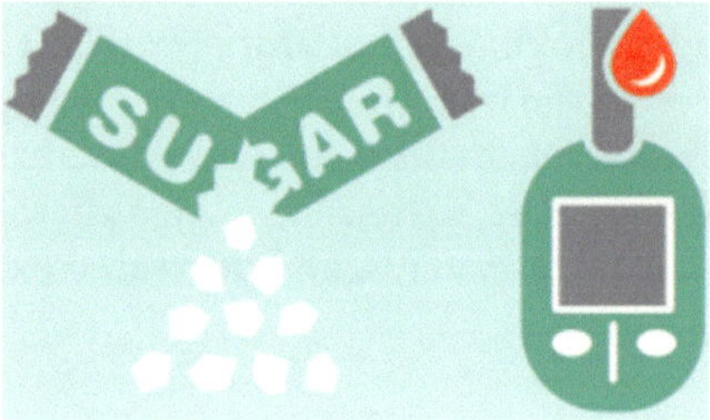

Figure 5.
There is a strong association between prediabetes/type 2 diabetes and NAFLD.

3.3.4 Dyslipidemia

Dyslipidemia is a significant risk factor for NAFLD and associated cardiovascular disease. The mechanism by which dyslipidemia increases the risk of NAFLD may be related to an increased accumulation of lipids in the hepatocytes [16].

3.3.5 Disrupted gut microbiome

Profound changes affecting the diversity and the abundance of gut microbiome (dysbiosis) are associated with several metabolic disorders including NAFLD [4, 10, 17–25, 83]. Gut microbiome plays a major role in the pathogenesis of NAFLD. Disrupted gut microbiome (e.g., increase in pro-inflammatory bacteria and decrease in protective bacteria) can promote or aggravate NAFLD through several mechanisms including change in intestinal permeability and change in the amount of absorbed energy (this can cause overweight/obesity, an important risk factor for NAFLD). Microbial metabolites and cell components contribute to the development of inflammation and hepatic steatosis.

Several clinical studies have shown the association of qualitative and quantitative changes in gut microbiome (e.g., increased *Lactobacillus* and Gram-negative bacteria) with NAFLD and its severity [4, 17–19, 24, 25]. The increased gut microbiome taxa may produce more short-chain fatty acids (SCFAs), alcohol, and lipopolysaccharides (LPS). Increased supply of SCFAs, alcohol, and LPS (endotoxins) into the portal circulation is implicated in the pathogenesis of NAFLD and its evolution to NASH (promotion of overweight/obesity and inflammation) [17, 20–23].

3.3.6 Impaired intestinal barrier function

Impaired intestinal barrier function causes increased intestinal permeability ("leaky gut") and is associated with several metabolic disorders including NAFLD [20, 23, 26, 27, 41–43, 70, 71].

Increased intestinal permeability is most likely caused by the disruption of intercellular tight junctions of the intestinal epithelium [26, 71]. It promotes translocation of bacteria-derived products (e.g., SCFAs, alcohol, and LPS) into the portal circulation, exposing the liver to substances capable of inducing hepatic steatosis and fibrosis [17, 20–23]. Several studies have reported that serum zonulin, a marker of intestinal permeability, correlates significantly with the severity of hepatic steatosis in subjects with NAFLD [43].

3.3.7 Miscellaneous endocrine disorders

Several miscellaneous endocrine disorders may contribute to the development of secondary NAFLD [75]. GH deficiency through different mechanisms including inflammation and insulin resistance may promote NAFLD. Hypothyroidism by causing impaired glucose and lipid metabolism and altered energy homeostasis can be linked to NAFLD. Polycystic ovary syndrome through multiple factors (e.g., obesity, inflammation, insulin resistance, and hyperandrogenism) may promote NAFLD. Hypogonadism can be associated with NAFLD through several mechanisms including obesity, insulin resistance, dyslipidemia, estrogen deficiency, and dehydroepiandrosterone deficiency.

3.3.8 Sirtuin 1 deficiency

Sirtuins are a group of proteins belonging to the family of silent information regulator 2. Humans have seven sirtuins. Sirtuin 1 is widely recognized as an important epigenetic regulator involved in multiple biological processes and its deficiency contributes to the pathogenesis of several diseases including NAFLD [76–79]. Exposure to sirtuin 1 inhibitors (e.g., fructose, alcohol, and LPS) leads to defective sirtuin 1 function and can promote NAFLD.

3.3.9 Genetic predisposition

Common genetic forms of NAFLD include variations in *PNPLA3*, *TM6SF2*, *MBOAT7*, and *GCKR* genes (**Figure 6**). These genetic forms of NAFLD are not associated with insulin resistance, type 2 diabetes, and dyslipidemia but can progress to NASH, cirrhosis, and hepatocellular cancer [5, 6].

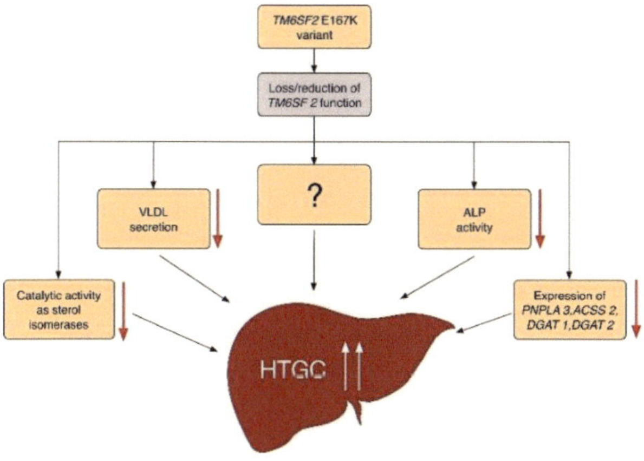

Figure 6.
Several gene variants can contribute to the pathogenesis of NAFLD.

3.3.10 Combination of several factors

Several of the above-mentioned factors can be present in subjects with NAFLD, especially when they are interrelated. For example, a subject with obesity may have inflammation, insulin resistance (with prediabetes or type 2 diabetes), gut microbiome dysbiosis, and leaky gut.

3.4 Diagnosis

NAFLD is a liver disease characterized by hepatic steatosis (≥ 5% fat deposit) on either imaging or histology. Several tests (non-invasive and invasive) can be performed to support and/or confirm the diagnosis of NAFLD and the presence of fibrosis, and optimize the intervention [1, 5, 6, 9, 84–88]. There are several national and international guidelines related to the diagnosis and the management of NAFLD (e.g., American Association for the Study of Liver Diseases "AASLD", National Institute for Health and Care Excellence "NICE", European Association for the Study of the Liver "EASL", Italian Association for the Study of the Liver "AISF", and Asia-Pacific guidelines) [1, 89].

3.4.1 Non-invasive tests

Non-invasive tests of NAFLD include liver biochemistry and imaging examination [1, 5, 6, 9, 84–88].

To establish the diagnosis of NAFLD, conventional liver biochemistry is used first. It may show an increase in liver enzymes including aspartate aminotransferase (AST), alanine aminotransferase (ALT), and gamma-glutamyl transpeptidase (GGT). However, up to approximately 75% of subjects with NAFLD may have normal liver enzymes. Additional biomarkers and scores have been proposed (e.g., cytokeratin-18 fragment, fatty liver index, Zhejiang University index, and NAFLD liver fat score) (non-exhaustive list).

Imaging of the liver can be obtained with several tools including ultrasound, computed tomography (CT), and magnetic resonance imaging (MRI) (**Figure 7**). Based on most guidelines, abdominal ultrasound should be the first-line examination for the identification of hepatic steatosis. Although ultrasound has some limitations in morbidly obese subjects and in subjects with liver fat content below 20%, it has the advantage of being widely available with low cost. MRI remains the gold standard for assessing and quantifying hepatic steatosis since it can detect a liver fat content as low as 5%. However, its use is limited due to high cost and a long time of execution. Another promising imaging technique is the ultrasonography-based transient elastography using continuous attenuation parameter.

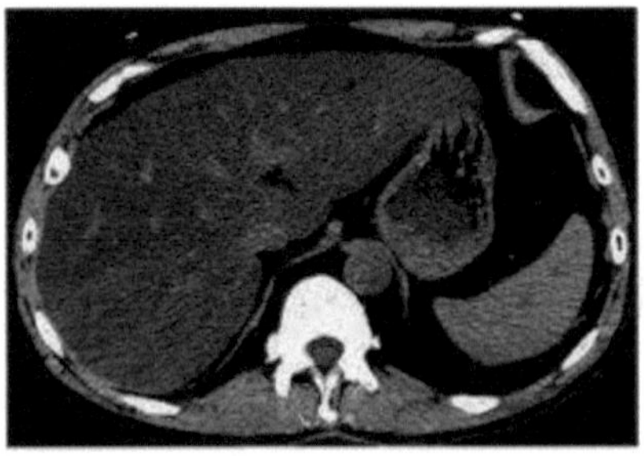

Figure 7.
Abdominal CT scan showing diffuse hepatic steatosis in a subject with NAFLD.

For the assessment of liver fibrosis, several biomarkers, scores, and imaging techniques have been proposed (e.g., AST/ALT ratio, AST to platelet ratio index, enhanced liver fibrosis score, NAFLD fibrosis score, and magnetic resonance elastography) (non-exhaustive list) [6, 84, 88].

All the non-imaging assessments of NAFLD have limitations and alone cannot replace liver biopsy.

3.4.2 Invasive tests

Liver biopsy is the gold standard test in the assessment of NAFLD to diagnose NASH and stage liver fibrosis. It is potentially harmful and carries a low risk of morbidity and extremely low risk of mortality. Therefore, it should be reserved to selected subjects (**Figure 8**) [1, 90]. One important limitation of liver biopsy is that it explores only a small portion of the liver (approximately 1/50,000), not representative of the entire organ.

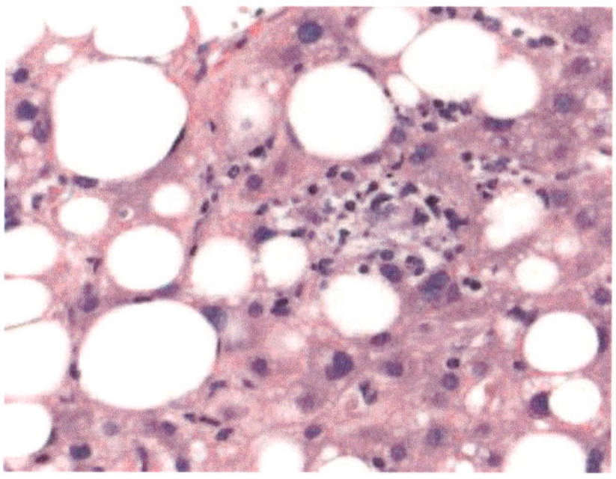

Figure 8.
Liver histology showing macrovesicular steatosis in a subject with NAFLD.

3.5 Treatment

Because NAFLD/NASH is associated with increased morbidity and higher risk of death mainly related to cardiovascular and liver diseases, it is essential to initiate a treatment as soon as the diagnosis is made. In the absence of approved pharmacotherapy for the treatment of NAFLD/NASH, the first-line therapy of NAFLD remains lifestyle intervention with weight loss (in case of excess body weight) [1, 2, 8, 28–30]. Gut microbiome and intestinal epithelial barrier are becoming promising targets for the treatment of several diseases including NAFLD [4, 17, 18, 20–22, 24, 25, 31–43]. When treating NAFLD/NASH, in addition to lifestyle changes and weight loss (in case of excess body weight), focus should also be on correcting gut microbiome and intestinal permeability directly and/or through gut microbiome modulation [4, 17, 18, 20–22, 24, 25, 35–40, 43]. Several drugs for the treatment of NAFLD/NASH are currently under investigation [6, 8, 91]. It is also important to treat the associated morbidities other than overweight/obesity (e.g., type 2 diabetes and dyslipidemia).

3.5.1 Lifestyle intervention

Lifestyle intervention which includes diet and exercise is the first-line therapy in NAFLD but is difficult to maintain (**Table 3**) [1, 2, 8, 28–30]. Diet is a powerful tool in the management of NAFLD. Diet relates to the amount and the composition of food that is consumed on a daily basis. There are several types of diets with different caloric content and different composition of macronutrients, fiber, minerals, and vitamins. They include hypocaloric diet, low-carbohydrate diet, low-fat, high-protein diet, high-fiber diet, and Mediterranean diet (non-exhaustive list) [8, 29, 30, 92]. In NAFLD subjects, hypocaloric diet is usually a deficit of 500–1,000 kcal/day. For macronutrient composition and according to most recommendations, carbohydrate intake should be between 40 and 50% (with exclusion of fructose from foods and beverages), fat intake no more than 30% (with saturated fat below 10%), and protein intake between 15 and 20% [28]. Even without significant weight loss, anti-inflammatory diets like Mediterranean diet (a mainly plant-based low-carbohydrate and high-unsaturated fat diet) have beneficial properties both in the prevention and treatment of NAFLD [8, 10, 25, 27–29, 93]. The omega-3 polyunsaturated fatty acids present in the Mediterranean diet may reduce hepatic steatosis. A diet containing sirtuin 1 activators (e.g., magnesium and zinc) can be beneficial in NAFLD subjects [79].

The objective in NAFLD subjects with excess body weight is a weight loss of 7–10%. To achieve weight loss, in addition to lifestyle intervention, other tools including drugs, medical devices, and bariatric surgery can also be used when needed and indicated [2, 28, 94–97]. Rapid sudden weight loss should be avoided (risk of aggravation of liver failure).

Lean NAFLD subjects may have visceral obesity that is not detected by BMI. These subjects may also benefit from diet and weight loss.

In addition to the type of diet, the timing and the frequency of the meals may also influence NAFLD. It is recommended to consume more daily calories in the morning versus the evening and avoid skipping meals [29].

Regular exercise including moderate intensity aerobic activities (3–5 weekly sessions with approximately 40 minutes per session) and resistance training can reduce hepatic steatosis even without significant weight loss [1, 8, 28, 29]. Combination of exercise and diet has greater benefit than exercise or diet alone.

Lifestyle Intervention	Description
Healthy diet	Low-carbohydrate diet, Low-fat diet, High-fiber diet, Mediterranean diet, etc.
Diet for weight loss (in case of excess body weight)	Hypocaloric diet
Exercise	Aerobic activities, Resistance training

Table 3.
Lifestyle intervention for the treatment of NAFLD.

3.5.2 Gut microbiome modulation

The prevention and management of NAFLD may benefit from modulation and correction of gut microbiome [4, 17, 18, 20–22, 24, 25, 35–40]. Gut microbiome can be modulated through diet, antibiotics, prebiotics, probiotics, synbiotics, and fecal microbiota transplantation [4, 17, 18, 20–22, 24, 25, 33–40, 58–65]. To optimize the efficacy of these therapies, focus should be on the altered gut microbiome (e.g., taxa responsible for high alcohol and LPS production) [17].

3.5.2.1 Diet

Diet is an important tool for the modulation of gut microbiome. The amount of daily caloric intake and the content of food significantly affect gut microbiome. A diet that is low in calories (when weight loss is needed), low in fat, and high in fiber has a favorable effect on weight control and gut microbiome (increase in richness, decrease in Firmicutes-to-Bacteroidetes phyla ratio) [58–64].

The diet, through the modulation of gut microbiome, could be beneficial in NAFLD subjects [4, 25].

3.5.2.2 Antibiotics

Antibiotics are medications used to fight local or systemic infection [98].

Antibiotics affect gut microbiome [4, 24, 59, 65]. They can deplete or alter gut microbiome (e.g., increase in Firmicutes phylum) and reduce liver disease development. However, their clinical use is limited since they may eliminate important beneficial bacterial species and cause antibiotic resistance.

3.5.2.3 Prebiotics

Prebiotics are chemicals (nondigestible food ingredients) inducing growth and/or activity of intestinal bacteria (e.g., inulin, lactulose, and resistant starch) [31, 69]. Some dietary fibers are prebiotics [25]. Prebiotics can be found in many foods (e.g., leek, asparagus, onion, soybean, apple, and banana) (**Figure 9**).

Prebiotics can positively modulate gut microbiome and improve NAFLD [4, 21, 24, 25, 35]. They lower the production of LPS. Treatment with oligofructose (16 g/day for 8 weeks) in subjects with NASH showed a significant decrease of AST [35].

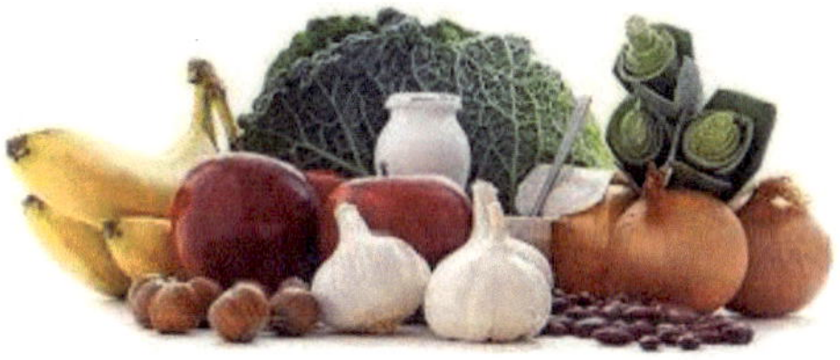

Figure 9.
Prebiotics can be beneficial in the treatment of NAFLD by modulating gut microbiome.

3.5.2.4 Probiotics

Probiotics are nonpathogenic living microorganisms with direct or indirect effect on gut microbiome [31, 32, 68]. Probiotics can be found in several foods (e.g., yogurt, cheese, and milk) (**Figure 10**).

Probiotics can positively impact gut microbiome and improve NAFLD [4, 21, 24, 36–39]. They reduce the production of LPS. Administration of *Lactobacillus rhamnosus* strain GG (12 billion CFU/day) for 8 weeks in children with NAFLD showed a significant decrease of ALT [36]. Treatment with VSL#3 (a mixture of 8 probiotic strains) for 4 months in children with NAFLD demonstrated a significant decrease of hepatic steatosis [38].

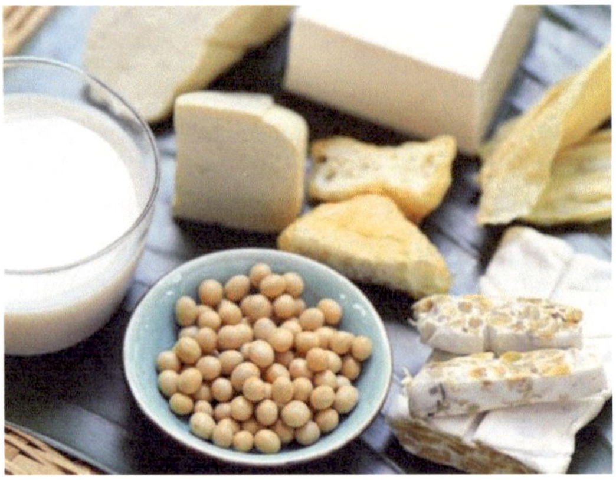

Figure 10.
Probiotics can be beneficial in the treatment of NAFLD by modulating gut microbiome.

3.5.2.5 Synbiotics

Synbiotics are combination of prebiotics and probiotics. They have the potential to induce more effects than prebiotics or probiotics used alone.

There are few studies assessing the effects of synbiotics on NAFLD subjects. They showed several beneficial effects including reduction of inflammation and hepatic steatosis [4, 24, 40]. Administration of *Bifidobacterium longum* with fructo-oligosaccharides for 24 weeks in subjects with NASH showed a significant decrease of AST, serum endotoxin, hepatic steatosis, and NASH activity index [40].

3.5.2.6 Fecal microbiota transplantation

Fecal microbiota transplantation consists of transfer of feces from a healthy donor to a recipient. The addition of healthy stool can be done through colonoscopy, orogastric tube, esophagogastroduodenoscopy, or oral capsule (**Figure 11**) [99].

Fecal microbiota transplantation is an exciting therapy with important potential indications. It was first approved by the United States Food and Drug Administration for the treatment of *Clostridium difficile* infection. Fecal microbiota transplantation can modify gut microbiome for the purpose of obesity and metabolic disorders management [33, 34]. Clinical studies using fecal microbiota transplantation in NAFLD subjects are currently ongoing.

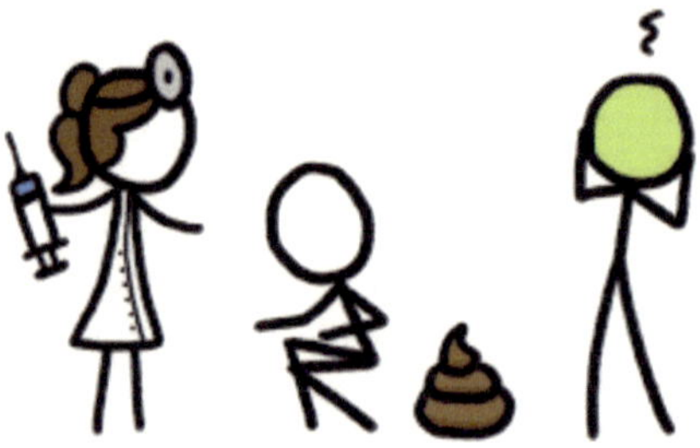

Figure 11.
Fecal microbiota transplantation has the potential to treat NAFLD by modifying gut microbiome.

3.5.3 Intestinal permeability correction

Restoring the intestinal epithelial barrier is an attractive therapeutic approach in NAFLD subjects. Currently, there is no approved drug for this indication. Intestinal permeability can be targeted and corrected directly (with diet) and/or through gut microbiome modulation [17, 18, 43].

A study using high-fiber diet for 6 months in subjects with NAFLD showed a decrease in intestinal permeability as demonstrated by a reduction of approximately 90% of serum zonulin, and a significant reduction of liver enzymes (e.g., AST, ALT, and GGT) and hepatic steatosis [43].

3.5.4 Drugs

There are no approved drugs for the treatment of NAFLD/NASH. Several investigational drugs are currently in various stages of clinical trials. They can impact at least four pathways related to NAFLD development and progression (hepatic fat accumulation, oxidative stress, gut microbiome, and hepatic fibrosis) [7, 8, 91]. Some of these investigational drugs have shown promising preliminary results (e.g., lanifibranor, cenicriviroc, and resmetirom) (non-exhaustive list) [6, 8, 91].

Any drug that is currently used in the treatment of NAFLD/NASH (e.g., antidiabetic drugs, lipid-lowering drugs, and vitamin E) should be considered as an off-label treatment [1, 2, 6–9, 14–16, 28, 91, 100]. Among the antidiabetic drugs, pioglitazone has shown a strong efficacy and became the first-line therapy in subjects who have type 2 diabetes and NAFLD [1, 2, 6, 14, 15, 28, 100].

The summary of different tools available in the United States of America (USA) or under investigation for the treatment of NAFLD/NASH is reported in **Table 4**.

Tool	Description
Lifestyle intervention	Diet, Exercise
Anti-obesity drug	Xenical®, Qsymia®, Contrave®, Saxenda®
Anti-obesity medical device	Lap-Band®, AspireAssist®, Orbera® Intragastric Balloon System, TransPyloric Shuttle®, Obalon® Balloon System, Plenity®
Bariatric surgery	Sleeve gastrectomy, Roux-en-Y gastric bypass
Gut microbiome modulation	Diet, Antibiotics, Prebiotics, Probiotics, Synbiotics, Fecal microbiota transplantation
Intestinal permeability correction	High-fiber diet, Gut microbiome modulation
Off-label drug	Antidiabetic drugs, Vitamin E, etc.
Investigational drug	Lanifibranor, Cenicriviroc, Resmetirom, etc.

Table 4.
Summary of different tools available in the USA or under investigation for the treatment of NAFLD/NASH.

3.5.5 Liver transplantation

NASH is becoming one of the leading causes of liver transplantation. Currently, in the USA, NASH ranks as the second most common reason for liver transplantation after hepatitis C [89].

4. Conclusions

NAFLD is the most common chronic liver disease worldwide. It is a spectrum of liver disorders ranging from simple steatosis to NASH. NAFLD subjects have overweight/obesity in the majority of cases and the disease can be associated with disrupted gut microbiome and impaired intestinal barrier function.

In the absence of approved pharmacotherapy for the treatment of NAFLD/NASH, in addition to lifestyle intervention with weight loss (in case of excess body weight), targeting gut microbiome and intestinal epithelial barrier with diet, prebiotics, probiotics, synbiotics, and fecal microbiota transplantation represents a promising novel therapeutic approach.

Conflict of interest

The author declares no conflict of interest.

Author details

Hassan M. Heshmati
Endocrinology Metabolism Consulting, LLC, Anthem, AZ, USA

*Address all correspondence to: hassanheshmati@yahoo.com

References

[1] Leoni S, Tovoli F, Napoli L, Serio I, Ferri S, Bolondi L. Current guidelines for the management of non-alcoholic fatty liver disease: A systematic review with comparative analysis. World Journal of Gastroenterology. 2018;**24**:3361-3373. DOI: 10.3748/wjg.v24.i30.3361

[2] Mundi MS, Velapati S, Patel J, Kellogg TA, Abu Dayyeh BK, Hurt RT. Evolution of NAFLD and its management. Nutrition in Clinical Practice. 2020;**35**:72-84. DOI: 10.1002/ncp.10449

[3] Younossi ZB, Koenig AB, Abdelatif D, Fazel Y, Henry L, Wymer M. Global epidemiology of nonalcoholic fatty liver disease – Meta-analytic assessment of prevalence, incidence, and outcomes. Hepatology. 2016;**64**:73-84. DOI: 10.1002/hep.28431

[4] Safari Z, Gérard P. The links between the gut microbiome and non-alcoholic fatty liver disease (NAFLD). Cellular and Molecular Life Sciences. 2019;**76**:1541-1558. DOI: 10.1007/s00018-019-03011-w

[5] Yki-Järvinen. Diagnosis of non-alcoholic fatty liver disease (NAFLD). Diabetologia. 2016;**59**:1104-1111. DOI: 10.1007/s00125-016-3944-1

[6] Drescher HK, Weiskirchen S, Weiskirchen R. Current status in testing for nonalcoholic fatty liver disease (NAFLD) and nonalcoholic steatohepatitis (NASH). Cells. 2019;**8**:845. DOI: 10.3390/cells8080845

[7] Oseini AM, Sanyal AJ. Therapies in non-alcoholic steatohepatitis (NASH). Liver International. 2017;**37** (Suppl 1): 97-103. DOI: 10.1111/liv.13302

[8] Pydyn N, Miękus K, Jura J, Kotlinowski J. New therapeutic strategies in nonalcoholic fatty liver disease: A focus on promising drugs for nonalcoholic steatohepatitis. Pharmacological Reports. 2020;**72**:1-12. DOI: 10.1007/s43440-019-00020-1

[9] Gharaibeh NE, Rahhal MN, Rahimi L, Ismail-Beigi F. SGLT-2 inhibitors as promising therapeutics for non-alcoholic fatty liver disease: Pathophysiology, clinical outcomes, and future directions. Diabetes, Metabolic Syndrome and Obesity: Targets and Therapy. 2019;**12**:1001-1012. DOI: 10.2147/DMSO.S212715

[10] Tilg H, Adolph TE, Moschen AR. Multiple parallel hits hypothesis in nonalcoholic fatty liver disease: Revisited after a decade. Hepatology. DOI: 10.1002/hep.31518

[11] Alisi A, Carpino G, Oliveira FL, Panera N, Nobili V, Gaudio E. The role of tissue macrophage-mediated inflammation on NAFLD pathogenesis and its clinical implications. Mediators of Inflammation. DOI: 10.1155/2017/8162421

[12] Vesa CM, Behl T, Nemeth S, et al. Prediction of NAFLD occurrence in prediabetes patients. Experimental and Therapeutic Medicine. 2020;**20**:190. DOI: 10.3892/etm.2020.9320

[13] Radaelli MG, Martucci F, Perra S, et al. NAFLD/NASH in patients with type 2 diabetes and related treatment options. Journal of Endocrinological Investigation. 2018;**41**:509-521. DOI: 10.1007/s40618-017-0799-3

[14] Tacelli M, Celsa C, Magro B, et al. Antidiabetic drugs in NAFLD: The accomplishment of two goals at once. Pharmaceuticals. 2018;**11**:121. DOI: 10.3390/ph11040121

[15] Kim KS, Lee BW. Beneficial effect of anti-diabetic drugs for nonalcoholic fatty liver disease. Clinical and

Molecular Hepatology. 2020;**26**:430-443. DOI: 10.3350/cmh.2020.0137

[16] Iqbal U, Perumpail BJ, John N, et al. Judicious use of lipid lowering agents in the management of NAFLD. Diseases. 2018;**6**:87. DOI: 10.3390/diseases6040087

[17] Zhu L, Baker RD, Baker SS. Gut microbiome and nonalcoholic fatty liver diseases. Pediatric Research. 2015;**77**:245-251. DOI: 10.1038/pr.2014.157

[18] Vespasiani-Gentilucci U, Gallo P, Picardi A. The role of intestinal microbiota in the pathogenesis of NAFLD: Starting points for intervention. Archives of Medical Science. 2018;**14**:701-706. DOI: 10.5114/aoms.2016.58831

[19] Grabherr F, Grander C, Effenberger M, Adolph TE, Tilg H. Gut dysfunction and non-alcoholic fatty liver disease. Frontiers in Endocrinology. 2019;**10**:611. DOI: 10.3389/fendo.2019.00611

[20] Kolodziejczyk AA, Zheng D, Shibolet O, Elinav E. The role of the microbiome in NAFLD and NASH. EMBO Molecular Medicine. 2019;**11**:e9302. DOI: 10.15252/emmm.201809302

[21] Durate SMB, Stefano JT, Oliveira CP. Microbiota and nonalcoholic fatty liver disease/nonalcoholic steatohepatitis (NAFLD/NASH). Annals of Hepatology. 2019;**18**:416-421. DOI: 10.1016/j.aohep.2019.04006

[22] Liu Q, Liu S, Chen L, et al. Role and effective therapeutic target of gut microbiota in NAFLD/NASH (review). Experimental and Therapeutic Medicine. 2019;**18**:1935-1944. DOI: 10.3892/etm.2019.7781

[23] Jadhav K, Cohen TS. Can you trust your gut? Implicating a disrupted intestinal microbiome in the progression of NAFLD/NASH. Frontiers in Endocrinology. 2020;**11**:592157. DOI: 10.3389/fendo.2020.592157

[24] Hu H, Lin A, Kong M, et al. Intestinal microbiome and NAFLD: Molecular insights and therapeutic perspectives. Journal of Gastroenterology. 2020;**55**:142-158. DOI: 10.1007/s00535-019-01649-8

[25] Pérez-Montes de Oca A, Julián MT, Ramos A, Puig-Domingo M, Alonso N. Microbiota, fiber, and NAFLD: Is there any connection? Nutrients. 2020;**12**:3100. DOI: 10.3390/nu12103100

[26] Luther J, Garber JJ, Khalili H, et al. Hepatic injury in nonalcoholic steatohepatitis contributes to altered intestinal permeability. Cellular and Molecular Gastroenterology and Hepatology. 2015;**1**:222-232. DOI: 10.1016/j.jcmgh.2015.01.001

[27] Biolato M, Manca F, Marrone G, et al. Intestinal permeability after Mediterranean diet and low-fat diet in non-alcoholic fatty liver disease. World Journal of Gastroenterology. 2019;**25**:509-520. DOI: 10.3748/wjg.v25.i4.509

[28] Hossain N, Kanwar P, Mohanty SR. A comprehensive updated review of pharmaceutical and nonpharmaceutical treatment for NAFLD. Gastroenterology Research and Practice. DOI: 10.1155/2016/7109270

[29] El-Agroudy NN, Kurzbach A, Rodionov RN, et al. Are lifestyle therapies effective for NAFLD treatment? Trends in Endocrinology & Metabolism. 2019;**30**:701-709. DOI: 10.1016/j.tem.2019.07.013

[30] Plaz Torres MC, Aghemo A, Lleo A, et al. Mediterranean diet and NAFLD: What we know and questions that still need to be answered. Nutrients. 2019;**11**:2971. DOI: 10.3390/nu11122971

[31] Dahiya DK, Renuka, Puniya M, et al. Gut microbiota modulation and its relationship with obesity using prebiotics fibers and probiotics: A review. Frontiers in Microbiology. 2017;**8**:563. DOI: 10.3389/fmicb.2017.00563

[32] Kobyliak N, Conte C, Cammarota G, et al. Probiotics in prevention and treatment of obesity: A critical view. Nutrition and Metabolism. 2016;**13**:14. DOI: 10.1186/s12986-016-0067-0

[33] Jayasinghe TN, Chiavaroli V, Holland DJ, Cutfield WS, O'Sullivan JM. The new era of treatment for obesity and metabolic disorders: Evidence and expectations for gut microbiome transplantation. Frontiers in Cellular and Infection Microbiology. 2016;**6**:15. DOI: 10.3389/fcimb.2016.00015

[34] Marotz CA, Zarrinpar A. Treating obesity and metabolic syndrome with fecal microbiota transplantation. Yale Journal of Biology and Medicine. 2016;**89**:383-388

[35] Daubioul CA, Horsmans Y, Lambert P, Danse E, Delzenne NM. Effects of oligofructose on glucose and lipid metabolism in patients with nonalcoholic steatohepatitis: Results of a pilot study. European Journal of Clinical Nutrition. 2005;**59**:723-726. DOI: 10.1038/sj.ejcn.1602127

[36] Vajro P, Mandato C, Licenziati MR, et al. Effects of *Lactobacillus rhamnosus* strain GG in pediatric obesity-related liver disease. Journal of Pediatric Gastroenterology and Nutrition. 2011;**52**:740-743. DOI: 10.1097/MPG.0b013e31821f9b85

[37] Ma YY, Li L, Yu CH, Shen Z, Chen LH, Li YM. Effects of probiotics on nonalcoholic fatty liver disease: A meta-analysis. World Journal of Gastroenterology. 2013;**19**:6911-6918. DOI: 10.3748/wjg.v19.i40.6911

[38] Alisi A, Bedogni G, Baviera G, et al. Randomized clinical trial: The beneficial effects of VSL#3 in obese children with non-alcoholic steatohepatitis. Alimentary Pharmacology and Therapeutics. 2014;**39**:1276-1285. DOI: 10.1111/apt.12758

[39] Lavekar AS, Raje DV, Manohar T, Lavekar AA. Role of probiotics in the treatment of nonalcoholic fatty liver disease: A meta-analysis. Euroasian Journal of Hepato-Gastroenterology. 2017;**7**:130-137

[40] Malaguarnera M, Vacante M, Antic T, et al. *Bifidobacterium longum* with fructo-oligosaccharides in patients with non alcoholic steatohepatitis. Digestive Diseases and Sciences. 2012;**57**:545-553. DOI: 10.1007/s10620-011-1887-4

[41] Bischoff SC, Barbara G, Buurman W, et al. Intestinal permeability – A new target for disease prevention and therapy. BMC Gastroenterology. 2014;**14**:189. DOI: 10.1186/s12876-014-0189-7

[42] Odenwald MA, Turner JR. The intestinal epithelial barrier: A therapeutic target? Nature Reviews. Gastroenterology & Hepatology. 2017;**14**:9-21. DOI: 10.1038/nrgastro.2016.169

[43] Krawczyk M, Maciejewska D, Ryterska K, et al. Gut permeability might be improved by dietary fiber in individuals with nonalcoholic fatty liver disease (NAFLD) undergoing weight reduction. Nutrients. 2018;**10**:1793. DOI: 10.3390/nu10111793

[44] Ozougwu JC. Physiology of the liver. International Journal of Research in Pharmacy and Biosciences. 2017;**4**:13-24

[45] The Human Microbiome Project Consortium. Structure, function and diversity of the healthy human

microbiome. Nature. 2012;**486**:207-214. DOI: 10.1038/nature11234

[46] Lozupone CA, Stombaugh JI, Gordon JI, Jansson JK, Knight R. Diversity, stability and resilience of the human gut microbiota. Nature. 2012;**489**:220-230. DOI: 10.1038/nature11550

[47] Kundu P, Blacher E, Elinav E, Pettersson S. Our gut microbiome: The evolving inner self. Cell. 2017;**171**:1481-1493. DOI: 10.1016/j.cell.2017.11.024

[48] Barko PC, McMichael MA, Swanson KS, Williams DA. The gastrointestinal microbiome: A review. Journal of Veterinary Internal Medicine. 2018;**32**:9-25. DOI: 10.1111/jvim.14875

[49] Schmidt TSB, Raes J, Bork P. The human gut microbiome: From association to modulation. Cell. 2018;**172**:1198-1215. DOI: 10.1016/j.cell.2018.02.044

[50] Heshmati HM. Gut microbiome in obesity management. In: Himmerich H, editor. Weight Management. London: IntechOpen; 2020. p. 255-268. DOI: 10.5772/intechopen.91974

[51] Conrad R, Vlassov AV. The human microbiota: Composition, functions, and therapeutic potential. Medical Science Review. 2015;**2**:92-103. DOI: 10.12659/MSRev.895154

[52] Ramakrishna BS. Role of the gut microbiota in human nutrition and metabolism. Journal of Gastroenterology and Hepatology. 2013;**28**(Suppl 4):9-17. DOI: 10.1111/jgh.12294

[53] Kovatcheva-Datchary P, Nilsson A, Akrami R, et al. Dietary fiber-induced improvement in glucose metabolism is associated with increased abundance of *Prevotella*. Cell Metabolism. 2015;**22**:971-982. DOI: 10.1016/j.cmet.2015.10.001

[54] Gerard C, Vidal H. Impact of gut microbiota on host glycemic control. Frontiers in Endocrinology. 2019;**10**:29. DOI: 10.3389/fendo.2019.00029

[55] Covasa M, Stephens RW, Toderean R, Cobuz C. Intestinal sensing by gut microbiota: Targeting gut peptides. Frontiers in Endocrinology. 2019;**10**:82. DOI: 10.3389/fendo.2019.00082

[56] Fu J, Bonder MJ, Cenit MC. The gut microbiome contributes to a substantial proportion of the variation in blood lipids. Circulation Research. 2015;**117**:817-824. DOI: 10.1161/CIRCRESAHA.115.306807

[57] Chen YC, Greenbaum J, Shen H, Deng HW. Association between gut microbiota and bone health: Potential mechanisms and prospective. The Journal of Clinical Endocrinology & Metabolism. 2017;**102**:3635-3646. DOI: 10.1210/jc.2017-00513

[58] Moschen AR, Wieser V, Tilg H. Dietary factors: Major regulators of the gut's microbiota. Gut and Liver. 2012;**6**:411-416. DOI: 10.5009/gnl.20126.4.411

[59] Voreades N, Kozil A, Weir TL. Diet and the development of the human intestinal microbiome. Frontiers in Microbiology. 2014;**5**:494. DOI: 10.3389/fmicb.2014.00494

[60] Graf D, Di Cagno R, Fåk F, et al. Contribution of diet to the composition of the human gut microbiota. Microbial Ecology in Health and Disease. 2015;**26**:26164. DOI: 10.3402/mehd.v26.26164

[61] Bibbò S, Ianiro G, Giorgio V, et al. The role of diet on gut microbiota composition. European Review for Medical and Pharmacological Sciences. 2016;**20**:4742-4749

[62] Singh RK, Chang HW, Yan D, et al. Influence of diet on the gut microbiome

and implications for human health. Journal of Translational Medicine. 2017;**15**:73. DOI: 10.1186/s12967-017-1175-y

[63] David LA, Maurice CF, Carmody RN, et al. Diet rapidly and reproducibly alters the human gut microbiome. Nature. 2014;**505**:559-563. DOI: 10.1038/nature12820

[64] Wu GD, Chen J, Hoffmann C, et al. Linking long-term dietary patterns with gut microbial enterotypes. Science. 2011;**334**:105-108. DOI: 10.1126/science.1208344

[65] Raymond F, Ouameur AA, Déraspe M, et al. The initial state of the human gut microbiome determines its reshaping by antibiotics. The ISME Journal. 2016;**10**:707-720. DOI: 10.1038/ismej.2015.148

[66] Le Bastard Q, Al-Ghalith GA, Grégoire M, et al. Systematic review: Human gut dysbiosis induced by non-antibiotic prescription medications. Alimentary Pharmacology & Therapeutics. 2018;**47**:332-345. DOI: 10.1111/apt.14451

[67] Maier L, Pruteanu M, Kuhn M, et al. Extensive impact of non-antibiotic drugs on human gut bacteria. Nature. 2018;**555**:623-628. DOI: 10.1038/nature25979

[68] Hill C, Guarner F, Reid G, et al. The International Scientific Association for Probiotics and Prebiotics consensus statement on the scope and appropriate use of the term probiotic. Nature Reviews. Gastroenterology & Hepatology. 2014;**11**:506-514. DOI: 10.1038/nrgastro.2014.66

[69] Carnahan S, Balzer A, Panchal SK, Brown L. Prebiotics in obesity. Panminerva Medica. 2014;**56**:165-175

[70] Citi S. Intestinal barriers protect against disease. Leaky cell-cell junctions contribute to inflammatory and autoimmune diseases. Science. 2018;**359**:1097-1098. DOI: 10.1126/science.aat0835

[71] Dai X, Wang B. Role of gut barrier function in the pathogenesis of nonalcoholic fatty liver disease. Gastroenterology Research and Practice. DOI: 10.1155/2015/287348

[72] Bianco C, Romeo S, Petta S, Long MT, Valenti L. MAFLD vs NAFLD: Let the contest begin. Liver International. 2020;**40**:2079-2081. DOI: 10.1111/liv.14620

[73] Ballestri S, Nascimbeni F, Baldelli E, Marrazzo A, Romagnoli D, Lonardo A. NAFLD as a sexual dimorphic disease: Role of gender and reproductive status in the development and progression of nonalcoholic fatty liver disease and inherent cardiovascular risk. Advances in Therapy. 2017;**34**:1291-1326. DOI: 10.1007/s12325-017-0556-1

[74] Wang L, Guo J, Lu J. Risk factor compositions of nonalcoholic fatty liver disease change with body mass index in males and females. Oncotarget. 2016;**7**:35632-35642

[75] Lonardo A, Mantovani A, Lugari S, Targher G. NAFLD in some common endocrine diseases: Prevalence, pathophysiology, and principles of diagnosis and management. International Journal of Molecular Sciences. 2019;**20**:2841. DOI: 10.3390/ijms20112841

[76] Lee IH. Mechanisms and disease implications of sirtuin-mediated autophagic regulation. Experimental & Molecular Medicine. 2019;**51**:102. DOI: 10.1038/s12276-019-0302-7

[77] Nassir F, Ibdah JA. Sirtuins and nonalcoholic fatty liver disease. World Journal of Gastroenterology. 2016;**22**:10084-10092. DOI: 10.3748/wjg.v22.i46.10084

[78] Martins I. The future of genomic medicine involves the maintenance of sirtuin I in global populations. International Journal of Molecular Biology. 2017;**2**:42-45. DOI: 10.15406/ijmboa.2017.02.00013

[79] Martins IJ. Nutrition therapy regulates caffeine metabolism with relevance to NAFLD and induction of type 3 diabetes. Journal of Diabetes and Metabolic Disorders. 2017;**4**:019. DOI: 10.24966/DMD-201X/100019

[80] Ye J. Mechanisms of insulin resistance in obesity. Frontiers of Medicine. 2013;**7**:14-24. DOI: 10.1007/s11684-013-0262-6

[81] Niriella MA, Kasturiratne A, Pathmeswaran A, et al. Lean non-alcoholic fatty liver disease (lean NAFLD): Characteristics, metabolic outcomes and risk factors from a 7-year prospective, community cohort study from Sri Lanka. Hepatology International. 2019;**13**:314-322. DOI: 10.1007/s12072-018-9916-4

[82] Ye Q, Zou B, Yeo YH, et al. Global prevalence, incidence, and outcomes of non-obese or lean non-alcoholic fatty liver disease: A systematic review and meta-analysis. Lancet Gastroenterology & Hepatology. 2020;**5**:739-752. DOI: 10.1016/S2468-1253(20)30077-7

[83] Holmes E, Li JV, Athanasiou T, Ashrafian H, Nicholson JK. Understanding the role of gut microbiome-host metabolic signal disruption in health and disease. Trends in Microbiolgy. 2011;**19**:349-359. DOI: 10.1016/j.tim.2011.05.006

[84] Cleveland E, Bandy A, VanWagner LB. Diagnostic challenges of nonalcoholic fatty liver disease/nonalcoholic steatohepatitis. Clinical Liver Disease. 2018;**11**:98-104

[85] Zhou JH, Cai JJ, She ZG, Li HL. Noninvasive evaluation of nonalcoholic fatty liver disease: Current evidence and practice. World Journal of Gastroenterology. 2019;**25**:1307-1326. DOI: 10.3748/wjg.v25.i11.1307

[86] Lee DH. Noninvasive evaluation of nonalcoholic fatty liver disease. Endocrinology and Metabolism. 2020;**35**:243-259. DOI: 10.3803/EnM.2020.35.2.243

[87] Fu CP, Ali H, Rachakonda VP, Oczypok EA, DeLany JP, Kershaw EE. The ZJU index is a powerful surrogate marker for NAFLD in severely obese North American women. Plos One. 2019;**14**:e0224942. DOI: 10.1371/journal.pone.0224942

[88] Kaswala DH, Lai M, Afdhal NH. Fibrosis assessment in nonalcoholic fatty liver disease (NAFLD) in 2016. Digestive Diseases and Sciences. 2016;**61**:1356-1364. DOI: 10.1007/s10620-016-4079-4

[89] Paul S, Davis AM. Diagnosis and management of nonalcoholic fatty liver disease. Journal of the American Medical Association. 2018;**320**:2474-2475

[90] Bedossa P. Histological assessment of NAFLD. Digestive Diseases and Sciences. 2016;**61**:1348-1355. DOI: 10.1007/s10620-016-4062-0

[91] Sumida Y, Yoneda M. Current and future pharmacological therapies for NAFLD/NASH. Journal of Gastroenterology. 2018;**53**:362-376. DOI: 10.1007/s00535-017-1415-1

[92] Freedman MR, King J, Kennedy E. Popular diets: A scientific review. Obesity Research. 2001;**9**(Suppl 1):1S–40S

[93] Tyrovolas S, Panagiotakos DB, Georgousopoulou EN, et al. The anti-inflammatory potential of diet and nonalcoholic fatty liver disease: The ATTICA study. Therapeutic Advances in

Gastroenterology. 2019;**12**:1-11. DOI: 10.1177/1756284819858039

[94] Gadde KM, Martin CK, Berthoud HR, Heymsfield SB. Obesity. Pathophysiology and management. Journal of the American College of Cardiology. 2018;**71**:69-84. DOI: 10.1016/j.jacc.2017.11.011

[95] Saxon DR, Iwamoto SJ, Mettenbrink CJ, et al. Antiobesity medication use in 2.2 million adults across eight large health care organizations: 2009-2015. Obesity. 2019;**27**:1975-1981. DOI: 10.1002/oby.22581

[96] Heshmati HM. Anti-obesity medical devices. In: Himmerich H, editor. Weight Management. London: IntechOpen; 2020. p. 239-253. DOI: 10.5772/intechopen.91697

[97] Radvinsky D, Iskandar M, Ferzli G. Bariatric surgery today: The good, the bad, and the ugly. Annals of Laparoscopic and Endoscopic Surgery. 2017;**2**:52. DOI: 10.21037/ales.2017.02.26

[98] Coates ARM, Halls G, Hu Y. Novel classes of antibiotics or more of the same? British Journal of Pharmacology. 2011;**163**:184-194. DOI: 10.1111/j.1476-5381.2011.01250.x

[99] Wang JW, Kuo CH, Kuo FC, et al. Fecal microbiota transplantation: Review and update. Journal of the Formosan Medical Association. 2019;**118**:S23-S31. DOI: 10.1016/j.jfma.2018.08.011

[100] Sawangjit R, Chongmelaxme B, Phisalprapa P, et al. Comparative efficacy of interventions on nonalcoholic fatty liver disease (NAFLD). A PRISMA-compliant systematic review and network meta-analysis. Medicine. 2016;**95**:32(e4529). DOI: 10.1097/MD.0000000000004529

Chapter 10

The Role of Bariatric Surgery in Fatty Liver

Anja Geerts and Sander Lefere

Abstract

Non-alcoholic fatty liver disease (NAFLD) is a crucial health problem with a prevalence that is increasing concurrently with the obesity epidemic on a global scale. Steatosis, nonalcoholic steatohepatitis (NASH), hepatocellular carcinoma (HCC), cirrhosis, and advanced fibrosis constitute the disease spectrum covered by NAFLD. NASH-related cirrhosis and HCC is currently the second most common indication for liver transplantation. Although lifestyle modifications, especially weight loss, effectively reduces the liver injury in NASH, adherence in the clinical setting is low. Potential treatments for NASH are still under investigation in phase 2–3 studies. Bariatric surgery can improve metabolic components and cause great weight loss. Therefore, bariatric surgery may reverse the pathological liver changes in NAFLD and NASH patients. However, complications such as liver failure after bariatric surgery can occur. This chapter will give an overview of the benefits and pitfalls of bariatric surgery in patients with NAFLD, liver transplant candidates and post-liver transplant patients.

Keywords: bariatric surgery, NAFLD, NASH, liver transplant, liver failure

1. Introduction

Over the last decades, there has been a drastic increase in obesity prevalence. Health statistics reports of 2018 showed that 40% of the total adult population of the United States were obese (BMI (body mass index) > 30 kg/m^2).

The obesity epidemic has led to a dramatic rise in the obesity-related liver disease non-alcoholic fatty liver disease (NAFLD). NAFLD currentlyaffects one quarter of the global population [1]. Steatosis or fatty liver, non-alcoholic steatohepatitis (NASH), fibrosis, cirrhosis, and hepatocellular carcinoma (HCC) make up the spectrum of conditions that NAFLD represents. The frequency of liver transplantation undertaken in patients with cirrhosis and HCC due to NASH has been increasing worldwide [2]. NAFLD has also been found to be associated with several health conditions like cardiovascular diseases which affect organs outside the liver and consititute the major cause of deaths in patients with NAFLD.

Lifestyle modification is the cornerstone of NAFLD therapy. As a matter of fact, reduced intake of calories combined with increased activity can make this achievable. The main driver of NAFLD improvement is the amount of actual weight loss, while the type of diet seems to be less important. Rrespective of how one achieves weight loss, the highest rates of steatohepatitis resolution (90%) as well as improvement of fibrosis (45%) can only be induced by >10% weight loss. A weight loss of >5% improves steatosis in about 64% and weight loss of >7% can resolve steatohepatitis in 72% [3]. Regrettably, the necessary weight loss goal of >7% to 10% is achieved only by a minority of the patients.

Currently, a vast array of drugs are being tested for NASH, and some of them are already in the third phase, but until now, there is no pharmacological therapy for NASH [4]. In our current understanding, any pharmacological treatment that is indicative for NASH should be prescribed only to patients with NASH and advanced liver fibrosis. The recommendations above result from data which show that fibrosis is the strongest prognostic predictor, with a decline in survival from fibrosis stage 2 onwards [5].

The use of bariatric surgery as a therapy for obesity is increasingly common, and evidence that also supports its therapeutic use for metabolic disturbances (so called "metabolic surgery") is increasing [6]. In addition, bariatric surgery is a promising therapeutic alternative for NAFLD as risk factors such as diabetes, inflammation, insulin resistance, and dyslipidemia that contribute to NAFLD pathogenesis can be reversed by it, and it is also effective for achieving long-term weight loss in patients [7].

According to current reimbursement guidelines, it is only administered to obese patients who are 18 years or over with a BMI > 40 kg/m^2 or BMI > 35 kg/m^2 with related co-morbidities such as diabetes mellitus, uncontrolled arterial high blood pressure and OSAS despite triple therapy. Consequently, NASH is not one of the co-morbidities regarded as an indication for bariatric surgery.

In this chapter, we will first elucidate the benefit of bariatric surgery in the field of NAFLD. Secondly, the possible role of bariatric surgery will be discussedin patients who are candidates for liver transplantation. Special considerationwill also be given to patients who develop recurrent or de novo NASH after liver transplantation. Finally, we outline the possible pitfalls with the risk of liver failure after bariatric surgery.

2. Types of bariatric surgery

A variety of procedures for bariatric surgery have been developed over the last decades. The 2 most frequently performed types of bariatric surgery are Roux-en-Y gastric bypass (RYGB) and Sleeve gastrectomy (SG). There has been a progressive decline in the use of the adjustable gastric banding procedure after sleeve gastrectomy was developed. Biliopancreatic diversion with duodenal switch (BPD–DS) is the procedure of choice for severe morbidly obese patients. Very low mortality and morbidity rates are associated with almost all bariatric operations performed laparoscopically [8]. In the USA and countries around the world, the currently most performed bariatric procedure is sleeve gastrectomy. The increase in popularity of the SG could be due to its relative technical simplicity, as there are no concerns for late complications such as internal herniation, ulcerations on anastomosis and no malabsorption of iron, calcium and vitamins. Malabsorptive surgery as jejunoileal bypass, biliopancreatic diversion (BDP), biliopancreatic diversion with duodenal switch (BDP-DS), and distal gastric bypass (D-GBP) can lead to large weight loss, yet can cause severe long-term complications.

Figure 1 shows the different types of surgery. The RYGB procedure consists of two components. First, a small gastric pouch of ~30 cm^3 in volume is constructed, secondly the small intestine is divided ~30–50 cm distal to the ligament of Treitz. The distal end of the small intestine that has been divided also known as the Roux limb is connected to the gastric pouch that was newly fabricated. The Roux limb ranges from 75–150 cm in length. SG is formed from a tubular gastric pouch (sleeve) that remains after ~80% of the lateral part of the stomach has

DOI: http://dx.doi.org/10.5772/intechopen.96975

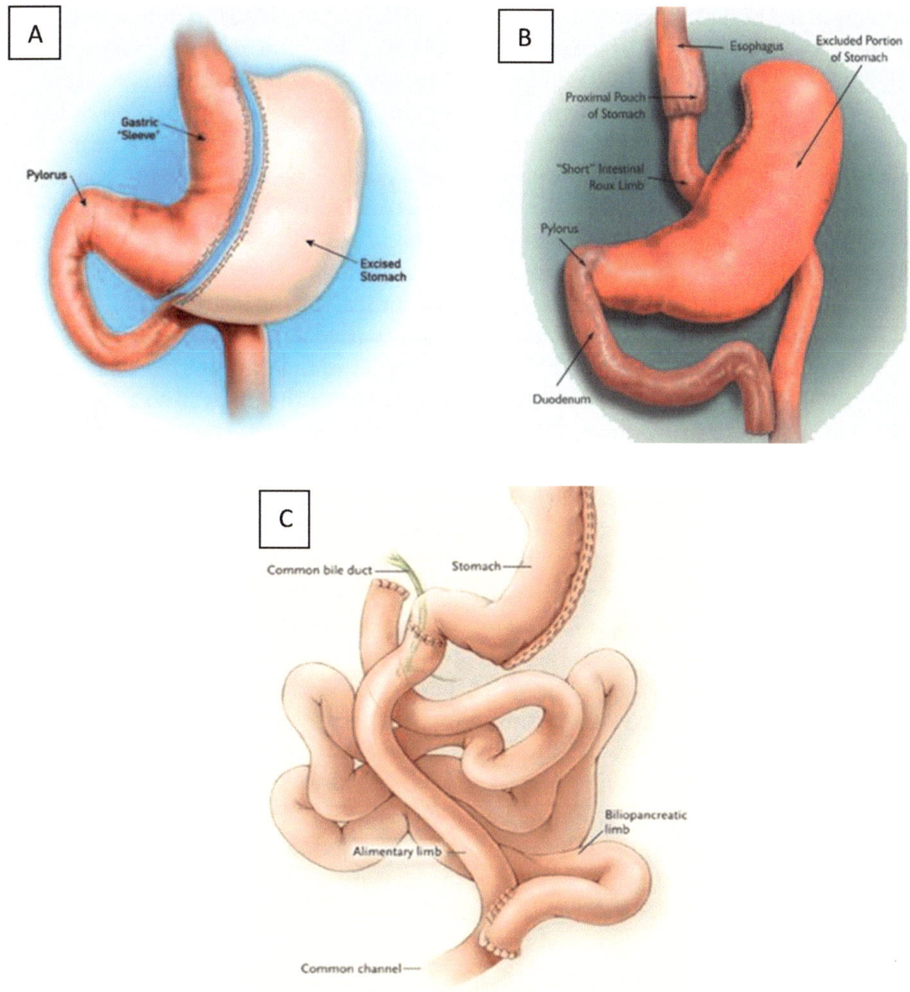

Figure 1.
Bariatric surgery procedures. (A) sleeve gastrectomy, (B) roux-en-Y gastric bypass, (C) biliopancreatic diversion with duodenal switch (reproduced with permission from www.uzgent.be).

been removed. The BPD–DS is a procedure where first a vertical gastrectomy is performed, similar to the SG. Next, a large portion (~50%) of the small intestine is bypassed, which creates malabsorption. The duodenum is divided immediately after the pylorus. At 250 cm proximal to the ileocecal valve, a portion of the distal ileum is divided and anastomosed to the duodenum in a Roux-en-Y configuration after bringing it up. Another anastomosis of the ileoileostomy is performed at 100 cm proximal to the ileocaecal valve to complete the operation [9].

3. Benefits of bariatric surgery in NAFLD patients

Already in 2008, Mathurin et al. published data showing animprovement of ste atosis, ballooning and NAS score 5 years after bariatric surgery in NAFLD patients. However they reporteda worsening of fibrosis in 19.8% of patients. This initial finding made the use of bariatric surgery questionable in the area of NASH. However, the worsening of fibrosis at 5 years was slight, 95% of the patients had a fibrosis score less than 1 and a lot of patients had no biopsy-proven NASH [10]. The same group reported recently data of a biopsy-proven cohort of NASH patients with liver samples 1 and 5 years after bariatric surgery [11, 12]. In this long-term prospective trial, NASH resolution was induced by bariatric surgery without fibrosis worsening in 84% of the patients at 5 years. Regression of fibrosis was seen in 70% of the patients, beginning to improve within 1 year and continued throughout 5 year follow-up. Also in patients with baseline fibrosis grade 3, there was an improvement seen in 68%.The non-responders (20%) to bariatric surgery were patients with low weight loss and less improvement in insulin resistance after their surgery. This large trial has demonstrated that there is an understandable benefit to consider bariatric surgery as a treatment option for patients with clinically significant NASH.

Lee et al. published in 2019 a systematic review with data of 32 cohort studies comprising 3093 biopsy-confirmed NAFLD patients and the effect of bariatric surgery [13]. The authors looked at complete resolution of the different features of NAFLD instead of improvement. The study results indicated that there was complete resolution of steatosis, inflammation, ballooning and fibrosis in 66%, 50%, 76% and 40%, respectively. A meta-analysis in 2008 of 15 cohort studies showed similar results [14]. By focusing on complete NAFLD resolution, these reviews provide further evidence that bariatric surgery is efficacious and that NAFLD as a comorbidity should prompt evaluation for bariatric surgery in patients with a BMI of 35 to 40 kg/m2.

Klebanoff et al. showed that bariatric surgery led to more QALY's for all obese patients and overweight patients regardless of fibrosis stage compared to lifestyle interventions. Their analysis also suggests that for patients in all obesity classes, bariatric surgery, as a therapy, is cost-effective and may even be considered cost-effective therapy for overweight individuals with advanced fibrosis [15]. The majority of the patients in the reported cohorts underwent RYGB, only 5 to 10% underwent Sleeve gastrectomy. A few studies have examined the effect other bariatric surgeries have on NASH. Caiazzo et al. showed that RYGB was associated with significantly greater improvement in the amount of steatosis and NASH at 1 and 5 years after surgery compared to adjustable gastric banding [16].

The use of comparative randomized trials that study the impact of bariatric surgery compared with current medical therapies should be the focus of future clinical studies. Data on new endoscopic bariatric therapies and the effect on NASH are also urgently needed.

4. Bariatric surgery related to liver transplantation

Candidates for transplantation with a BMI > 40 kg/m^2havea significantly higher mortality on the waiting list compared with candidates with a BMI > 30 kg/m^2. The reason is a faster progression of liver detioration among obese patients versus nonobese [17]. The most frequently used BMI cutoffs in the literature as relative and absolute contra-indication for livertransplantation were 40 and 45, respectively. This is mainly based on the fact that studies reported a higher risk of perioperative complications, mostly wound-related infections, in obese patients. Morbid obesity cannot be considered as an absolute contra-indication for liver transplant despite the presence of associated complications in these patients. This observation leads us to the need to address obesity before and after liver transplantation.

4.1 Bariatric surgery in pre-liver transplant candidates

Treating obesity before transplantation can reduce the risk of decompensation and reduce co-morbiditities such infections and metabolic syndrome in the post-operative period [18, 19].

The first issue to consider is whether bariatric surgery is safe in cirrotic patients. Data are mostly coming from retrospective incidental findings at the time of bariatric surgery with a prevalence between 0.14% to 1.5% [20, 21]. Younus et al. described a cohort of 26 patients with incidental finding of cirrhosis (proven with biopsy) at the time of bariatric surgery [20]. The type of procedure was mainly RYGB (55%). A higher risk of immediate complications postoperative (38.5% versus 16.7% in non-cirrhotic group) was seen, probably also dueto a high BMI in this study (median BMI of 52 kg/m^2). No long-term cirrhosis-related complications or increased mortality were noted in this cohort. Jan et al. published a review with pooled data of nine similar studies with a total of 122 cirrhotic patients. The characteristics of the patients were mainly Child Pugh A patients, a few Child Pugh B and 7 patients with portal hypertension. The type of procedure was again predominantly RYGB. There was an overall complication rate of 22.5% with also a 6.5% liver decompensation rate and a late mortality rate of 2.45%. A lower complication rate in cirrhotic patientswas seen in the group who underwent SG or gastric banding when compared with malabsorptive bariatric procedures including RYGB [22].

Bariatric surgery can be done in a carefully selected patient group with cirrhosis, especially Child Pugh A patients without significant portal hypertension. It is important to recognize and diagnose cirrhosis, estimate liver function and the presence or absence of portal hypertension pre-operatively. This can help in deciding the type of procedure and anticipatingcomplications. Most of the data currently available indicatethat sleeve gastrectomy can be done safely in compensated liver cirrhosis patients [23, 24].

The risk of 30-day mortality in decompensated cirrotic patients undergoing bariatric surgery was noted to be 16.7% versus 0.9% in compensated cirrhosis. So, bariatric surgery is absolutely contra-indicated in patients with a decompensated liver disease.

4.2 Bariatric surgery simultaneously with liver transplantation

For patients who are too sick before transplant, a simultaneous bariatric surgery and liver transplantation is another approach to manage obesity in this population. Small series of patients who underwent combined sleeve gastrectomy and liver transplantation has been published from the group of the Mayo Clinic [25]. Death, graft loss, operative complications were similar between the two groups, however post-liver transplantation metabolic outcomes were superior in the group who underwentthe combined SG and transplantation. Long-term outcomes were described recently with demonstrating efficacy and maintaining wieght loss and favorable metabolic profiles [26]. So far, there are only two other case reports of sleeve gastrectomy and liver transplantation combined that have been reported [27, 28].

The main disadvantage of this approach can be the impact on the nutritional state in the immediate post-operative period. More data and experience in is needed before promoting this approach.

4.3 Bariatric surgery after liver transplantation

Long-term weight gain and development of metabolic syndrome are the main concerns post-liver transplantation. Up to 46% of the patients will develop themetabolic syndrome, especially those with a BMI > 30 kg/m^2 or higherpre-liver transplant BMI. Recently it has been shown that NASH liver transplant recipients have a 10 year graft survival of 61% which is significantly lower than primary sclerosing cholangitis, auto-immuun hepatitis and primary biliary cholangitisrecipients (respectively 74%, 71,7% and 71%) [29]. Probably the outcomes of NASH cirrhosis liver transplant recipients are not as good as previously thought and this is due to the development of metabolic risk factors. The bulk of weight gain appears to occur within the first year, with studies reporting a median weight gain of 5 to 10 kg at 12 months after liver transplantation. Recurrent NAFLD/NASH after transplantation is very common, ranging in cohorts from respectively 10 to 100% and 4 to 28%. Risk factors are older age, higher BMI at the time of liver transplantation, presence of diabetes mellitus type 2 pre-livertransplant and dislipidemia [30–32].

The development of de novo NAFLD is also frequent after liver transplantation. There are reports that described 78% de novo NAFLD and 4% NASH in 2378 liver transplant recipients at 5 year follow-up [33]. A very important finding is the faster progression of fibrosis in patients with de novo NASH after liver transplantation [30–33].

Case reports and series of bariatric surgery in post transplant recipients showed no difference in mortality with the general population [34–36]. Sleeve gastrectomy is the most performed procedure with lack of malabsorption and no interference of immuunsuppressive drugs. Optimal timing of bariatric surgery post liver transplantation need to be defined, because delaying too long can cause fibrosis and reduce patient survival.

5. Liver failure as a result of prior bariatric surgery

Decompensated cirrhosis that results from an earlier bariatric surgery, is a clinical condition that is far more demanding. Complications including severely impaired hepatic function are mostly described after jejunoileal bypass (JIB) and biliopancreatic diversion (BPD) procedures. They occurred in up to 10% of the patients. The occurrence of these and other complications resulted in abandonment of JIB surgery. The frequency of hepatic complications after BPD is unclear, but hepatocellular failure has been reported in small series and case reports. In 1992, the first case of chronic end-stage liver disease after BPD was reported [37]. We published a multicenter Belgian Survey on liver transplantation for hepatocellular failure after bariatric surgery. 10 patients who underwent bariatric surgery and developed liver failure afterward were reported in the Belgian survey: 1 after JIB and 9 after BPD. Patients who underwent JIB or BPD subsequently became candidates for liver transplantation, even >20 years after bariatric surgery [38]. Probably, the real incidence of hepatic complications after BPD surgery is underreported in the current literature; so we are still unaware of the real incidence of Scopinaro procedure-induced liver failure. The pathogenesis of post-BPD steatohepatitis remains poorly understood. One important factor implicated in the pathogenesis of liver injury after JIB or BPD was intestinal bacterial overgrowth in the excluded small intestine segment. As we see no liver failure after equivalent intestinal resection, this may explain the role of excluded segment. Bacterial overgrowth leads to mucosal injury and increases gut permeability toespecially endotoxins. When these toxins are absorbed via the portal vein to the liver, they can induce hepatocellular damage. Another factor in the pathogenesis of liver failure postbypass surgery is protein and amino acid malnutrition, which can perpetuate or increase lipid accumulation in the liver.

Mahawar et al. confirmed that the lenght of the biliopancreatic limb (BPL) matters [39]. A long BPL (100–150 cm) results in better weight loss, intensifies the antidiabetic effect in RYGB compared with a shorter BPL of 50–75 cm. The increased risk of insufficiency of protein with successive malnutrition constitute the drawback of using a long BPL with a shorter alimentary limb lenght (TALL). Recent data suggests that at least 350–400 cm of TALL must remain [40, 41].

Although liver transplantation and intestinal anatomy restoration have been regarded as the standard therapy for liver failure that results from BDP or JIB surgery, the use of these measures has been reported to be unsuccessful in some cases [42, 43]. We reported a case of refractory subacute steatohepatitis after BPD [43]. There may be a significant improvement when surgery is used to achieve a gastric bypass-like anatomy, however, its feasibility is directly related to the severity of liver decompensation as well as effects of nutritional correction. Correction of vitamine depletion, malnutrition and aggressive nutrition is warranted and might already significantly improve the patient's condition. In case of incipient deterioration, early referral to a liver transplant center is necessary.

The exact magnitude of liver failure after RYGB, which is not associated with much malabsorption, has not yet been fully established. There are some case reports. Mahawar et al. found10 reports of liver failure after RYGB in the entire surgical literature [39]. In view of the fact that RYGB is the most common performed bariatric procedure worldwide, potentially millions have been carried out, this means that only a minuscule proportion of patients undergoing this operation would suffer from liver failure.

4 out of the 10 reports were seen in cirrhotic patients, 2 had extended limb RYGB, 1 distal RYGB, 2 had early or late complication. Extended limb or distal versions of RYGB can behave like biliopancreatic diversion with higher potential for malabsorption. These versions of RYGB may hence be more likely to predispose to liver failure.

High risk groups of patients undergoing RYGB, such as patients with incidental finding of cirrhosis, extented limb or distal versions of RYGB, complications of surgery and alcohol abuse, should be follow up carefully withroutine lifelong monitoring of liver function tests.

6. Conclusions

Bariatric surgery provides effective treatment for obesity and metabolic complications. Lifestyle modification with weight loss is currently the most important treatment in NAFLD patients, but this is hard to achieve in clinical practice. Recent reports showed that bariatric surgery could resolve NASH in 84%of the patients without worsening of fibrosis. These findings support the notionthat bariatric surgery is an effective treatment for NASH patients. Bariatric surgery, especially sleeve gastrectomy, also seems to be feasible in compensated cirrhotic patients. Special attention should be paid to recurrent and de novo NAFLD after liver transplantation. It is worthy of note that, on a case-by-case basis and prior to liver transplantation, the feasibility of bariatric surgery as well as interventions and how they are timed and sequenced should be discussed in a broad multidisciplinary discussion.

Liver decompensation or failure hardly occurs in patients undergoing RYGB without pre-existing cirrhosis. Potentially fatal liver complications are described with severe malabsorptive bariatric procedures such as biliopancreatic diversion or distal versions of RYGB. Closely monitoring of liver function is recommended in this high risk group and early referral for surgical conversion is necessary.

Conflict of interest

The authors declare no conflict of interest.

Author details

Anja Geerts* and Sander Lefere
Hepatology Research Unit, Department of Internal Medicine and Pediatrics, Liver Research Center Ghent, Ghent University, Ghent, Belgium

*Address all correspondence to: anja.geerts@uzgent.be

References

[1] Younossi Z, Anstee Q, Marietti M, Hardy T, Henry L et al. Global burden of NAFLD and NASH; trends, predictions, risk factors and prevention. Nat Rev Gastroenterol Hepatol 2018;15:11-20.

[2] Younossi ZM. Non-alcoholic fatty liver disease – a global health perspective. J Hepatol 2019; 70:531-544.

[3] Villar-Gomez E, Martinez-Perez Y, Calzadilla-Bertot L, Torres-Gonzales A, Gra-Oramas B et al. Weight loss through lifestyle modification significantly reduces features of nonalcoholic steatohepatitis. Gastroenterology 2017;149:367-378.

[4] Younossi ZM, Ratziu V, Loomba R, Rinella M, Anstee QM et al. Obeticholic acid for the treatment of non-alcoholic steatohepatitis: interim analysis from a multicentre, randomised, placebo-controlled phase 3 trial. Lancet 2019;394:2184-2196.

[5] Dulai PS, Singhi S, Patel J, Soni M, Prokop LJ et al. Increased risk of mortality by fibrosis stage in nonalcoholic fatty liver disease:systematic review and meta-analysis. Hepatology 2017;65:1557 1565.

[6] Sjostrom L, Peltonen M, Jacobson P et al. Bariatric surgery and long-term cardiovascular events. JAMA 2012;307:56-65

[7] Sjostrom L, Lindroos AK, Peltonen M, Torgerson J, Bouchard C et al. Lifestyle, diabetes, and cardiovascular risk factors 10 years after bariatric surgery. N Engl J Med 2004;351:2683-93.

[8] Cardoso L, Rodrigues D, Gomes L, Carrilho F. Short-and long-term mortality after bariatric surgery: a systematic review and meta-analysis. Diabetes Obes Metab 2017;19:1223-1232.

[9] Nguyen N, Varela J. Bariatric surgery for obesity and metabolic disorders: state of the art. Nat Rev Gastroenterol Hepatol 2017;14:160-169.

[10] Mathurin P, Hollebecque A, Arnalsteen L, Buob D, Leteurtre E et al. Prosepctive study of the long-term effects of bariatric surgery on liver injury in patients without advanced disease. Gastroenterology 2009;137:532-540.

[11] Lassailly G, Caiazzo R, Buob D, Pigeyre M, Verkindt H et al. Bariatric surgery reduces features of nonalcoholic steatohepatitis in morbidly obese patients. Gastroenterology 2015;149:379-388.

[12] Lassailly G, Caiazzo R, Ntandja-Wandji LC, Gnemmi V, Baud G et al. Bariatric surgery provides long-term resolution of nonalcoholic steatohepatitis and regression of fibrosis. Gastroenterology 2020;159:1290-1301.

[13] Lee Y, Doumouras AG, Yu J, Brar K, Banfield L, Gmora S, Anvari M, Hong D. Complete resolution of nonalcoholic fatty liver disease after bariatric surgery: a systematic review and meta-analysis. Clinical gastroenterology and Hepatology 2019;17:1040-1060

[14] Mummadi R, Kasturi K, Chennareddygari S, Sood G. Effect of bariatric surgery on nonalcoholic fatty liver disease: systematic review and meat-analysis. Clin Gastroenterol Hepatol 2008;12:1396-402.

[15] Klebanoff MJ, Corey KE, Chhatwal J, Kaplan LM, Chung RT et al.Bariatric surgery for nonalcoholic steatohepatitis in morbidly obese patients. Gastroenterology 2015;149:379-388.

[16] Caiazzo R, Lassailly G, Leteurtre E, Baud G, Verkindt H et al. Roux-en-Y gastric bypass versus adjustable gastric banding to reduce nonalcoholic fatty liver disease: a 5 year controlled longitudinal study. Ann Surg 2014;260:893-8

[17] Berzigotti A, Garcia-Tsao G, Bosch J, Grace ND, Burroughs AK et al. Obesity is an independent risk factor for clinical decompensation in patients with cirrhosis. Hepatology 2011;54:555-61.

[18] Takata MC, Campos G, Ciovia R, Rabl C, Rogers S et al. Laparoscopic bariatric surgery improves candidacy in morbidly obese patients awaiting transplantation. Surg Obes Relat Dis 2008;4:159-164

[19] Lin MY, Tavakol MM, Sarin A, Amirkiai S, Rogers S et al. Laparscopic sleeve gastrectomy is safe and efficacious for pretransplant candidates. Surg Obes Relat Dis 2013;9:653-8

[20] Younus H, Sharma A, Miquel R, Uaglia A, Kanchustambam S et al. Bariatric surgery in cirrhotic patients: is it safe? Obes Surg 2020;30:1241-1248

[21] Spengler E, O'Leary J, Te H, Rogal S, Pillai A et al. Liver transplantation in the obese cirrhotic patient. Transplantation 2017;101:2288-2296.

[22] Jan A, Narwaria M, Mahawar K. A systematic review of bariatric surgery in patients with liver cirrhosis. Obes Surg 2015;25:1518-26

[23] Garcia-Sesma A, Calvo J, Manrique A, Cambra F, Justo I et al. Morbidly obese patients awaiting liver transplantation-sleeve gastrectomy: safety and efficacy from a liver transplant unit experience. Transplantation Proceddings 2019:51; 33-37

[24] Ayloo S, Guss C, Pentakota SR, Hanna J, Molinan M. Minimally invasive sleeve gastrectomy as a surgical treatment for nonalcoholic fatty liver disease in liver transplant recipients. Transplantation proceedings 2020;52:276-283

[25] Heimbach J, Watt K, Poterucha J, Francisco-Ziller N, Cecco S et al. Combined liver transplantation and gastric sleeve resection for patients with medically complicated obesity and end-stage liver disease. Am J Transplant 2013;13:363-8.

[26] Zamora-Valdes D, Watt K, Kellogg T, Poterucha J, Di Cecco S et al. Long-term outcomes of patients undergoing simultaneous liver transplantation and sleeve gastrectomy. Hepatology 2018;68: 485-495.

[27] Nesher E, Mor E, Shlomai A, Naftaly-Cohen M, Yemini R et al. Simultaneous liver transplantation and sleeve gastrectomy: prohibitive combination or a necessity? Obes Surg 2017;27:1387-1390.

[28] Tariciotti L, D'Ugo S, Manzia T, Tognoni V, Sica G et al. Combined liver transplantation and sleeve gastrectomy for end-stage liver disease in a bariatric patient; First European case-report. Int J Surg Case Rep 2016;28:38-41.

[29] Cotter T, Charlton M. Nonalcoholic steatohepatitis after liver transplantation. Liver Transplantation 2020;26:141-159.

[30] Dumortier J, Giostra E, Belbouab S, Morard I, Guillaud O et al. Non-alcoholic fatty liver disease in liver transplant recipients: another story of "seed and soil". Am J Gastroenterol 2010;105:613-20.

[31] Narayanan P, Mara K, Izzy M, Dierkhising R, Heimbach J et al. Recurrent or de novo allograft steatosis and long-term outcomes after liver transplantation. Transplantation 2019;103:e14-e21.

[32] Saeed N, Glass L, Sharma P, Shannon C, Sonnenday C, Tincopa M. Incidence and risks for nonalcoholic fatty liver disease and steatohepatitis post-liver transplant: systematic review and meta-analysis. Transplantation 2019;103

[33] Galvin Z, Rajakumar R, Chen E, Adeyi O, Selzner M et al. Predictors of de novo nonalcoholic fatty liver disease after liver transplantation and associated fibrosis. Liver transplantation 2019;25:56-67.

[34] Morris M, Jung A, Kim Y, Lee T, Kaiser T et al. Delayed sleeve gastrectomy following liver transplantation: a 5 year experience. Liver Transpl 2019;25:1673-1681.

[35] Elli EF, Gonzalez-Heredia R, Sanchez-Johnsen L, Patel N, Garcia-Roca R et al. Sleeve gastrectomy surgery in obese patients post-organ transplantation. Surg Obes Relat Dis 2016;12:528-534.

[36] Khoraki J, Katz MG, Funk LM, Greenberg JA, Fernandez LA et al. Feasibility and outcomes of laparoscopic sleeve gastrectomy after solid organ transplantation. Surg Obes Relat Dis 2016;12:75-83.

[37] Grimm IS, Schindler W, Haluszka O. Steatohepatitis and fatal hepatic failure after biliopancreatic diversion. Am J Gastroenterol 1992; 87:775.

[38] Geerts A, Darius T, Chapelle T, Roeyen G, Francque S et al. The multicenter belgian survey on liver transplantation for hepatocellular failure after bariatric surgery. Transplant Proc 2010, 42:4395-4398.

[39] Mahawar K, Parmar C, Graham Y, De Alwis N, Carr W et al. Monitoring of liver function tests after Roux-en-Y gastric bypass: an examination of evidence base. Obes Surg 2016;26:2516-2522.

[40] Shah K, Nergard BJ, Fagerland MW, Gislason H. Limb lenght in gastric bypass in super-obese patients importance of lenght of total almentary small bowel tract. Obes surg 2019 Jul:29(7):2012-21.

[41] Kraljevic M, Kostler T, Susstrunk J, Lazaridis I, Taheri A et al. Revisional surgery for insufficient loss or regain of weight after Roux-en-Y gastric bypass:biliopancreatic limb lenght matters. Obes Surg 2020; 30:804-811.

[42] D'Albuquerque MA, Gonzalez AM, Wahle RC, de Oliveira Souza E, Mancero JM et al.Liver transplantation for subacute hepatocellular failure due to massive steatohepatitis after bariatri surgery. Liver Transpl 2008;14:881-885.

[43] Lefere S, Hoorens A, Raevens S, Troisi R, Verhelst X,et al. Refractory subacute steatohepatitis after biliopancreatic diversion. Hepatology 2017;66:289-291.

Section 8

Liver Cirrhosis and Complications

Chapter 11

Spontaneous Bacterial Peritonitis: Physiopathological Mechanism and Clinical Manifestations

Rebeca Pérez-Cabeza De Vaca, Balasubramaniyan Vairappan, Tomás Cortés Espinoza, Juan Antonio Suárez Cuenca, Cuauhtemoc Licona Cassani, Brenda Maldonado Arriaga, Chrisitan Navarro Gerrard, Diana Selene Morgan Penagos, Paul Mondragón Terán and Victoria Chagoya De Sanchez

Abstract

Changes in intestinal permeability have been determined to influence secondary inflammatory reactions and clinical manifestations such as spontaneous bacterial peritonitis (SBP) secondary to cirrhosis. As of yet, no in-depth exploration of the changes in the microbiota and how this influences cirrhosis to differ from clinically more severe cases than others has not begun. However, at the level of pathophysiological mechanism, it must be taken into account that due to the abuse of substances such as alcohol and chronic fatty liver disease, changes in the bacterial composition and intestinal permeability are induced. This set of changes in the bacterial composition (microbiome) and modification of the intestinal permeability could be related to the presence of ascites and spontaneous peritonitis secondary to cirrhosis, being of relevance the knowledge of the mechanisms underlying this phenomenon, as well as clinical manifestation. Prophylaxis and antibiotic treatment of SBP requires clinical knowledge for the treatment decisions based mainly on the presence of ascitic fluid, accompanied of risk factors, laboratory indexes such as PMN count and culture results, in order to determine the kind of molecule that will help to the SBP recovery or to amelioration symptoms, always taking care of not exceed the antibiotic consumption and restoring the microbiome imbalance.

Keywords: bacteria, peritonitis, microbiome, cirrhosis, gut permeability

1. Introduction

In cirrhotic patients with ascites, spontaneous bacterial peritonitis (SBP), an ominous complication, occurs recurrently with an annual increase rate of 69% [1]. Furthermore, in cirrhosis with portal hypertension, SBP is a key hallmark feature in developing hepatic encephalopathy, variceal bleeding, hepatorenal syndrome and increased mortality [2]. Also, intestinal barrier dysfunction is pondered central in the pathogenesis of cirrhotic complications. In health, intestinal barrier function is

IntechOpen

crucial against extensive and continuous exposure of the liver to the gut microbiota and their products and metabolites. Thus, gut microbiome sets the stage for the gut-liver axis [3]. Nevertheless, in cirrhosis, intestinal barrier dysfunction, increased permeability and extensive inflammation occurs due to SBP. The intestinal barrier consists of several layers, including mucus layer, intestinal epithelial cells, lamina propria and Peyer's patches. They determine the extent to which gut microbes and their products (endotoxin) can access the host vasculature [4].

Therefore, the intestinal vascular barrier is considered an important layer controlling the entry of gut bacterial products into the portal circulation and liver [5]. Gut microbiota may therefore have a prime role in a pathologic loop, which regulates portal hypertension, and thus have a role in the cirrhosis development.

SBP is a frequent and severe complication in cirrhotic patients with ascites. On the other hand, cirrhotic complication initiates dysregulation of intestinal AMP and bacterial overgrowth, which triggers mucosal inflammation. The proinflammatory cytokine milieu in the intestinal lumen plays a critical role in disrupting the tight junction protein integrity, leading to BT. Bacterial endotoxin and harmful pathogenic bacterial species translocate to the liver through portal vein further exacerbate the already prevalent hepatic inflammation and fibrosis in the liver, causing a cyclic progression of liver injury. Pathogenic bacteria and endotoxins also translocate to blood causes systemic inflammatory responses induced by cytokines, chemokines and interferons resulting cytokine storm syndrome and hemodynamic abnormalities, thereby promotes liver injury followed by multiorgan failure and eventually it causes death.

2. The pathophysiological mechanism involved in spontaneous bacterial peritonitis in cirrhosis: loss of permeability and gut microbiota

Peritonitis occurs in patients with cirrhosis and ascites, in the absence of any other intra-abdominal cause of infection, such as an abscess or intestinal perforation. The spontaneous bacterial peritonitis (SBP) is defined as an infection of the ascites fluid, which produces an inflammatory reaction of the peritoneum and as previously described. It has been associated with intestinal dysbiosis, since it leads to dysfunction of the intestinal barrier that can cause bacterial translocation of very small quantities of viable or dead bacteria, constituting a physiologically important reinforcement for the immune system. Bacterial translocation is defined as the passage of bacteria or bacterial products that go from the intestine to the mesenteric lymph nodes.

2.1 Bacterial translocation

Due to the close anatomical and physiological connections between the liver and gut, barrier dysfunction results in translocation of viable bacteria and its product to the liver via the portal circulation, thereby causing liver dysfunction. Several experimental studies showed that cirrhotic patients had increased intestinal permeability which might be a critical contributing factor to cirrhosis development [6, 7]. In addition, microbial overgrowth has been observed in intrahepatic cholestatic patients [8]. Bacterial infections such as SBP and bacteraemia are associated with the four-fold increased death rate in cirrhotic patients [9]. In this context, it was observed that the presence of bacterial DNA in the blood and ascitic fluid of cirrhotic patients developed poor prognosis compared to cirrhotic patients who had negative for bacterial DNA [10]. Bacterial translocation (BT) initiates a cycle of dysfunctional immune activation, and systemic inflammatory response, facilitating the worsening of pre-existing hepatic and hemodynamic abnormalities in cirrhosis [11]. Identification of bacterial DNA has been associated with worsening of intrahepatic endothelial dysfunction and extra-hepatic (peripheral) vasodilation [12]. Further, lipopolysaccharide-binding protein (LBP) is a surrogate marker for BT, correlated with systemic hemodynamic abnormalities in cirrhotic patients [13]. Endotoxemia has been closely associated with hyperdynamic circulation, coagulopathy, portal hypertension, renal and cardiac dysfunction in cirrhosis [14]. Furthermore, systemic inflammatory response syndrome (SIRS) with bacterial infection shows an increased risk of 67% in cirrhotic patients suggesting that SIRS also contributing to cirrhosis prognosis **Figure 1** [15].

2.2 Gut dysbiosis

Bacterial dysbiosis is characterized by the pathogenic shift in quantity or quality from the symbiotic state existing between the host and indigenous bacteria [16, 17]. A marked alteration has been observed in the small intestinal microbiota in patients with cirrhosis compared to normal individuals. A ratio of autochthonous to non-autochthonous bacterial taxa is referred to as cirrhosis dysbiosis ratio (CDR). Patients with cirrhosis were shown to exhibit a lower CDR [16]. The pathogenic shift in the proportion of bacterial taxa is also associated with decompensation of cirrhosis. The disruption of microbial balance in cirrhosis leads to accumulation of harmful bacterial metabolites that damage the intestinal epithelial barrier [16]. Gut dysbiosis also leads to intestinal immune system dysregulation by changing the composition of short-chain fatty acids produced by the microbiota [17]. This immune dysregulation with functional proinflammatory switch

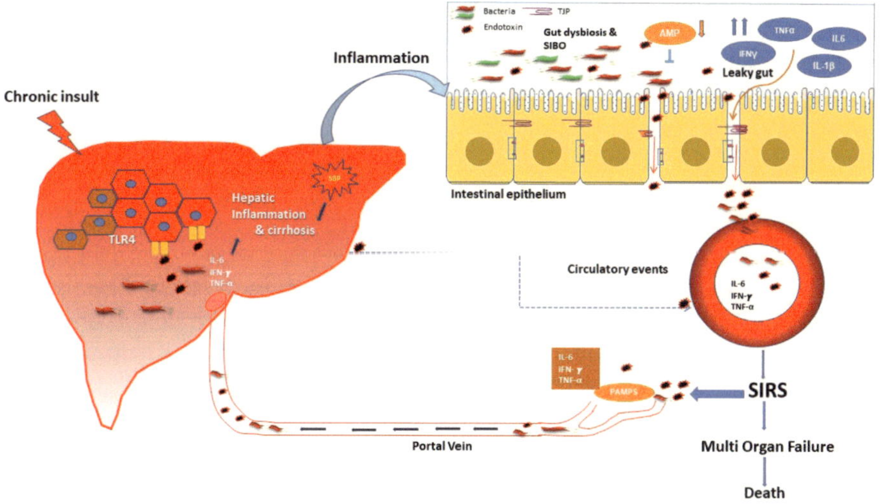

Figure 1.
The pathophysiological mechanism associated with BT and SBP in decompensated cirrhosis. SBP is a frequent and severe complication in cirrhotic patients with ascites. On the other hand, cirrhotic complication initiates dysregulation of intestinal AMP and bacterial overgrowth, which triggers mucosal inflammation. The proinflammatory cytokine milieu in the intestinal lumen plays a critical role in disrupting the tight junction protein integrity, leading to BT. Bacterial endotoxin and harmful pathogenic bacterial species translocate to the liver through portal vein further exacerbate the already prevalent hepatic inflammation and fibrosis in the liver, causing a cyclic progression of liver injury. Pathogenic bacteria and endotoxins also translocate to blood causes systemic inflammatory responses induced by cytokines, chemokines and interferons resulting cytokine storm syndrome and hemodynamic abnormalities, thereby promotes liver injury followed by multiorgan failure and eventually it causes death. Note: AMP-anti microbial peptides; BT-bacterial translocation; IFN-Interferon; IL-interleukin; IJP-tight junction protein; SBP-spontaneous bacterial peritonitis; TLR-toll-like receptor; TNF-tumor necrosis factor.

contributes to mucosal barrier dysfunction and BT [17] and thus, bile acids (BA) derangement, which plays a causal role in the gut dysbiosis.

In cirrhotic patients, intraluminal BA reduction was shown to increase deconjugation by enteric bacteria [18]. Moreover, defect in intestinal BA concentration accelerates BT and develops susceptibility to bacterial endotoxin [19]. Intestinal dysmotility is another important contributor to the development of SBP in cirrhotic patients [20].

2.3 Tight junctions and intestinal permeability

Increased intestinal permeability exerts a pivotal role in the pathogenesis of SBP in cirrhosis following elevated systemic endotoxemia. Moreover, a significant association was found between elevated portal pressure and gastro-duodenal and intestinal permeability in cirrhosis [21]. Specific ultrastructural and functional alterations in the intestinal mucosa have been identified in cirrhosis patients associated with increased intestinal permeability to BT [22]. The intestinal barrier comprises tight junction (TJ) proteins that allow specific passage of gut bacterial products and metabolites, thus maintaining intestinal structural integrity and regulating intestinal permeability following SBP [23]. Zona occludens (ZO-1), occludin and claudins are the major integral transmembrane proteins composed of TJ and maintaining the intestinal permeability [24]. The TJ proteins expression and turnover are predisposed by oxidative stress and inflammation following SBP in cirrhosis, consequently, disruption of the intestinal barrier allows bacterial endotoxin from the intestinal lumen to pass into the portal circulation and thus reaches the liver culminating hepatic complications (**Figure 1**). Significant alterations in occludin were observed in intestine of both compensated decompensated cirrhotic patients compared to healthy subjects [6, 7]. Notably, the reduction in intestinal occludin expression was associated with elevated endotoxins levels and severe variceal bleeding [6]. We found significantly decreased hepatic ZO 1 levels in patients with cirrhosis and HCC [25]. Furthermore, our rodent experimental data show evidence that in cirrhosis and HCC, diminished hepatic expression of ZO-1 and occludin was correlated with BT [25, 26].

2.4 Small intestinal bacterial overgrowth (SIBO)

Small intestinal bacterial overgrowth (SIBO) induced by prolonged gastric and small intestinal transit of bacterial products and metabolites. It is a condition in which colonic bacterial translocate into the small intestine [27]. The process of bacterial dysbiosis, coupled with SIBO, is well documented in cirrhosis [16, 28]. Increased proportion of the gram-negative Bacteroides species and the gram-positive *Enterococcus spp.* were identified in the small intestine of patients with alcoholic liver disease [28]. SIBO is also accompanied by a decrease in *Lactobacillus spp.*, which is regarded as beneficial to the host [29]. SIBO coupled with bacterial dysbiosis (**Figure 1**) leads to accumulation of bacterial endotoxins such as LPS, an specific PAMP (Pathogen Associated Molecular Patterns), which in turn results in the induction of inflammatory response culminating in intestinal epithelial damage and gut permeability [30] this mechanism will be explained deeply ahead in this chapter. Cirrhotic patients who use proton pump inhibitors are vulnerable to SBP, due to intestinal overgrowth of *Enterococcus spp*. [31, 32]. Antimicrobial peptides (AMP) are considered the first line of defence to counter bacterial overgrowth and maintain bacterial symbiosis, which are primarily produced by paneth cells and intestinal epithelial cells [33]. Decreased AMP was pronounced in the ileum, which was associated with increased BT in cirrhosis [34]. Also, human and experimental

ALD attributed to decreased AMP expression [33, 35]. Regenerating family member 3 alpha [Reg3A] belongs to the C-type lectin family is one of the important AMP in regulating intestinal inflammation [36] and facilitating the repair of gut mucosa in rodent models. Moreover, our recent study shows that Reg3A protein expression was significantly reduced in cirrhotic mice small intestine [37]. We also found significantly decreased Lactobacillus and increased *Bacteroides* and *Enterococcus* 16 s rRNA levels in the liver and small intestine of cirrhotic mice [37]. This reduced intestinal Reg3A expression was associated with an increased E*nterococcus* translocation to rodent cirrhotic liver. Similarly, Darnaud et al., observed that Reg3A overexpression in colitis mice attenuated intestinal inflammation and restricted BT [36]. Moreover, Reg3A expression protected against dextran sulphate sodium (DSS)-induced intestinal inflammation, intestinal permeability and BT in mice [36]. In addition, intestinal Reg3A has been reported to promote the enrichments of *Lactobacilli sp* [38] and depletion of *Bacteroidetes* population [36], indicating Reg3A could be a critical factor in restricting BT by averting bacterial dysbiosis. Cathelin-related antimicrobial peptide (CRAMP) is an AMP produced by intestinal epithelial cells exhibits potent antibiotic activity against various strains of gram-negative bacteria [39]. Deficiency of CRAMP expression correlated with impaired microbial clearance and elevated proinflammatory cytokine response in glial cells exposed to bacterial endotoxins [40]. We found CRAMP cellular expression in the small intestine of cirrhotic mice albeit, no significant difference between control and cirrhotic mice [37].

2.5 Inflammation in spontaneous bacterial peritonitis

Inflammation and oxidative stress are other key players contributing to mucosal damage and cirrhosis progression by triggering cytokine productions. Activation of Kupffer cells and the recruitment of proinflammatory monocyte subsets could propagate both intra-hepatic and extra-hepatic (systemic) inflammation [41, 42]. Of note, the cirrhotic patients with bacterial infections exhibited elevated systemic levels of inflammatory and pyrogenic cytokines IL-6 and TNF-α compared to septicemia patients without cirrhosis [43]. IL-6 levels in cirrhotic patients correlated with immune cell activation, organ failure, and portal hypertension [14, 44]. Moreover, soluble TNF-α receptor levels in hepatic venous and portal venous blood correlated with endotoxin concentration as well as hemodynamic derangements in cirrhosis [45]. Hence endotoxin-induced proinflammatory cytokines serve as important mediators of SIRS induced-hemodynamic abnormalities in cirrhosis. In this context, our experimental data show evidence that significantly elevated ascitic fluid cytokine concentrations in cirrhotic mice [37]. Gastrointestinal tract inflammation was contemplated as a major mediator of TJ disruption. Decreased TJ proteins ZO-1 and occludin were reported in gastric carcinoma with inflammation [46]. In cirrhosis with SBP, intestinal barrier disruption has been precipitated by inflammation [26]. Proinflammatory cytokines such as TNF alpha, IL-I beta and IFN gamma trigger barrier damage on the gut epithelium by inducing endocytosis of TJ proteins and increased expression of myosin light chain kinase protein, thereby causing TJ permeability [17, 26]. Intestinal mucosa covered by the mucus layer provides a first line of defence mechanism against harmful bacteria and endotoxin from invading the microvillus environment [30]. Inflammatory mediators, LPS and growth factors affect the secretion of mucin, which is present in the mucus layer. In particular, nuclear factor-κB [NF-κB] binds with the specific site of the promoter region of mucin and affect its secretion [47]. Therefore, modulation of bacterial adherence to the gut mucosal surface by intestinal mucus results in loss of gut barrier function [48]. In this context, a previous experimental study shows evidence in cirrhotic rats ileum that increased mucin 2&3 mRNA expression compared to control [49]. Moreover, increased mucus content in the small intestine was found following chronic alcohol supplementation to rats [30].

In cirrhosis, SBP is a major precipitating factor initiates gut-liver axis dysfunction. It is mainly due to the fact that intestinal microbiota dysbiosis, bacterial overgrowth and bacterial translocation [4], which originates intestinal mucosal dysfunction and damage at the systemic immune cell functions [50]. Moreover, inflammation and oxidative stress are other contributing factors that can influence the barrier function of both the small and the large intestine and probably result in the occurrence of SBP in cirrhosis.

2.6 Microbiota in spontaneous bacterial peritonitis consequence

The gut microbiota plays a key role in spontaneous bacterial peritonitis due to intestinal dysbiosis and bacterial translocation. A study conducted by Lachar & Bajaj, 2016, demonstrated that patients with spontaneous bacterial peritonitis presented intestinal dysbiosis, and thus concluded that it can be a useful quantitative index to describe the microbiome alterations that accompany the progression and complications of cirrhosis [51].

The term microbiota refers to the community of living microorganisms that reside in a specific ecological niche. In the gastrointestinal tract, the microbiota is a dynamic system that maintains a symbiotic relationship with the intestinal mucosa. This relationship imparts metabolic, protective and immune functions that contribute to the well-being of the host, which are modified by environmental factors. Additionally, it participates in metabolic processes that connect the intestine with liver, muscle and brain [52, 53]. The eubiosis microbiota comprises a balance between symbiotic microorganisms [bacteria with homeostasis-promoting functions] and pathobionts [commensal bacteria with the ability to induce pathology]. However, the dysregulation of this balance can determine a state of dysbiosis [54] (**Figure 2A**). Therefore, alterations in the intestinal microbiota are important in the pathogenesis of several complications that arise in liver disease, such as spontaneous bacterial peritonitis. This is usually caused by the presence of one or more species of aerobic and anaerobic enteric bacteria that act in synergy [55–59] (**Figure 2B**).

The most common microorganisms associated with this disorder are Gram-negative bacteria, such as *Escherichia coli* and *Klebsiella* species, and infections by Gram-positive bacteria such as *Staphylococcus*. Gram negative bacilli, especially *Escherichia coli*, which are found in low concentrations in the small intestine of healthy subjects, these are increased as jejunal microbiota in many cirrhotic patients, especially in those patients with more advanced cirrhosis and a greater decrease in the intestinal motility. *Escherichia coli* is known to be the main cause of SBP and is more frequently isolated in ascites fluid, in previous studies it has been described that the isolation rate is 66.6%. An increase in endotoxin levels in patients with advanced cirrhosis has been shown to promote the production of multiple pro-inflammatory elements, so the activation of this cytokine cascade in spontaneous bacterial peritonitis has been associated with greater complications leading to death [60–62].

In recent years the prevalence of Gram-positive bacteria in SBP has increased. In addition, there is a growing resistance to multiple drugs such as quinolones, which is of particular importance since norfloxacin represents the antimicrobial of choice for SBP. But this has changed dramatically, as multidrug resistant organisms (MDRO) have been described [63]. A study carried out by Mücke *et al.*

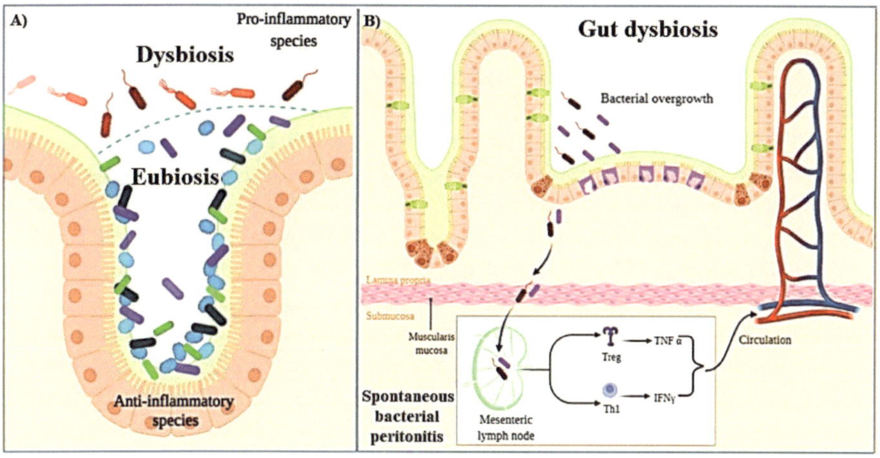

Figure 2.
The role of the gut microbiota in spontaneous bacterial peritonitis. (A) Ecology of the gut microbiota. Ecological community in balance of symbiotic microorganisms (anti-inflammatory species) and pathobionts (pro-inflammatory species) that share a certain niche and are considered an important factor in health or disease. (B) Bacterial translocation in spontaneous bacterial peritonitis. From the intestinal lumen, in a state of dysbiosis, bacteria (gram-negative bacilli of enteric origin and to a lesser extent gram-positive) cross the intestinal barrier and infect the mesenteric lymph nodes, a process known as bacterial translocation, and from there they reach the blood circulation through of the lymphatic pathway leading to the hepatosplenic and systemic circulation. Which leads to the development of an inflammatory reaction in the mesenteric lymph nodes themselves with the release of pro-inflammatory cytokines. TRL-4 is responsible for the production of TNF-α in response to endotoxin, while Th1 cells release interferon γ.

demonstrated that the presence of MDRO and quinolone-resistant Gram-negative bacteria (QR-GNB) has been associated with the failure of antimicrobial prophylaxis [64].

There is great concern worldwide about the increase in antimicrobial resistance, which has now been associated with SBP. Appropriate antimicrobial therapy should be administered as soon as possible, as inappropriate administration increases hospital mortality. Unfortunately, it has been reported that treatment protocols still support the use of third-generation cephalosporins as a first line of therapy [65–67]. In a meta-analysis carried out by Iogna *et al.*, showed that there is significant uncertainty about the choice of antimicrobial therapy that is best in people with SBP. It is important to highlight that the short-term mortality from spontaneous bacterial peritonitis (SBP) is high, approximately 25% [68]. Therefore, having the result of the culture, and an antimicrobial regimen with a narrower spectrum should be started. Based on these findings, it is essential to perform a microbiological surveillance for the use of the correct use of antimicrobials.

3. Clinical manifestations of spontaneous bacterial peritonitis and diagnostic

Patients with liver cirrhosis (LC) and ascites are at a high risk of developing bacterial infections, spontaneous bacterial peritonitis [SBP] can be a life-threatening infection in these patients [69]. The diagnosis of SBP is based on the patient's signs and symptoms, in addition to the findings at diagnostic paracentesis in a patient with ascites fluid. The patient with peritonitis may have symptoms such as abdominal pain, nausea, vomiting, diarrhea and signs of a systemic inflammatory response (hyper or hypothermia, chills, altered white blood cell count, tachycardia, and/or tachypnea), also presenting with worsening of liver function, hepatic encephalopathy, shock, kidney failure and gastrointestinal bleeding. However, it is important to note that SBP can be asymptomatic particularly in outpatients [70].

Diagnostic paracentesis should be performed in all patients who present symptoms is extremely important, as the PMN count in the ascitic fluid plays an essential role in obtaining a diagnosis of SBP [71]. However, clinical signs and symptoms are occasionally absent in patients with SBP [72]. The diagnosis of SBP is confirmed based on a PMN count of >250 cells/mm3 in the ascitic fluid cell analysis (**Figure 3**). The cutoff value of 250 PMN cells/mm3 has the greatest sensitivity, whereas 500 PMN cells/mm3 exhibits the greatest specificity [73].

The gold standard for ascitic neutrophil count is manual microscopy, but it is labor intensive and associated with interobserver variability, time and costs. In most places this has been substituted with automated counts based on flow cytometry for counting and differentiating cells. This technique has been documented to have high linearity with manual microscopy and thus sensitivity and specificity close to 100% [74].

3.1 Clinical manifestations of spontaneous bacterial peritonitis.

For Spontaneous bacterial peritonitis (SBP) the diagnosis is established based on positive ascitic fluid bacterial cultures and the detection of an elevated absolute fluid polymorphonuclear neutrophil (PMN) count in the ascites (>250/mm^3) without an evident intra-abdominal surgically treatable source of infection (**Figure 3**). In addition, ascitic fluid cultures are negative in approximately 10–60% of patients with clinical manifestations of SBP [75].

The Secondary Bacterial Peritonitis, that differs of Spontaneous bacterial peritonitis (SBP) consists of ascitic fluid infection due to intraabdominal infections, for example, perforation of gastrointestinal tract or abscess. It is much less frequent, but has still high mortality rate compared with SBP in patients with LC [76].

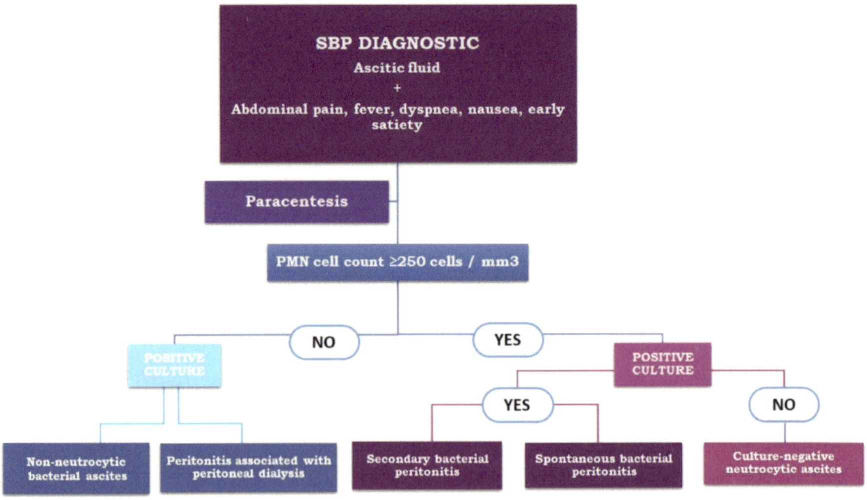

Figure 3.
*Recommended empirical antibiotic treatment for SBP. Community-acquired agents are treated with 3rd generation Cephalosporins, Amoxicilin/Clavulanic acid, Ciprofloxacin, Ofloxacin or Piperacilin/Tazobactam. Health care associated and nosocomial agents are treated with Piperacilin/Tazobactam or a Carbapenem antibiotic. For profilaxis of SPB, Norfloxacin is the agent of choice. (Figure adapted from [66]). *In case of multidrug resistant organism.*

Non-neutrocytic bacterial ascites or Bacterascites: is an ascitic fluid polymorphonuclear -neutrophil (PMN) count below 250/μL and a positive ascitic fluid culture results in the absence of an evident intra-abdominal, surgically treatable source of infection. It is a different clinical entity than spontaneous bacterial peritonitis (SBP), which is characterized by a neutrophil reaction in ascites regardless of the bacterial culture result. Bacterascites is prevalent in 8–11% of all patients with cirrhosis and ascites, and the clinical significance seems to vary according to how the infection was acquired [77].

3.2 Treatment of spontaneous bacterial peritonitis

Even though the spectrum of this chapter does not contemplate treatment modalities we thought it best to give an updated brief view of the treatment involved in SBP in an easy diagram (**Figure 4**). First step is to acknowledge and apply the indication of a paracentesis, which are the following according to multiple clinical practice guidelines: All patients with new onset grade 2 or 3 of ascites, in those hospitalized for worsening of ascites or any complication of cirrhosis. Other indications are new onset of ascites, any patient admitted to the hospital with preexisting ascites, regardless of the reason for admission and ascites who has signs of clinical deterioration [78]. Once the diagnosis of SBP is made the treatment modalities must be applied as soon as possible (**Figure 4**). These empiric treatment schemes should also be administered if the patient has a diagnosis of culture-negative neutrocyte ascites and monomicrobial non-neutrocytic bacterial ascites or bacterial ascites. Particularly the treatment decision differs from the community acquired SBP from the nosocomial one, considering the risk factors, other comorbidities treatment and the previous use of antibiotic (3 months at least) to prescribe the specific drug, because the microbiome involucrate in each case requires a different antibiotic. For example, the use of 3rd. generation cephalosporines in community acquired SBP, not such as the treatment suggested in the nosocomial acquired SPB that the carbapenem is indicated as first therapeutic option.

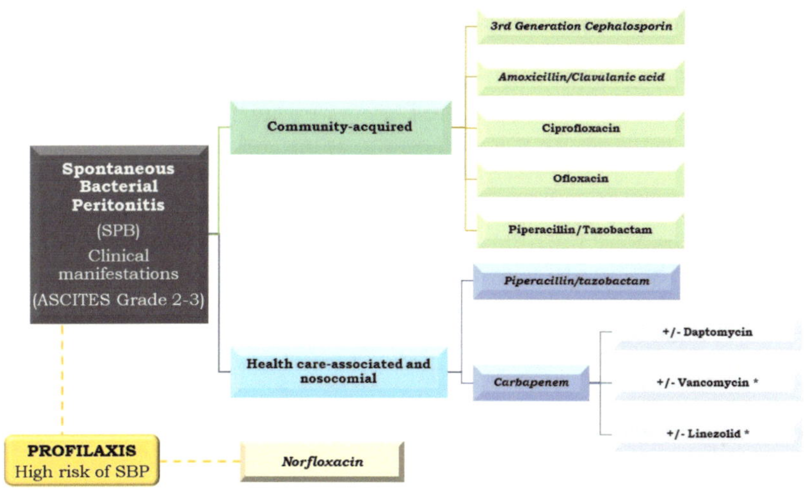

Figure 4.
Diagnostic algorithm of SBP. The diagnosis of SBP is established based on positive ascitic fluid bacterial cultures and the detection of an elevated absolute fluid polymorphonuclear neutrophil (PMN) count in the ascites (>250/mm³) without an evident intra-abdominal surgically treatable source of infection, except in peritonitis associated with peritoneal dialysis, where bacteria can enter the body through the open ends of the PD catheter during exchanges.

The efficacy of antibiotic therapy should ideally be revised doing a second paracentesis at 48 hours from the starting treatment. One should suspect either resistance to antibiotics, secondary bacterial peritonitis or fungal peritonitis if the patient exhibits worsening clinical signs and symptoms or does not have a marked reduction in the leucocyte count of at least 25% [78, 79]. In addition to the antibiotics administered it is vital to administer albumin 1.5 g/kg body weight at diagnosis followed by 1 g/kg on day three. This in order to significantly decrease the incidence of type 1 Hepatorenal syndrome and mortality in up to 30% of the cases [78].

Another important topic is the prophylaxis of SBP in high risk patients which in which in summary are three: (1) Patients with acute gastrointestinal hemorrhage; (2) Patients with less than 15 g/L of ascitic fluid protein; (3) Patients with previous history of SBP. For the prophylaxis of SBP in high risk patients the recommended prophylaxis schemes are with norfloxacin [79]. Healthcare providers must be very conscious when they are considering the use of prophylactic antibiotics balancing the risks of generating gastrointestinal complications secondary to gut dysbiosis *vs* the benefits of preventing an event of SBP. As healthcare workers one must avoid the abuse of antibiotic use, it is important to know and apply these indications, and imperative to be clear in which antibiotic can be used in these specific cases, and avoid the use of broad spectrum antibiotics.

4. Conclusions

In cirrhotic patients, the intestinal barrier dysfunction increased permeability, and extensive inflammation occurs due to Spontaneous Bacterial Peritonitis. Clinically, the SBP is a frequent and severe complication in cirrhotic patients with ascites. It is well documented that bacterial endotoxin and harmful pathogenic bacterial species translocate to the liver through portal vein further exacerbate the already prevalent hepatic inflammation and fibrosis driven by hepatocytes destruction and loss of biochemical functionality, thereby these phenomena promote liver injury followed by multiorgan failure and eventually death in a high percentage of cirrhotic patients.

In this analysis were described that microbiota plays an essential role in this pathological process, but it is also related to gut permeability loss due to previous treatments or the inflammation sustained signalling by hepatic lesion immunological response.

Clinically, a flux for diagnostic and treatment was proposed for SBP, that includes de analysis of ascitic fluid and polymorphonuclear cells as consequence.

It is suggested that there is a lot of task to do in public health, in order to control the self-medication and the excess of antibiotic therapy, in order to avoid microbiota dysbiosis and SBP.

Acknowledgements

Programa Presupuestal E015 de Investigación y Desarrollo Tecnológico en Salud, ISSSTE.

Conflict of interest

The authors declare no conflict of interest.

Author details

Rebeca Pérez-Cabeza De Vaca[1,6*], Balasubramaniyan Vairappan[2], Tomás Cortés Espinoza[3], Juan Antonio Suárez Cuenca[4], Cuauhtemoc Licona Cassani[5], Brenda Maldonado Arriaga[4], Chrisitan Navarro Gerrard[3], Diana Selene Morgan Penagos[3], Paul Mondragón Terán[4] and Victoria Chagoya De Sanchez[6]

1 Biomedical Research Division, Centro Médico Nacional “20 de Noviembre” ISSSTE, Mexico City, Mexico

2 Department of Biochemistry, Jawaharlal Institute of Postgraduate Medical Education and Research (JIPMER), Pondicherry, India

3 Department of Gastroenterology, Clínica de Enfermedad Inflamatoria Intestinal, Centro Médico Nacional “20 de Noviembre” ISSSTE, Mexico City, Mexico

4 Laboratorio de Metabolismo Experimental e Investigación Clínica, Coordinación de Investigación, Centro Médico Nacional “20 de Noviembre” ISSSTE, Mexico City, Mexico

5 Centro de Biotecnología-FEMSA, Tecnológico de Monterrey, Monterrey, Mexico

6 Departamento de Biología Celular y Desarrollo, Laboratorio 305-Sur, Instituto de Fisiología Celular, UNAM, Mexico City, Mexico

*Address all correspondence to: esderebk@gmail.com

References

[1] Trad D, Sabbah M, Jlassi H, Ouakaa A, Bibani N, Elloumi H and Gargouri D. Spontaneous Bacterial Peritonitis in Cirrhotic Patients: Predictive Factors of Recurrence and Survival. Annals of Clinical Hepatology. Remedy Publications LLC. 2019; 3[2];1013: 1-6

[2] Dever JB, Sheikh MY. Review article: spontaneous bacterial peritonitis--bacteriology, diagnosis, treatment, risk factors and prevention. Aliment Pharmacol Ther. 2015;41[11]:1116-31.

[3] Tripathi A, Debelius J, Brenner DA, Karin M, Loomba R, Schnabl B, et al. The gut-liver axis and the intersection with the microbiome. Nat Rev Gastroenterol Hepatol. 2018;15[7]:397-411.

[4] Riva A, Gray EH, Azarian S, Zamalloa A, McPhail MJW, Vincent RP, et al. Faecal cytokine profiling as a marker of intestinal inflammation in acutely decompensated cirrhosis. JHEP Rep. 2020;2[6]:100151.

[5] Spadoni I, Zagato E, Bertocchi A, Paolinelli R, Hot E, Di Sabatino A, et al. A gut-vascular barrier controls the systemic dissemination of bacteria. Science. 2015;350[6262]:830-4.

[6] Assimakopoulos SF, Tsamandas AC, Tsiaoussis GI, Karatza E, Triantos C, Vagianos CE, et al. Altered intestinal tight junctions' expression in patients with liver cirrhosis: a pathogenetic mechanism of intestinal hyperpermeability. Eur J Clin Invest. 2012;42[4]:439-46.

[7] Pijls KE, Koek GH, Elamin EE, de Vries H, Masclee AA, Jonkers DM. Large intestine permeability is increased in patients with compensated liver cirrhosis. Am J Physiol Gastrointest Liver Physiol. 2014;306[2]:G147-53.

[8] Lisowska A, Kobelska-Dubiel N, Jankowska I, Pawlowska J, Moczko J, Walkowiak J. Small intestinal bacterial overgrowth in patients with progressive familial intrahepatic cholestasis. Acta Biochim Pol. 2014;61[1]:103-7.

[9] Arvaniti V, D'Amico G, Fede G, Manousou P, Tsochatzis E, Pleguezuelo M, et al. Infections in patients with cirrhosis increase mortality four-fold and should be used in determining prognosis. Gastroenterology. 2010;139[4]:1246-56, 56 e1-5.

[10] Zapater P, Frances R, Gonzalez-Navajas JM, de la Hoz MA, Moreu R, Pascual S, et al. Serum and ascitic fluid bacterial DNA: a new independent prognostic factor in noninfected patients with cirrhosis. Hepatology. 2008;48[6]:1924-31.

[11] Bruns T, Zimmermann HW, Stallmach A. Risk factors and outcome of bacterial infections in cirrhosis. World J Gastroenterol. 2014;20[10]:2542-54.

[12] Bellot P, Garcia-Pagan JC, Frances R, Abraldes JG, Navasa M, Perez-Mateo M, et al. Bacterial DNA translocation is associated with systemic circulatory abnormalities and intrahepatic endothelial dysfunction in patients with cirrhosis. Hepatology. 2010;52[6]:2044-52.

[13] Albillos A, de la Hera A, Gonzalez M, Moya JL, Calleja JL, Monserrat J, et al. Increased lipopolysaccharide binding protein in cirrhotic patients with marked immune and hemodynamic derangement. Hepatology. 2003;37[1]:208-17.

[14] Fukui H. Gut-liver axis in liver cirrhosis: How to manage leaky gut and endotoxemia. World J Hepatol. 2015;7[3]:425-42.

[15] Cazzaniga M, Dionigi E, Gobbo G, Fioretti A, Monti V, Salerno F. The systemic inflammatory response syndrome in cirrhotic patients: relationship with their in-hospital outcome. J Hepatol. 2009;51[3]:475-82.

[16] Bajaj JS, Heuman DM, Hylemon PB, Sanyal AJ, White MB, Monteith P, et al. Altered profile of human gut microbiome is associated with cirrhosis and its complications. J Hepatol. 2014;60[5]:940-7.

[17] Munoz L, Borrero MJ, Ubeda M, Conde E, Del Campo R, Rodriguez-Serrano M, et al. Intestinal Immune Dysregulation Driven by Dysbiosis Promotes Barrier Disruption and Bacterial Translocation in Rats With Cirrhosis. Hepatology. 2019;70[3]:925-38.

[18] Ridlon JM, Alves JM, Hylemon PB, Bajaj JS. Cirrhosis, bile acids and gut microbiota: unraveling a complex relationship. Gut Microbes. 2013;4[5]:382-7.

[19] Parks RW, Clements WD, Smye MG, Pope C, Rowlands BJ, Diamond T. Intestinal barrier dysfunction in clinical and experimental obstructive jaundice and its reversal by internal biliary drainage. Br J Surg. 1996;83[10]:1345-9.

[20] Guarner C, Soriano G. Bacterial translocation and its consequences in patients with cirrhosis. Eur J Gastroenterol Hepatol. 2005;17[1]:27-31.

[21] Arab JP, Martin-Mateos RM, Shah VH. Gut-liver axis, cirrhosis and portal hypertension: the chicken and the egg. Hepatol Int. 2018;12 [Suppl 1]:24-33.

[22] Bhonchal S, Nain CK, Prasad KK, Nada R, Sharma AK, Sinha SK, et al. Functional and morphological alterations in small intestine mucosa of chronic alcoholics. J Gastroenterol Hepatol. 2008;23[7 Pt 2]:e43-8.

[23] Kim S, Goel R, Kumar A, Qi Y, Lobaton G, Hosaka K, et al. Imbalance of gut microbiome and intestinal epithelial barrier dysfunction in patients with high blood pressure. Clin Sci [Lond]. 2018;132[6]:701-18.

[24] Vairappan B, Sundhar M, Srinivas BH. Resveratrol Restores Neuronal Tight Junction Proteins Through Correction of Ammonia and Inflammation in CCl4-Induced Cirrhotic Mice. Mol Neurobiol. 2019;56[7]:4718-29.

[25] Ram AK, Balasubramaniyan V, Srinivas BH. Nimbolide inhibits tumor growth by restoring hepatic tight junction protein expression and reduced inflammation in an experimental hepatocarcinogenesis. World J Gastroenterol. 2020;26[45]:7131-52.

[26] Mohandas S, Vairappan B. Pregnane X receptor activation by its natural ligand Ginkgolide-A improves tight junction proteins expression and attenuates bacterial translocation in cirrhosis. Chem Biol Interact. 2020;315:108891.

[27] Bernardi M. Spontaneous bacterial peritonitis: from pathophysiology to prevention. Intern Emerg Med. 2010;5 Suppl 1:S37-44.

[28] Bauer TM, Steinbruckner B, Brinkmann FE, Ditzen AK, Schwacha H, Aponte JJ, et al. Small intestinal bacterial overgrowth in patients with cirrhosis: prevalence and relation with spontaneous bacterial peritonitis. Am J Gastroenterol. 2001;96[10]:2962-7.

[29] Hartmann P, Seebauer CT, Schnabl B. Alcoholic liver disease: the gut microbiome and liver cross talk. Alcohol Clin Exp Res. 2015;39[5]:763-75.

[30] Tsiaoussis GI, Assimakopoulos SF, Tsamandas AC, Triantos CK, Thomopoulos KC. Intestinal barrier

dysfunction in cirrhosis: Current concepts in pathophysiology and clinical implications. World J Hepatol. 2015;7[17]:2058-68.

[31] Goel GA, Deshpande A, Lopez R, Hall GS, van Duin D, Carey WD. Increased rate of spontaneous bacterial peritonitis among cirrhotic patients receiving pharmacologic acid suppression. Clin Gastroenterol Hepatol. 2012;10[4]:422-7.

[32] Llorente C, Jepsen P, Inamine T, Wang L, Bluemel S, Wang HJ, et al. Gastric acid suppression promotes alcoholic liver disease by inducing overgrowth of intestinal Enterococcus. Nat Commun. 2017;8[1]:837.

[33] Hendrikx T, Schnabl B. Antimicrobial proteins: intestinal guards to protect against liver disease. J Gastroenterol. 2019;54[3]:209-17.

[34] Teltschik Z, Wiest R, Beisner J, Nuding S, Hofmann C, Schoelmerich J, et al. Intestinal bacterial translocation in rats with cirrhosis is related to compromised Paneth cell antimicrobial host defense. Hepatology. 2012;55[4]:1154-63.

[35] Wang L, Fouts DE, Starkel P, Hartmann P, Chen P, Llorente C, et al. Intestinal REG3 Lectins Protect against Alcoholic Steatohepatitis by Reducing Mucosa-Associated Microbiota and Preventing Bacterial Translocation. Cell Host Microbe. 2016;19[2]:227-39.

[36] Darnaud M, Dos Santos A, Gonzalez P, Augui S, Lacoste C, Desterke C, et al. Enteric Delivery of Regenerating Family Member 3 alpha Alters the Intestinal Microbiota and Controls Inflammation in Mice With Colitis. Gastroenterology. 2018;154[4]:1009-23 e14.

[37] Mohandas S, Vairappan B. Ginkgolide-A attenuates bacterial translocation through activating PXR and improving antimicrobial peptide Reg 3A in experimental cirrhosis. Life Sci. 2020;257:118111.

[38] Qi H, Li Y, Yun H, Zhang T, Huang Y, Zhou J, et al. Lactobacillus maintains healthy gut mucosa by producing L-Ornithine. Commun Biol. 2019;2:171.

[39] Gallo RL, Kim KJ, Bernfield M, Kozak CA, Zanetti M, Merluzzi L, et al. Identification of CRAMP, a cathelin-related antimicrobial peptide expressed in the embryonic and adult mouse. J Biol Chem. 1997;272[20]:13088-93.

[40] Kress E, Merres J, Albrecht LJ, Hammerschmidt S, Pufe T, Tauber SC, et al. CRAMP deficiency leads to a pro-inflammatory phenotype and impaired phagocytosis after exposure to bacterial meningitis pathogens. Cell Commun Signal. 2017;15[1]:32.

[41] Kakinuma Y, Kimura T, Watanabe Y. Possible Involvement of Liver Resident Macrophages [Kupffer Cells] in the Pathogenesis of Both Intrahepatic and Extrahepatic Inflammation. Can J Gastroenterol Hepatol. 2017;2017:2896809.

[42] Pérez-Cabeza de Vaca R, Domínguez-López M, Guerrero-Celis N, Rodríguez-Aguilera JR, Chagoya de Sánchez V. Inflammation is regulated by the adenosine derivative molecule, IFC-305, during reversion of cirrhosis in a CCl4 rat model. Int Immunopharmacol. 2018 Jan;54:12-23. doi: 10.1016/j.intimp.2017.10.019. Epub 2017 Oct 28. PMID: 29100033.

[43] Byl B, Roucloux I, Crusiaux A, Dupont E, Deviere J. Tumor necrosis factor alpha and interleukin 6 plasma levels in infected cirrhotic patients. Gastroenterology. 1993;104[5]:1492-7.

[44] Lee FY, Lu RH, Tsai YT, Lin HC, Hou MC, Li CP, et al. Plasma interleukin-6 levels in patients with

cirrhosis. Relationship to endotoxemia, tumor necrosis factor-alpha, and hyperdynamic circulation. Scand J Gastroenterol. 1996;31[5]:500-5.

[45] Trebicka J, Krag A, Gansweid S, Appenrodt B, Schiedermaier P, Sauerbruch T, et al. Endotoxin and tumor necrosis factor-receptor levels in portal and hepatic vein of patients with alcoholic liver cirrhosis receiving elective transjugular intrahepatic portosystemic shunt. Eur J Gastroenterol Hepatol. 2011;23[12]:1218-25.

[46] Jiang Y, Guo C, Zhang D, Zhang J, Wang X, Geng C. The altered tight junctions: an important gateway of bacterial translocation in cachexia patients with advanced gastric cancer. J Interferon Cytokine Res. 2014;34[7]:518-25.

[47] Li JD, Feng W, Gallup M, Kim JH, Gum J, Kim Y, et al. Activation of NF-kappaB via a Src-dependent Ras-MAPK-pp90rsk pathway is required for Pseudomonas aeruginosa-induced mucin overproduction in epithelial cells. Proc Natl Acad Sci U S A. 1998;95[10]:5718-23.

[48] Katayama M, Xu D, Specian RD, Deitch EA. Role of bacterial adherence and the mucus barrier on bacterial translocation: effects of protein malnutrition and endotoxin in rats. Ann Surg. 1997;225[3]:317-26.

[49] Xie YR, Liu SL, Liu X, Luo ZB, Zhu B, Li ZF, et al. Intestinal microbiota and innate immunity-related gene alteration in cirrhotic rats with liver transplantation. Transplant Proc. 2011;43[10]:3973-9.

[50] Wiest R, Lawson M, Geuking M. Pathological bacterial translocation in liver cirrhosis. J Hepatol. 2014;60[1]:197-209.

[51] Lachar, J., & Bajaj, J. S. Changes in the Microbiome in Cirrhosis and Relationship to Complications: Hepatic Encephalopathy, Spontaneous Bacterial Peritonitis, and Sepsis. Seminars in liver disease. 2016;36[4]:327-330. DOI:10.1055/s-0036-1593881

[52] Ding S, Chi MM, Scull BP, Rigby R, Schwerbrock NM, Magness S, et al. High-fat diet: bacteria interactions promote intestinal inflammation which precedes and correlates with obesity and insulin resistance in mouse. PLoS One. 2010;5[8]:e12191.

[53] Quigley E. Microbiota-Brain-Gut Axis and Neurodegenerative Diseases. Current neurology and neuroscience reports. 2017;17[12]:94. DOI:10.1007/s11910-017-0802-6

[54] Ghaisas, S., Maher, J., & Kanthasamy, A. Gut microbiome in health and disease: Linking the microbiome-gut-brain axis and environmental factors in the pathogenesis of systemic and neurodegenerative diseases. Pharmacology & therapeutics. 2016;158:52-62. DOI:10.1016/j.pharmthera.2015.11.012

[55] Arab, J. P., Martin-Mateos, R. M., & Shah, V. H. Gut-liver axis, cirrhosis and portal hypertension: the chicken and the egg. *Hepatology international*. 2018;12[Suppl 1]:24-33. DOI:10.1007/s12072-017-9798-x

[56] Tudorașcu, D. R., Bărbulescu, A. L., Cârțână, E. T., Petrescu, I. O., Ciurea, R. N., Ciobanu, D., Forțofoiu, M. C., Pădureanu, V., Tica, O. S., Tudorache, S., & Petrescu, F. Study of the Etiological Spectrum of Spontaneous Bacterial Peritonitis in a Group of Patients Suffering from Liver Cirrhosis. Current health sciences journal. 2016;42[4]:365-371. DOI:10.12865/CHSJ.42.04.06

[57] Velkey, B., Vitális, E., & Vitális, Z. Spontán bakteriális peritonitis [Spontaneous bacterial peritonitis].

Orvosi hetilap. 2017;158[2]:50-57. DOI:10.1556/650.2017.30637

[58] Dever, J. B., & Sheikh, M. Y. Review article: spontaneous bacterial peritonitis--bacteriology, diagnosis, treatment, risk factors and prevention. Alimentary pharmacology & therapeutics. 2015;41[11]:1116-1131. DOI:10.1111/apt.13172

[59] Gómez-Hurtado, I., Such, J., & Francés, R. Microbiome and bacterial translocation in cirrhosis. Microbioma y traslocación bacteriana en la cirrosis. Gastroenterologia y hepatología. 2016;39[10]:687-696. DOI:10.1016/j.gastrohep.2015.10.013

[60] Ascione, T., Di Flumeri, G., Boccia, G., & De Caro, F. Infections in patients affected by liver cirrhosis: an update. Le infezioni in medicina. 2017;25[2]:91-97.

[61] Kajihara, M., Koido, S., Kanai, T., Ito, Z., Matsumoto, Y., Takakura, K., Saruta, M., Kato, K., Odamaki, T., Xiao, J. Z., Sato, N., & Ohkusa, T. Characterisation of blood microbiota in patients with liver cirrhosis. European journal of gastroenterology & hepatology. 2019;31[12]:1577-1583. DOI:10.1097/MEG.0000000000001494

[62] Duah, A., & Nkrumah, K. N. Prevalence and predictors for spontaneous bacterial peritonitis in cirrhotic patients with ascites admitted at medical block in Korle-Bu Teaching Hospital, Ghana. *The Pan African medical journal*. 2019;33:35. DOI:10.11604/pamj.2019.33.35.18029

[63] De Mattos, A. A., Costabeber, A. M., Lionço, L. C., & Tovo, C. V. Multi-resistant bacteria in spontaneous bacterial peritonitis: a new step in management?. World journal of gastroenterology. 2014;20[39]:14079-14086. DOI:10.3748/wjg.v20.i39.14079

[64] Mücke, M. M., Mayer, A., Kessel, J., Mücke, V. T., Bon, D., Schwarzkopf, K., Rüschenbaum, S., Queck, A., Göttig, S., Vermehren, A., Weiler, N., Welker, M. W., Reinheimer, C., Hogardt, M., Vermehren, J., Herrmann, E., Kempf, V., Zeuzem, S., & Lange, C. M. Quinolone and Multidrug Resistance Predicts Failure of Antibiotic Prophylaxis of Spontaneous Bacterial Peritonitis. *Clinical infectious diseases : an official publication of the Infectious Diseases Society of America*. 2020;70[9]:1916-1924. DOI:10.1093/cid/ciz540

[65] Friedrich, K., Nüssle, S., Rehlen, T., Stremmel, W., Mischnik, A., & Eisenbach, C. Microbiology and resistance in first episodes of spontaneous bacterial peritonitis: implications for management and prognosis. Journal of gastroenterology and hepatology. 2016;31[6]:1191-1195. DOI:10.1111/jgh.13266

[66] Li, Y. T., Yu, C. B., Huang, J. R., Qin, Z. J., & Li, L. J. Pathogen profile and drug resistance analysis of spontaneous peritonitis in cirrhotic patients. World journal of gastroenterology. 2015;21[36]:10409-10417. DOI:10.3748/wjg.v21.i36.10409

[67] Fiore, M., Gentile, I., Maraolo, A. E., Leone, S., Simeon, V., Chiodini, P., Pace, M. C., Gustot, T., & Taccone, F. S. Are third-generation cephalosporins still the empirical antibiotic treatment of community-acquired spontaneous bacterial peritonitis? A systematic review and meta-analysis. European journal of gastroenterology & hepatology. 2018;30[3]:329-336. DOI:10.1097/MEG.0000000000001057

[68] Iogna Prat, L., Wilson, P., Freeman, S. C., Sutton, A. J., Cooper, N. J., Roccarina, D., Benmassaoud, A., Plaz Torres, M. C., Hawkins, N., Cowlin, M., Milne, E. J., Thorburn, D., Pavlov, C. S., Davidson, B. R., Tsochatzis, E., & Gurusamy, K. S. Antibiotic treatment for spontaneous bacterial peritonitis in people with decompensated liver cirrhosis: a network meta-analysis.

The Cochrane database of systematic reviews. 2019;9[9]:CD013120. DOI:10.1002/14651858.CD013120.pub2

[69] Shizuma T. Spontaneous bacterial and fungal peritonitis in patients with liver cirrhosis: A literature review. World J Hepatol 2018; 10[2]: 254-266.

[70] The European Association for the Study of the Liver. EASL Clinical Practice Guidelines for the management of patients with decompensated cirrhosis. J Hepatol [2018].

[71] Wiest R., Krag A., Gerbes A. "Spontaneous bacterial peritonitis: recent guidelines and beyond," Gut, vol. 61, no. 2, pp. 297-310, 2012.

[72] Moore K. P., Aithal G. P. "Guidelines on the management of ascites in cirrhosis," Gut, vol. 55, no. S6, pp. vi1–vi12, 2006.

[73] Garcia-Tsao G., Conn H. O., Lerner E. "The diagnosis of bacterial peritonitis: comparison of pH, lactate concentration and leukocyte count," Hepatology, vol. 5, no. 1, pp. 91-96, 1985.

[74] Van de Geijn GM, Van Gent M, Van Pul-Bom N, Beunis MH, van Tilburg AJ, Njo TL. A new flow cytometric method for differential cell counting in ascitic fluid. Cytometry B Clin Cytom 2016;90:506-511.

[75] Enomoto H., Shin-ichi I., Matsuhisa A., Nishiguchi S. Diagnosis of Spontaneous Bacterial Peritonitis and an In Situ Hybridization Approach to Detect an "Unidentified" Pathogen, International Journal of Hepatology, Volume 2014, Article ID 634617, 7 pages.

[76] Krastev N, Djurkov V, Murdjeva M, Akrabova P, Karparova T, Penkov V, Kiprin G, Asenov K. Diagnosis of spontaneous and secondary bacterial peritonitis in patients with hepatic cirrhosis and ascites. Khirurgiia [Sofiia] 2013; [3]: 20-25

[77] Oey RC, Van Buuren HR, De Jong DM, Erler NS, De Man RA. Bacterascites: A study of clinical features, microbiological findings, and clinical significance. Liver Int. 2018;38:2199-2209.

[78] Angeli P, Bernardi M, Villanueva C, Francoz C, Mookerjee RP, Trebicka J, et al. EASL Clinical Practice Guidelines for the management of patients with decompensated cirrhosis. J Hepatol. 2018;69[2]:406-60.

[79] Xu X, Duan Z, Ding H, Li W, Jia J, Wei L, et al. Chinese guidelines on the management of ascites and its related complications in cirrhosis. Hepatol Int. 2019;13[1]:1-21.

Chapter 12

Hepatorenal Syndrome

Arshpal Gill, Ra'ed Nassar, Ruby Sangha, Mohammed Abureesh, Dhineshreddy Gurala, Zeeshan Zia, Rachelle Hamadi and Suzanne El-Sayegh

Abstract

Hepatorenal Syndrome (HRS) is an important condition for clinicians to be aware of in the presence of cirrhosis. In simple terms, HRS is defined as a relative rise in creatinine and relative drop in serum glomerular filtration rate (GFR) alongside renal plasma flow (RPF) in the absence of other competing etiologies of acute kidney injury (AKI) in patients with hepatic cirrhosis. It represents the end stage complication of decompensated cirrhosis in the presence of severe portal hypertension, in the absence of prerenal azotemia, acute tubular necrosis or others. It is a diagnosis of exclusion. The recognition of HRS is of paramount importance for clinicians as it carries a high mortality rate and is an indication for transplantation. Recent advances in understanding the pathophysiology of the disease improved treatment approaches, but the overall prognosis remains poor, with Type I HRS having an average survival under 2 weeks. Generally speaking, AKI and renal failure in cirrhotic patients carry a very high mortality rate, with up to 60% mortality rate for patients with renal failure and cirrhosis and 86.6% of overall mortality rates of patients admitted to the intensive care unit. Of the various etiologies of renal failure in cirrhosis, HRS carries a poor prognosis among cirrhotic patients with acute kidney injury. HRS continues to pose a diagnostic challenge. AKI can be either pre-renal, intrarenal or postrenal. Prerenal causes include hypovolemia, infection, use of vasodilators and functional due to decreased blood flow to the kidney, intra-renal such as glomerulopathy, acute tubular necrosis and post-renal such as obstruction. Patients with cirrhosis are susceptible to developing renal impairment. HRS may be classified as Type 1 or rapidly progressive disease, and Type 2 or slowly progressive disease. There are other types of HRS, but this chapter will focus on Type 1 HRS and Type 2 HRS. HRS is considered a functional etiology of acute kidney injury as there is an apparent lack of nephrological parenchymal damage. It is one several possibilities for acute kidney injury in patients with both acute and chronic liver disease. Acute kidney injury (AKI) is one of the most severe complications that could occur with cirrhosis. Up to 50% of hospitalized patients with cirrhosis can suffer from acute kidney injury, and as mentioned earlier an AKI in the presence of cirrhosis in a hospitalized patient has been associated with nearly a 3.5-fold increase in mortality. The definition of HRS will be discussed in this chapter, but it is characterized specifically as a form of acute kidney injury that occurs in patients with advanced liver cirrhosis which results in a reduction in renal blood flow, unresponsive to fluids this occurs in the setting of portal hypertension and splanchnic vasodilation. This chapter will discuss the incidence of HRS, recognizing HRS, focusing mainly on HRS Type I and Type II, recognizing competing etiologies of renal impairment in cirrhotic patients, and the management HRS.

IntechOpen

Keywords: Hepatorenal Syndrome, Cirrhosis, Kidney Injury

1. Introduction

Hepatorenal Syndrome (HRS) is an important condition for clinicians to be aware of in the presence of cirrhosis. In simple terms, HRS is defined as a relative rise in creatinine and relative drop in serum glomerular filtration rate (GFR) alongside renal plasma flow (RPF) in the absence of other competing etiologies of acute kidney injury (AKI) in patients with hepatic cirrhosis [1–7]. It represents the end stage complication of decompensated cirrhosis in the presence of severe portal hypertension, in the absence of prerenal azotemia, acute tubular necrosis or others. It is a diagnosis of exclusion [2]. The recognition of HRS is of paramount importance for clinicians as it carries a high mortality rate. Recent advances in understanding the pathophysiology of the disease improved treatment approaches, but the overall prognosis remains poor, with Type I HRS having an average survival under 2 weeks [3]. Generally speaking, AKI and renal failure in cirrhotic patients carry a very high mortality rate, with up to 60% mortality rate for patients with renal failure and cirrhosis and 86.6% of overall mortality rates of patients admitted to the intensive care unit [4, 5]. Of the various etiologies of renal failure in cirrhosis, HRS carries a poor prognosis among cirrhotic patients with AKI.

HRS continues to pose a diagnostic challenge. AKI is relatively frequent, seen in about 20% of patients with cirrhosis [8]. AKI can be either pre-renal, intrarenal or postrenal. Prerenal causes include hypovolemia, infection, use of vasodilators and functional due to decreased blood flow to the kidney, intra-renal such as glomerulopathy, acute tubular necrosis and post-renal such as obstruction. Patients with cirrhosis are susceptible to developing renal impairment. HRS may be classified as type 1 or rapidly progressive disease, and type 2 or slowly progressive disease. There are other types of HRS [9], but this chapter will focus on type 1 HRS and type 2 HRS. HRS is considered a functional etiology of AKI as there is an apparent lack of nephrological parenchymal damage. This is one of several possibilities of AKI in patients with both acute and chronic liver disease.

AKI is one of the most severe complications that could occur with cirrhosis. Up to 50% of hospitalized patients with cirrhosis can suffer from AKI, and as mentioned earlier an AKI in the presence of cirrhosis in a hospitalized patient has been associated with nearly a 3.5-fold increase in mortality [6].

The definition of HRS will be discussed in this chapter, but it is characterized specifically as a form of AKI that occurs in patients with advanced liver cirrhosis which results in a reduction in renal blood flow, unresponsive to fluids this occurs in the setting of portal hypertension and splanchnic vasodilation [7].

This chapter will discuss the incidence, definitions and management of HRS, focusing mainly on HRS type I and type II.

2. Frequency of acute kidney injury in cirrhosis

AKI is a common entity in cirrhotic patients at baseline. It is also commonly seen in general hospitalized patients, both with and without cirrhosis. This fundamentally means that a clinician should be able to distinguish various etiologies of AKI establish the reason for AKI in each cirrhotic patient so that management can be conducted appropriately.

As mentioned before, the frequency of AKI in patients with underlying liver pathology can be as high as 50%. One study looked at hospitalized patients with cirrhosis. Of these patients, 19% found to have an AKI, out of these 23% found to have HRS [10]. "The AKI was divided into pre-renal, intrinsic, and post-renal. Pre-renal injury was the most common form of AKI which represented 68% of patients with AKI. The pre-renal injury was usually volume responsive, while HRS is non-volume responsive. In most cases, the injury was volume responsive and therefore less likely HRS [11, 12]. Although HRS is not always the most common cause of renal impairment in cirrhosis; renal impairment itself is commonly seen as the frequency of AKI in cirrhosis can vary in the literature from approximately 15–40% [13–15].

The etiologies of AKI in cirrhosis vary, and the prognosis that each etiology carries also varies. One large prospective study found that hypovolemia and infections were in fact the most common culprits of AKI in cirrhosis, with HRS being identified in 13% of cases [16]. The definition of HRS is important as it can guide clinicians into decision making. For instance, if the etiology of an AKI in cirrhosis is reversible and will not cause significant long-term impairment, the urgency for immediate transplantation dissipates. Conversely, if there is the development of HRS, there may be urgent indication for transplantation.

While there are varying figures reported in the literature on the frequency of AKI in the cirrhotic population, it is evident that it is a common entity. Not all AKI in cirrhosis is considered HRS and defining HRS as the specific cause of renal impairment in cirrhosis represents another challenge for clinicians.

3. Defining hepato-renal syndrome

As stated previously, HRS is defined as renal impairment that occurs in patients who have clinically established cirrhosis or have significant liver impairment. The most widely used definition is the relative rise in creatinine and the relative drop in serum GFR and renal plasma flow in the absence of other causes of AKI like prerenal, renal or post-renal. Given its poor prognosis, HRS was formerly associated with the term terminal functional renal failure [17]. In theory, since there is no intrinsic kidney pathology, upon reversing the hepatic dysfunction either medically or via transplantation, there should be resolution of HRS. In intrinsic renal pathologies, this would not be the case. Before considering HRS, clinicians should rule out other competing etiologies.

4. Competing etiologies of hepatorenal syndrome

Differentiating HRS from other etiologies of AKI in cirrhotic patients is clinically of high importance because of the pronounced difference in management and prognosis. Patients with liver cirrhosis are prone to have acute, subacute and chronic kidney disease through a variety of mechanisms. Clinicians should have a broad differential diagnosis when approaching patients with AKI as there is no definitive test for HRS yet [18]. It is therefore necessary to rule out other differential diagnosis before a diagnosis of HRS is made. Identification of risk factors and careful assessment of the renal system are the mainstay to make such a diagnosis.

Cirrhotic patients may have a certain level of renal insufficiency at baseline since some etiologies of cirrhosis can directly or indirectly lead to renal insufficiency. For instance, patients with non-alcoholic fatty liver disease have higher incidence of obesity and associated diabetes and diabetic nephropathy. Also, both glomerulonephritis and vasculitis can occur in patients with liver cirrhosis secondary to viral hepatitis [2]. These are just a few examples of how one pathology can affect both the hepatic and renal system.

Given the wide spectrum of possibilities, when approaching a renal impairment in a patient with cirrhosis, a systematic approach can be of benefit to clinicians to assess the nature of renal impairment. Causes of AKI and renal failure in cirrhotic patients can be summarized in four main categories.

4.1 Hypovolemia-induced renal failure

This is usually due to hemorrhage related to gastrointestinal bleed or fluid loss associated with excessive diuresis or diarrhea induced by excessive laxatives use [19]. Also, can be secondary to different infectious etiologies including spontaneous bacterial peritonitis. In any of these cases, renal failure will occur soon after any of the mentioned hypovolemic events [16, 19]. Due to the fact that patients with worsening liver cirrhosis will have decreased intravascular volume and mean arterial resistance [17], hypovolemia should be considered as a frequent component of AKI in those patients [16]. The management of hypovolemia induced renal failure is to address the volume status.

4.2 Parenchymal renal disease

By definition HRS is a purely functional disease and it does not induce renal parenchymal damage. However, any parenchymal renal disease can occur in both cirrhotic patients and non-cirrhotic patients. The presence of proteinuria, hematuria or both is associated with glomerular disease. Differentiating HRS from acute Tubular Necrosis (ATN) remains difficult. While the presence of muddy brown casts favors ATN, other urinary indexes like fractional excretion of sodium (FeNa) can be misleading due to the prolonged use of diuretics in cirrhotic patients. Granular casts can be seen in both ATN and HRS [19].

4.3 Drug induced renal disease

Drug-induced tubular/tubulointerstitial injury is a common cause of AKI especially with the consideration ill patients such as those with cirrhosis will inevitably need medications. There are various pathways and in which a drug can cause renal injury [20]. Some examples can include aminoglycosides, vancomycin, and even administration of contrast needed for imaging studies.

4.4 Hepatorenal syndrome

HRS is a diagnosis of exclusion based on the previously mentioned criteria. This chart simplifies the definition based on the criteria set forth by the International Ascites Club [21, 22].

The key factor in diagnosing HRS is the absence of improvement of kidney function despite discontinuation of potential nephrotoxic agents, and a trial of fluid repletion. Essentially HRS appears as a non-volume responsive pre-renal injury. This is why it is essential to rule out all other possible AKI systematically (**Table 1**).

4.4.1 Diagnosis

AKI stage 1 is defined as the increase in serum creatinine (sCr) of >0.3 mg/dl within 48 hours or a > 50% percentage increase in sCr from a known or presumed

Defining hepatorenal syndrome
• Chronic or acute liver failure with signs of portal hypertension
• Low GFR
• Exclusion of shock
• Protienuria less than 0.5 grams per day with exclusion of obsrtuvtive uropathy and exclusion of parecnyhmal disease
• Failure of renal function improve with 1.5 liter isotonic volume - exapnsion and/or with discontiuation of diuretic
Additional criteria
• Urine volume less than 0.5 liters per day
• Low urine sodium (<10mmol/l), serum sodium <130mmol/l
• Less than 50 red blood cells per hpf on urine microscopy

Table 1.
Defining Hepatorenal Syndrome. Adopted from International Ascites Club and in [21, 22].

baseline in the past 3 months which occurred within the past 7 days or urine volume < 0.5 cc/kg for 6 hours.

Changes in the definition of AKI in patients with cirrhosis has changed over time and has been replaced by the ICA (International Club of Ascites) AKI criteria [4, 23]. One of the most important changes was the removal of cutoff values of sCr for diagnosis of HRS in the setting of AKI, allowing earlier recognition and treatment of HRS.

Major diagnostic criteria include cirrhosis with ascites, presence of renal failure which helps differentiate HRS type I and HRS type II.

4.4.1.1 HRS type I

HRS type 1, renal failure is acute based on the KDIGO guidelines, increase in serum creatinine by ≥0.3 mg/dL within 48 hours; Increase in serum creatinine to ≥1.5 times baseline (i.e. 50% above baseline), which is known or presumed to have occurred within the prior 7 days; or urine volume < 0.5 mL/kg/h over a 6-hour period [23].

4.4.1.2 HRS type II

Type 2 HRS renal failure decline in renal function progresses more slowly, usually Cr >1.5. Diagnosis of HRS-type 2 be made either in the context of chronic kidney disease (CKD), that is, in a patient with cirrhosis and a GFR <60 ml/min per 1.73 m2 for >3 months (HRS-CKD) in whom other causes have been excluded, or in the context of AKI, defined as a renal dysfunction that does not meet criteria for AKI and lasts for less than 90 days.

KDIGO guidelines define CKD as abnormalities in kidney structure or function (GFR <60 ml/min/1.72 m2) that persist for more than 90 days, and acute kidney disease (AKD), as AKI or as abnormalities in kidney structure or function that persist for more than 90 days [9, 23].

A recent proposal in the European association for the study of the liver guide lines suggested that HRS-2 should be referred to as HRS-NAKI (hepato-renal syndrome non-acute kidney injury) [24]. This is due to many reasons. HRS 2 is poorly defined and is more of an assumption that chronic abnormalities in serum creatinine without a definite timeline, thus arriving at a new definition of HRS-2 is more challenging than expected.

It is proposed that the diagnosis of HRS-NAKI be made either in the context of CKD, that is in a patient with cirrhosis and a decrease in GFR greater than 3 months (HRS-CKD) or in the context of AKD, defined as a renal dysfunction that does not meet criteria for AKI and lasts for less than 90 days underlying factors such as diabetes, arterial hypertension causing nonalcoholic steatohepatitis which eventually lead to cirrhosis can simultaneously affect the kidneys causing CKD as well [23].

The new nomenclature may enable clinicians to define the presence of HRS-AKI superimposed on CKD in a patient with structural damage of the kidney, as evidenced by previous abnormal biopsy, renal ultrasonography or by significant proteinuria.

In the context of the new definition of HRS-AKI on CKD: HRS-AKI, there would be no evidence of chronic structural damage. For HRS-AKI on CKD in which there would be evidence of chronic structural damage such as chronic proteinuria and/or abnormal renal ultrasonography but with a high suspicion of HRS-AKI.

Other diagnostic criteria for hepatorenal syndrome include:

1. Failure of response to 48-hour volume expansion with albumin and discontinuation of diuretics.

2. Absence of current use of nephrotoxic medications.

3. Absence of macroscopic indication of structural kidney injury such as of proteinuria less than 500 mg per day, microhematuria (less than 50 red blood cells per high powered field) and normal kidney ultrasound [9, 21, 23] (**Table 2**).

4.4.2 Challenges in diagnosing hepatorenal syndrome

Although the definition of HRS appears straightforward, there are many clinical challenges to consider when making a diagnosis. For instance, the usefulness of creatinine measurement in patients with cirrhosis may be limited for many reasons such as assay interference with bilirubin, reduced creatinine production in liver failure patients, muscle wasting and malnutrition [25].

Also using the urine output in patients with cirrhosis is limited as it can affected by other factors, for example decreased urine can be a normal in hypovolemic patients as they retain sodium or it can be simply increased secondary to the use of diuretics, [26, 27] despite that urine output remain a factor to look for, as was demonstrated by, Amathieu et al. who showed that reduction in urine output is associated with worse prognosis and 3-fold increased in hospital mortality [28].

These are just a few examples of how clinicians must use sound judgment when attempting to make a diagnosis of HRS. As mentioned earlier, it is important to stratify causes as it would impact both management and possibly the urgency for transplantation.

4.5 ATN versus HRS

Differentiating ATN and HRS can also pose a challenge to clinicians. Pre-renal azotemia represents the leading cause of AKI in patients with cirrhosis, good history and physical examination of patients warranted to exclude causes of hypovolemia as discussed above.

Urine studies have been also sought to be helpful, with structural etiologies such as ATN, tubular injury limits sodium reabsorption and fraction excretion of sodium (FENa) is increased, typically by greater than 2–3%, using these cutoffs has been challenging owing to the fact that all patients with advanced cirrhosis have chronic

Hepatorenal syndrome type 1	Hepatorenal syndrome type II
Rapid, progressive	Insidious
Median survival <2 weeks	Median survival 6 months

Table 2.
Comparing Types of Hepatorenal Syndrome. Adopted from KDIGO guidelines [9, 21, 23].

renal hypoperfusion and have an FENa less than 1%, even in the absence of AKI [29]. Other studies such as urinary sodium (less than 40 milliequivalents per liter), low urine osmolality are suggestive of ATN although their use in HRS has been limited.

The fraction excretion of urea (FEUrea) is superior to FeNA in differentiating AKI-HRS from ATN, obtaining such tests is very important in HRS as most patients with HRS are on diuretics. Urinary sodium is known to be affected by use of diuretic which can falsely elevate the urine sodium. That is one main reason why FeNa has been excluded from HRS definitions.

4.6 The role of biomarkers in diagnosing HRS

Novel urine biomarkers of tubular injury have long been sought to differentiate AKI-HRS and ATN in patients with cirrhosis [30].

There are many biomarkers released by tubular injury. Among these, NGAL has been the most widely studied biomarker in patients with cirrhosis and showed the greatest diagnostic accuracy in differentiating ATN from AKI-HRS [9]. Cut-off of 0.2% has been widely used in distinguishing HRS from ATN [9]. Urinary NGAL seems to be superior to plasma concentrations and performs better when measured after the two-day volume challenge recommended in the management of any AKI including HRS [31].

At the current time human studies rely on expert adjudication for differentiating ATN from AKI-HRS owing to the limited availability of renal biomarkers and restricted use of kidney biopsies in such a high risk population.

5. Management of hepatorenal syndrome

HRS is one of the many causes of AKI in individuals with both acute and chronic liver disease. After correctly making a diagnosis of HRS, clinicians must address the underlying etiology of HRS. Patients that develop usually have cirrhosis, alcoholic hepatitis, liver failure, or fulminant hepatic failure from any etiology. Management of HRS is usually supportive, with the definitive treatment being reversal of the underlying liver pathology. In several patients, this means liver transplantation.

First line treatment of supportive management for HRS is using vasoconstrictors in combination with albumin to combat splanchnic arterial vasodilation [32]. The goal of treatment is to improve hemodynamic dysfunction by combatting the decreased circulating volume and increasing mean arterial pressure. The most common vasoconstrictors used are vasopressin analogues (terlipressin), norepinephrine, and somatostatin analogues such as octreotide and midodrine.

6. Vasopressin analogues (terlipressin)

The vasopressin analogue Terilpressin is noted to have a greater affinity for the vasopressin 1 receptors in the splanchnic bed, it has been found to improve kidney function in patients with HRS with a decreased incidence of ischemia as compared to vasopressin [33]. Studies have demonstrated that continuous administration of Terlipressin is better tolerated and associated with fewer adverse effects as compared to intermittent bolus administration [34]. Continuous infusion of terlipressin in an outpatient setting has also been reported to be an effective, safe option of HRS treatment as a bridge to transplant [35, 36]. Terlipressin is considered as the first treatment of choice of HRS in Europe. Despite this fact, it is not currently approved by the Food and Drug Administration for use in the United States and Canada as a clear benefit of treatment in HSR has not been established.

Terlipressin was proven to be more effective than placebo in treating HRS type 1 although terlipressin use was associated with more adverse events such abdominal pain, nausea, diarrhea and respiratory failure [37].

7. Norepinephrine

While Terilpressin is the traditional first choice for HRS, norepinephrine is another option clinician can use as vasoconstrictive therapy. One large meta-analysis looking at randomized control trials in HRS compared the efficacy of various constrictive therapies. Terlipressin did demonstrate the most effective pressor to reverse HRS, but had an increased risk of adverse events. Norepinephrine was nearly as efficacious as Terlipressin, and although it was not able to provide the survival benefit as Terlipressin did have a better safety profile [38, 39].

8. Role of albumin

Albumin has a role in maintaining plasma oncotic pressure and detoxification. One of the few indications for albumin administration is HRS; with existing studies in the literature that report the efficacy of albumin in the treatment of HRS [40]. Although albumin has been proven to help in HRS, the optimal treatment dose has not yet been established in guidelines. One large meta-analysis study did demonstrate a benefit with albumin, but optimal treatment dose with albumin has yet to be established. The study did demonstrate that a cumulative dose predicts a successful response to therapy [41].

Current recommendation is to use both albumin with Terlipressin as it has been shown that it improves its beneficial effect when compared to using terlipressin alone or placebo [34, 42].

9. Transjugular intrahepatic portosystemic shunt

Transjugular intrahepatic portosystemic shunt (TIPS) is a treatment option for those patients who fail to respond to pharmacologic therapy. TIPS reduces portal pressures by placing a stent between the portal and hepatic vein. This decreases portal pressure and vascular resistance by reducing endothelin-1 [43, 44]. This procedure has shown to improve kidney function in patients with HRS with a reduction in serum blood urea nitrogen, serum creatinine, and urinary sodium excretion [45, 46]. Although the TIPS procedure does improve elements of HRS, it was shown that there is limited evidence of survival benefit in patients with HRS [47] in addition to risk of development of hepatic encephalopathy which remains the greatest concern for clinicians. This is due to the portosystemic bypass shunt which results in bypassing the livers detoxifying function.

10. Renal replacement therapy

Renal replacement therapy (RRT) is an option for patients with HRS who progress to kidney failure and is most commonly done in patients awaiting liver transplant, or those with an acute reversible event. The role of RRT remains unclear due to lack of survival benefits as similar short term and long-term survival rates have been demonstrated as compared with non RRT treated patients [48].

11. Liver transplantation

HRS is an important entity in liver transplantation. Firstly, many patients waiting for liver transplant will develop HRS. This is owing to the fact that the indication for liver transplant is often advanced cirrhosis or decompensated cirrhosis with ascites. These conditions may also predispose for HRS. The 1-year probability of developing HRS in the presence of ascites is 20%, and the 5-year probability is 40%. The patient population at highest risk of complications are those with fluid retention, which is seen in advanced and decompensated cirrhosis [49, 50].

Secondly, in patients who have HRS the therapies mentioned above such as vasoconstrictors are used often as a bridge to transplantation. Therapies discussed above including vasoconstrictors may help, but the definitive treatment in HRS patients is often a transplant. Aggressive supportive care is unable to improve the recovery of kidney function in less than 50% of patients with HRS [50].

12. Simultaneous liver and kidney transplant

The concept of addressing HRS with a Simultaneous Liver and Kidney Transplant (SLKT) would seem to address both organ dysfunctions. However, HRS has the potential to be reversed by liver transplantation alone, and thus SLKT is not routinely considered in HRS. As mentioned in earlier sections, HRS is associated with many renal pathologies and it is possible for patients with HRS to develop end-stage renal disease after liver transplant alone. Long wait times for liver transplantation has led to a rise in the incidence of pre-transplantation renal dysfunction. The prolonged HRS and long-term RRT can lead to permanent renal damage. The permanent renal injury may lead to a decline in renal function that may not be adequate after liver transplant alone [42, 50].

13. Conclusion

HRS is not an uncommon entity in cirrhotic patients. It remains a challenge both diagnostically and in terms of management. Although there are many causes of renal impairment in the setting of cirrhosis, HRS is unique as the kidneys do not have an organic injury; rather they are a victim of poor circulation seen in advanced liver disease. Any renal impairment has the potential to increase mortality in the cirrhosis population, but HRS in particular is endangering to patients. There are two common forms of HRS, type 1 and type 2, and they can be generally distinguished based on acuity. There appears to be promise in the ease of diagnosis, with the advent of possible biomarkers; however, the present diagnosis is one of exclusion and can often be of challenge for clinicians. The management is mostly supportive care, with albumin and pressor playing a prominent role. The definitive treatment is addressing the underlying liver pathology, which often means liver transplantation. In some instances, there may be a simultaneous transplantation of the kidney and liver.

Abbreviations

HRS	hepatorenal syndrome
GFR	glomerular filtration rate
AKI	acute kidney injury
ATN	acute tubular necrosis
CKD	chronic kidney disease
HRS-NAKI	hepato-renal syndrome non-acute kidney injury
AKD	acute kidney disease
FENa	fraction excretion of sodium
FEUrea	The fraction excretion of urea
RRT	Renal replacement therapy
SLKT	Simultaneous Liver and Kidney Transplant

Author details

Arshpal Gill[1]*, Ra'ed Nassar[1], Ruby Sangha[2], Mohammed Abureesh[1], Dhineshreddy Gurala[1], Zeeshan Zia[1], Rachelle Hamadi[1] and Suzanne El-Sayegh[1]

1 Hofstra/Northwell School of Medicine, Staten Island University Hospital, Staten Island, New York, United States

2 Upstate Medical University, New York, United States

*Address all correspondence to: arshgillmd@gmail.com

References

[1] Pillebout E. Syndrome hépatorénal [Hepatorenal syndrome]. Nephrol Ther. 2014 Feb;10(1):61-8. French. doi: 10.1016/j.nephro.2013.11.005. Epub 2014 Jan 1. PMID: 24388293.

[2] Morales JM, Kamar N, Rostaing L. Hepatitis C and renal disease: epidemiology, diagnosis, pathogenesis and therapy. Contrib Nephrol. 2012;176:10-23. doi: 10.1159/000333772. Epub 2012 Jan 30. PMID: 22310777.

[3] Ranasinghe IR, Sharma B, Bashir K. Hepatorenal Syndrome. 2020 Aug 12. In: StatPearls [Internet]. Treasure Island (FL): StatPearls Publishing; 2021 Jan–. PMID: 28613606.

[4] Amin AA, Alabsawy EI, Jalan R, Davenport A. Epidemiology, Pathophysiology, and Management of Hepatorenal Syndrome. Semin Nephrol. 2019 Jan;39(1):17-30. doi: 10.1016/j.semnephrol.2018.10.002. PMID: 30606404.

[5] Chen YC, Tsai MH, Ho YP, Hsu CW, Lin HH, Fang JT, Huang CC, Chen PC. Comparison of the severity of illness scoring systems for critically ill cirrhotic patients with renal failure. Clin Nephrol. 2004 Feb;61(2):111-118. doi: 10.5414/cnp61111. PMID: 14989630.

[6] Tandon P, James MT, Abraldes JG, Karvellas CJ, Ye F, Pannu N. Relevance of New Definitions to Incidence and Prognosis of Acute Kidney Injury in Hospitalized Patients with Cirrhosis: A Retrospective Population-Based Cohort Study. PLoS One. 2016 Aug 9;11(8):e0160394. doi: 10.1371/journal.pone.0160394. PMID: 27504876; PMCID: PMC4978466.

[7] Mindikoglu AL, Pappas SC. New Developments in Hepatorenal Syndrome. Clin Gastroenterol Hepatol. 2018 Feb;16(2):162-177.e1. doi: 10.1016/j.cgh.2017.05.041. Epub 2017 Jun 7. Erratum in: Clin Gastroenterol Hepatol. 2018 Jun;16(6):988. PMID: 28602971; PMCID: PMC5831376.

[8] Garcia-Tsao G, Parikh CR, Viola A. Acute kidney injury in cirrhosis. Hepatology. 2008 Dec;48(6):2064-2077. doi: 10.1002/hep.22605. PMID: 19003880.

[9] Angeli P, Garcia-Tsao G, Nadim MK, Parikh CR. News in pathophysiology, definition and classification of hepatorenal syndrome: A step beyond the International Club of Ascites (ICA) consensus document. J Hepatol. 2019 Oct;71(4):811-822. doi: 10.1016/j.jhep.2019.07.002. Epub 2019 Jul 11. PMID: 31302175.

[10] Garcia-Tsao, G., Parikh, C. R., & Viola, A. (2008). Acute kidney injury in cirrhosis. *Hepatology (Baltimore, Md.)*, *48*(6), 2064-2077. https://doi.org/10.1002/hep.22605

[11] Low G, Alexander GJ, Lomas DJ. Renal impairment in cirrhosis unrelated to hepatorenal syndrome. Can J Gastroenterol Hepatol. 2015 Jun-Jul;29(5):253-7. doi: 10.1155/2015/967683. Epub 2015 Apr 15. PMID: ; PMCID: .

[12] Fang JT, Tsai MH, Tian YC, Jenq CC, Lin CY, Chen YC, Lien JM, Chen PC, Yang CW. Outcome predictors and new score of critically ill cirrhotic patients with acute renal failure. Nephrol Dial Transplant. 2008 Jun;23(6):1961-1969. doi: 10.1093/ndt/gfm914. Epub 2008 Jan 10. PMID: 18187499.

[13] Péron JM, Bureau C, Gonzalez L, Garcia-Ricard F, de Soyres O, Dupuis E, Alric L, Pourrat J, Vinel JP. Treatment of hepatorenal syndrome as defined by the international ascites club by albumin and furosemide infusion according to the central venous pressure: a prospective pilot study. Am J

Gastroenterol. 2005 Dec;100(12):2702-2707. doi: 10.1111/j.1572-0241.2005.00271.x. PMID: 16393223.

[14] Piano S, Rosi S, Maresio G, Fasolato S, Cavallin M, Romano A, Morando F, Gola E, Frigo AC, Gatta A, Angeli P. Evaluation of the Acute Kidney Injury Network criteria in hospitalized patients with cirrhosis and ascites. J Hepatol. 2013 Sep;59(3):482-489. doi: 10.1016/j.jhep.2013.03.039. Epub 2013 May 7. PMID: 23665185.

[15] du Cheyron D, Bouchet B, Parienti JJ, Ramakers M, Charbonneau P. The attributable mortality of acute renal failure in critically ill patients with liver cirrhosis. Intensive Care Med. 2005 Dec;31(12):1693-1699. doi: 10.1007/s00134-005-2842-7. Epub 2005 Oct 22. PMID: 16244877.

[16] Martín-Llahí M, Guevara M, Torre A, Fagundes C, Restuccia T, Gilabert R, Solá E, Pereira G, Marinelli M, Pavesi M, Fernández J, Rodés J, Arroyo V, Ginès P. Prognostic importance of the cause of renal failure in patients with cirrhosis. Gastroentero logy. 2011 Feb;140(2):488-496.e4. doi: 10.1053/j.gastro.2010.07.043. Epub 2010 Aug 1. PMID: 20682324.

[17] Wadei HM, Mai ML, Ahsan N, Gonwa TA. Hepatorenal syndrome: pathophysiology and management. Clin J Am Soc Nephrol. 2006 Sep;1(5):1066-1079. doi: 10.2215/CJN.01340406. Epub 2006 Jul 12. PMID: 17699328.

[18] Martín-Llahí M, Guevara M, Torre A, Fagundes C, Restuccia T, Gilabert R, Solá E, Pereira G, Marinelli M, Pavesi M, Fernández J, Rodés J, Arroyo V, Ginès P. Prognostic importance of the cause of renal failure in patients with cirrhosis. Gastroentero logy. 2011 Feb;140(2):488-496.e4. doi: 10.1053/j.gastro.2010.07.043. Epub 2010 Aug 1. PMID: 20682324.

[19] Ginès P, Schrier RW. Renal failure in cirrhosis. N Engl J Med. 2009 Sep 24;361(13):1279-90. doi: 10.1056/NEJMra0809139. Erratum in: N Engl J Med. 2011 Jan 27;364(4):389. PMID: 19776409.

[20] Wu H, Huang J. Drug-Induced Nephrotoxicity: Pathogenic Mechanisms, Biomarkers and Prevention Strategies. Curr Drug Metab. 2018;19(7):559-567. doi: 10.2174/1389200218666171108154419. PMID: 29119923.

[21] Ng CK, Chan MH, Tai MH, Lam CW. Hepatorenal syndrome. Clin Biochem Rev. 2007 Feb;28(1):11-7. PMID: 17603637; PMCID: PMC1904420.

[22] Arroyo V, Ginès P, Gerbes AL, Dudley FJ, Gentilini P, Laffi G, Reynolds TB, Ring-Larsen H, Schölmerich J. Definition and diagnostic criteria of refractory ascites and hepatorenal syndrome in cirrhosis. International Ascites Club. Hepatology. 1996 Jan;23(1):164-176. doi: 10.1002/hep.510230122. PMID: 8550036.

[23] Angeli P, Gines P, Wong F, Bernardi M, Boyer TD, Gerbes A, Moreau R, Jalan R, Sarin SK, Piano S, Moore K, Lee SS, Durand F, Salerno F, Caraceni P, Kim WR, Arroyo V, Garcia-Tsao G; International Club of Ascites. Diagnosis and management of acute kidney injury in patients with cirrhosis: revised consensus recommendations of the International Club of Ascites. Gut. 2015 Apr;64(4):531-537. doi: 10.1136/gutjnl-2014-308874. Epub 2015 Jan 28. PMID: 25631669.

[24] European Association for the Study of the Liver (2010). EASL clinical practice guidelines on the management of ascites, spontaneous bacterial peritonitis, and hepatorenal syndrome in cirrhosis. Journal of hepatology, *53*(3), 397-417. https://doi.org/10.1016/j.jhep.2010.05.004

[25] Caregaro L, Menon F, Angeli P, Amodio P, Merkel C, Bortoluzzi A, Alberino F, Gatta A. Limitations of serum creatinine level and creatinine clearance as filtration markers in cirrhosis. Arch Intern Med. 1994 Jan 24;154(2):201-5. PMID: 8285815. Nov;2(3):363-74. doi: 10.1016/s0272-6386(82)80096-6. PMID: 7148828.

[26] Angeli P, Gatta A, Caregaro L, Menon F, Sacerdoti D, Merkel C, Rondana M, de Toni R, Ruol A. Tubular site of renal sodium retention in ascitic liver cirrhosis evaluated by lithium clearance. Eur J Clin Invest. 1990 Feb;20(1):111-117. doi: 10.1111/j.1365-2362.1990.tb01800.x. PMID: 2108033.

[27] Angeli P, Gatta A, Caregaro L, Menon F, Sacerdoti D, Merkel C, Rondana M, de Toni R, Ruol A. Tubular site of renal sodium retention in ascitic liver cirrhosis evaluated by lithium clearance. Eur J Clin Invest. 1990 Feb;20(1):111-117. doi: 10.1111/j.1365-2362.1990.tb01800.x. PMID: 2108033.

[28] Amathieu R, Al-Khafaji A, Sileanu FE, Foldes E, DeSensi R, Hilmi I, Kellum JA. Significance of oliguria in critically ill patients with chronic liver disease. Hepatology. 2017 Nov;66(5):1592-1600. doi: 10.1002/hep.29303. Epub 2017 Sep 26. PMID: 28586126.

[29] Alsaad AA, Wadei HM. Fractional excretion of sodium in hepatorenal syndrome: Clinical and pathological correlation. World J Hepatol. 2016 Dec 8;8(34):1497-1501. doi: 10.4254/wjh.v8.i34.1497. PMID: 28008340; PMCID: PMC5143430.

[30] Belcher JM, Sanyal AJ, Peixoto AJ, Perazella MA, Lim J, Thiessen-Philbrook H, Ansari N, Coca SG, Garcia-Tsao G, Parikh CR; TRIBE-AKI Consortium. Kidney biomarkers and differential diagnosis of patients with cirrhosis and acute kidney injury. Hepatology. 2014 Aug;60(2):622-32. doi: 10.1002/hep.26980. Epub 2014 Jun 26. PMID: 24375576; PMCID: PMC4065642.

[31] Verna EC, Brown RS, Farrand E, Pichardo EM, Forster CS, Sola-Del Valle DA, Adkins SH, Sise ME, Oliver JA, Radhakrishnan J, Barasch JM, Nickolas TL. Urinary neutrophil gelatinase-associated lipocalin predicts mortality and identifies acute kidney injury in cirrhosis. Dig Dis Sci. 2012 Sep;57(9):2362-70. doi: 10.1007/s10620-012-2180-x. Epub 2012 May 6. PMID: 22562534; PMCID: PMC3979299.

[32] Arroyo V, García-Martinez R, Salvatella X. Human serum albumin, systemic inflammation, and cirrhosis. J Hepatol. 2014 Aug;61(2):396-407. doi: 10.1016/j.jhep.2014.04.012. Epub 2014 Apr 18. PMID: 24751830.

[33] Ortega R, Ginès P, Uriz J, Cárdenas A, Calahorra B, De Las Heras D, Guevara M, Bataller R, Jiménez W, Arroyo V, Rodés J. Terlipressin therapy with and without albumin for patients with hepatorenal syndrome: results of a prospective, nonrandomized study. Hepatology. 2002 Oct;36(4 Pt 1):941-948. doi: 10.1053/jhep.2002.35819. PMID: 12297842.

[34] Fabrizi F, Aghemo A, Messa P. Hepatorenal syndrome and novel advances in its management. Kidney Blood Press Res. 2013;37(6):588-601. doi: 10.1159/000355739. Epub 2013 Dec 5. PMID: 24356549.

[35] Robertson M, Majumdar A, Garrett K, Rumler G, Gow P, Testro A. Continuous outpatient terlipressin infusion for hepatorenal syndrome as a bridge to successful liver transplantation. Hepatology. 2014 Dec;60(6):2125-2126. doi: 10.1002/hep.27154. Epub 2014 May 19. PMID: 24687396.

[36] Vasudevan A, Ardalan Z, Gow P, Angus P, Testro A. Efficacy of outpatient continuous terlipressin

infusions for hepatorenal syndrome. Hepatology. 2016 Jul;64(1):316-318. doi: 10.1002/hep.28325. Epub 2015 Dec 22. PMID: 26524479.

[37] Wong, F., Pappas, S. C., Curry, M. P., Reddy, K. R., Rubin, R. A., Porayko, M. K., Gonzalez, S. A., Mumtaz, K., Lim, N., Simonetto, D. A., Sharma, P., Sanyal, A. J., Mayo, M. J., Frederick, R. T., Escalante, S., Jamil, K., & CONFIRM Study Investigators (2021). Terlipressin plus Albumin for the Treatment of Type 1 Hepatorenal Syndrome. The New England journal of medicine, *384*(9), 818-828. https://doi.org/10.1056/NEJMoa2008290

[38] Zheng JN, Han YJ, Zou TT, Zhou YJ, Sun DQ, Zhong JH, Braddock M, Zheng MH. Comparative efficacy of vasoconstrictor therapies for type 1 hepatorenal syndrome: a network meta-analysis. Expert Rev Gastroenterol Hepatol. 2017 Nov;11(11):1009-1018. doi: 10.1080/17474124.2017.1356223. Epub 2017 Jul 27. PMID: 28708431.

[39] Nanda A, Reddy R, Safraz H, Salameh H, Singal AK. Pharmacological Therapies for Hepatorenal Syndrome: A Systematic Review and Meta-Analysis. J Clin Gastroenterol. 2018 Apr;52(4): 360-367. doi: 10.1097/MCG.0000000000000913. PMID: 28991106.

[40] Valerio C, Theocharidou E, Davenport A, Agarwal B. Human albumin solution for patients with cirrhosis and acute on chronic liver failure: Beyond simple volume expansion. World J Hepatol. 2016 Mar 8;8(7):345-54. doi: 10.4254/wjh.v8.i7.345. PMID: 26981172; PMCID: PMC4779163.

[41] Salerno F, Navickis RJ, Wilkes MM. Albumin treatment regimen for type 1 hepatorenal syndrome: a dose-response meta-analysis. BMC Gastroenterol. 2015 Nov 25;15:167. doi: 10.1186/s12876-015-0389-9. PMID: 26606982; PMCID: PMC4660686.

[42] Zhang, J., Rössle, M., Zhou, X., Deng, J., Liu, L., & Qi, X. (2019). Terlipressin for the treatment of hepatorenal syndrome: an overview of current evidence. Current medical research and opinion, *35*(5), 859-868. https://doi.org/10.1080/03007995.2018.1552575

[43] Rössle M. TIPS: 25 years later. J Hepatol. 2013 Nov;59(5):1081-1093. doi: 10.1016/j.jhep.2013.06.014. Epub 2013 Jun 25. PMID: 23811307.

[44] Umgelter A, Reindl W, Geisler F, Saugel B, Huber W, Berger H, Schmid RM. Effects of TIPS on global end-diastolic volume and cardiac output and renal resistive index in ICU patients with advanced alcoholic cirrhosis. Ann Hepatol. 2010 Jan-Mar;9(1):40-45. PMID: 20308721.

[45] Brensing KA, Textor J, Perz J, Schiedermaier P, Raab P, Strunk H, Klehr HU, Kramer HJ, Spengler U, Schild H, Sauerbruch T. Long term outcome after transjugular intrahepatic portosystemic stent-shunt in non-transplant cirrhotics with hepatorenal syndrome: a phase II study. Gut. 2000 Aug;47(2):288-95. doi: 10.1136/gut.47.2.288. PMID: 10896924; PMCID: PMC1727992.

[46] Guevara M, Ginès P, Bandi JC, Gilabert R, Sort P, Jiménez W, Garcia-Pagan JC, Bosch J, Arroyo V, Rodés J. Transjugular intrahepatic portosystemic shunt in hepatorenal syndrome: effects on renal function and vasoactive systems. Hepatology. 1998 Aug;28(2):416-422. doi: 10.1002/hep.510280219. PMID: 9696006.

[47] Song, T., Rössle, M., He, F., Liu, F., Guo, X., & Qi, X. (2018). Transjugular intrahepatic portosystemic shunt for hepatorenal syndrome: A systematic review and meta-analysis. Digestive and liver disease : official journal of the Italian Society of Gastroenterology and the Italian Association for the Study of

the Liver, *50*(4), 323-330. https://doi.org/10.1016/j.dld.2018.01.123

[48] Zhang Z, Maddukuri G, Jaipaul N, Cai CX. Role of renal replacement therapy in patients with type 1 hepatorenal syndrome receiving combination treatment of vasoconstrictor plus albumin. J Crit Care. 2015 Oct;30(5):969-974. doi: 10.1016/j.jcrc.2015.05.006. Epub 2015 May 19. PMID: 26051980.

[49] Garcia-Tsao G, Parikh CR, Viola A. Acute kidney injury in cirrhosis. Hepatology. 2008 Dec;48(6):2064-2077. doi: 10.1002/hep.22605. PMID: 19003880.

[50] Modi RM, Patel N, Metwally SN, Mumtaz K. Outcomes of liver transplantation in patients with hepatorenal syndrome. World J Hepatol. 2016 Aug 28;8(24):999-1011. doi: 10.4254/wjh.v8.i24.999. PMID: 27648152; PMCID: PMC5002501.

Chapter 13

Treatment Approach in Patients with Decompensated Liver Cirrhosis

Anıl Delik and Yakup Ülger

Abstract

Chronic liver disease and decompensated cirrhosis are the major causes of morbidity and mortality in the world. According to current data, deaths due to liver cirrhosis constitute 2.4% of the total deaths worldwide. Cirrhosis is characterized by hepatocellular damage that leads to fibrosis and regenerative nodules in the liver. The most common causes of cirrhosis include alcohol consumption, hepatitis C, hepatitis B, and non-alcoholic fatty liver disease. Dysbiosis and intestinal bacterial overgrowth play a role in the development of complications of cirrhosis through translocation. In liver cirrhosis, ascites, gastrointestinal variceal bleeding, spontaneous bacterial peritonitis infection, hepatic encephalopathy, hepatorenal syndrome, hepatocelluler carcinoma are the most common complications. In addition, there are refractory ascites, hyponatremia, acute on-chronic liver failure, relative adrenal insufficiency, cirrhotic cardiomyopathy, hepatopulmonary syndrome and portopulmonary hypertension. In the primary prophylaxis of variceal bleeding, non-selective beta blockers or endoscopic variceal ligation are recommended for medium and large variceal veins. In current medical treatment, vasoactive agents, antibiotics, blood transfusion, endoscopic band ligation are the standard approach in the treatment of acute variceal bleeding. Sodium-restricted diet, diuretics and large-volume paracentesis are recommended in the management of ascites. In the treatment of hepatic encephalopathy, lactulose, branched chain amino acids, rifaximin and L-ornithine L-aspartate can be used. New therapeutic approaches such as ornithine phenyl acetate spherical carbon and fecal microbiota transplantation have shown beneficial effects on hepatic encephalopathy symptoms. In addition to their antioxidative, anti-proliferative and anti-inflammatory properties, statins have been shown to reduce the risk of decompensation and death by reducing portal pressure in compensated cirrhosis. In the treatment of liver failure, some artificial liver devices such as molecular adsorbent recirculating system, the single albumin dialysis system, fractionated plasma separation and adsorption are used until transplantation or regeneration. The purpose of this chapter is to review the most up-to-date information on liver cirrhosis and to explain the complications assessment, current management and potential treatment strategies in decompensated cirrhosis.

Keywords: advanced liver disease, ascites, gastrointestinal bleeding, hepatic encephelopathy, acute on chronic liver failure, therapy

1. Introduction

Decompensated cirrhosis is characterized by the development of complications related to portal hypertension (PHT) such as variceal bleeding, ascites, spontaneous bacterial peritonitis (SBP), hepatic encephalopathy (HE), hepatorenal syndrome (HRS), or hepatopulmunary syndrome (HPS) in the presence of cirrhosis [1]. The mortality rate in patients with decompensated cirrhosis is 10 times higher than in the normal population. In cirrhosis, PHT occurs due to increased plasma volume, cardiac output and imbalance of biochemical parameters (such as vasoconstrictors, vasodilators, vascular endothelial growth factor, and nitric oxide) [2]. The incidence of cirrhosis is 26 per 100,000 in Europe, and the incidence in Asia ranges from 16.5 per 100,000 in East Asia to 23.6 per 100,000 in Southeast Asia [3]. It causes 1.2 million deaths due to complications of cirrhosis and 790.000 deaths due to liver cancer, accounting for 3.5% of all deaths worldwide [4]. Chronic liver disease epidemiology, hepatitis B (HBV) incidence and complications decrease with HBV vaccination and antiviral treatment programs. In addition, chronic hepatitis C (HCV) infection reduces the risk of cirrhosis and HCC development with direct-acting antiviral (DAA) treatment. Non-alcoholic fatty liver disease (NAFLD) increases due to obesity and metabolic syndrome. Similarly, alcohol consumption accounts for approximately 27% of liver-related death causes in the world. NAFLD has the highest mortality rate in western countries [5]. Asymptomatic cirrhotic patients develop decompensated cirrhosis at a rate of 5–7% each year [6]. The development of decompensation causes dysfunction in multiple organs and systems, leading to systemic disease [7]. Although many factors play a role in the background of cirrhosis pathophysiology, mainly according to the peripheral vasodilation hypothesis, arterial vasodilation in the splanchnic circulatory system in cirrhosis leads to the activation of compensatory vasoconstrictor systems (such as renal angiotensin aldosterone axis, sympathetic nervous system and activation of water retention systems). Changes in saliva and intestinal microbiome in cirrhosis have been found to be associated with the development of intestinal bacterial overgrowth, dysbiosis, increased intestinal permeability, and decompensating complications from portal tract intestinal translocation [8]. Treatment strategy in decompensated cirrhosis patients should be aimed at preventing the progression of cirrhosis before complications occur. The ultimate treatment for decompensated cirrhosis should be aimed at regressing fibrosis by suppressing inflammation, normalizing liver cell number and function by regulating portal and arterial circulation, and restoring liver integrity [9].

2. Treatment of complications in decompensated cirrhosis

2.1 Ascites

Ascites is the abnormal accumulation of fluid in the abdominal cavity and is the most common cause of decompensation in cirrhosis. The basis for the formation of ascites is renal sodium uptake due to activation of sodium-sparing systems such as the renin angiotensin aldosterone system (RAAS) and the sympathetic nervous system [10]. Extra cellular volume increase and decreased effective volume secondary to splanchnic arterial vasodilation are the main determinants of these changes. There are 5 different phases of the ascites development process. The first phase pre-ascites does not cause a decrease in effective blood volume due to hyperdynamic circulation accompanying splanchnic arterial vasodilation, cardiac output and increase in plasma volume. Blood pressure, kidney function, renin activity, noradrenaline and anti-diuretic hormone (ADH) levels remain normal. In the second phase, there is a moderate decrease in sodium excretion unrelated to the sympathetic nervous system and RAAS activation [11]. In the third phase, RAAS and activation of the sympathetic nervous system cause sodium retention as a result of an increase in splanchnic arterial vasodilation. In the fourth phase, plasma renin activity, noradrenaline and ADH levels increase significantly, decreasing the renal perfusion and glomerular filtration rate (GFR) and decreasing the osmotic free water excretion ability of the kidneys leads to dilutional hyponatremia. In the fifth phase, severe systemic vasodilation and a decrease in cardiac output cause left ventricular systolic dysfunction in cirrhosis patients and type 2 hepatorenal syndrome develops [12, 13].

2.1.1 Classification of ascites

It is classified as uncomplicated ascites and refractory ascites according to the recommendation of the international ascites club (IAC). Ascites is considered uncomplicated if not associated with infection or hepatorenal syndrome (**Table 1**).

Refractory ascites are defined as non-regressing at least one degree of regression with diuretic therapy and dietary sodium restriction, or early recurrence after large-volume paracentesis. There are two subtypes, diuretic resistance and diuretic intractable. Type 1 subtype has resistance to optimal dose diuretics. The second subtype is due to insufficient diuretic dose [14].

2.1.2 Ascites treatment in cirrhosis patients

2.1.2.1 Uncomplicated ascites treatment

The management of uncomplicated acids according to the European association for the study of the liver (EASL) guidelines depends on the degree of clinical symptoms. Diuretics and low sodium diet are not needed in patients with grade 1 ascite. Grade 2 ascite patients can be treated on an outpatient basis using sodium restriction and diuretics. Daily sodium intake should be determined as 80–120 mmol/d. A very low sodium restrictive diet should be avoided (<40 mmol/d). Bed rest is not required due to the lack of data on the activation of sodium-sparing systems and the negative effect of vertical posture on renal perfusion. It can lead to the progression of muscle atrophy [15]. The diuretic agents preferred in the treatment of ascites are aldosterone antagonists (spironolactone, carnenone, potassium canrenoate etc). They not only inhibit sodium and water retention, but also suppress potassium excretion and reduce the synthesis of permeases in the collecting tubules and distal tubules of the aldosterone-sensitive kidney. In addition, loop diuretics are used. It inhibits sodium reabsorption along the emerging branch of the henle ring. Loop diuretics are not recommended as monotherapy because of their lower efficacy and higher number of complications compared to aldosterone antagonists [16].

Grading of ascites	Findings
Grade 1	A small amount of acid that can only be demonstrated by ultrasonography
Grade 2	Moderate acid in the abdomen
Grade 3	Massive, common acid

Table 1.
Grading ascites according to the amount of intraabdominal ascites.

Sequential administration of aldosterone antagonists and loop diuretics in the first phase of acid therapy and a combination of these drugs if recurrence occurs. Initial treatment starts with 100–200 mg/d spironolactone administration, then 20–40 mg furosemide is added within two weeks in case of no effect. In the follow-up, daily doses can be increased to 400 mg and 160 mg, respectively. The second recommended method is the combination of diuretic agents and it is recommended to increase the dose of spironolactone and furosemide gradually to 400 mg and 160 mg/d [17]. Daily diuresis and weight monitoring is required to prevent hypovolemia, hyponatremia and acute kidney damage. The reduction in body weight should not exceed 500 g/day in patients without peripheral edema and 1000 g/day in patients with this [18]. In cirrhosis patients with second degree uncomplicated acid, it is possible to achieve 90% success with a combination of diuretic therapy and low sodium diet. Even if a small amount of fluid remains in the abdomen, the effect is considered sufficient, but peripheral edema should not be. It is recommended that the dose of diuretic be reduced to the lowest effective dose after the treatment goal is reached [19]. Diuretic-related side effects may occur during the first weeks of treatment. It often causes fluid electrolyte imbalance such as dehydration, hypovolemic hypoosmolar hyponatremia, hypokalemia or hyperkalemia. It can also cause possible complications such as HE, gynecomastia, muscle cramps, and acute kidney damage. Aldosterone antagonists may cause hypovolemic hypoosmolar hyponatremia, especially with the use of thiazide group diuretics in elderly patients with cirrhotic acid. This group of agents inhibit reabsorption of sodium and chlorine in distal folded tubules. Hypovolemic hypoosmolar hyponatremia is characterized by a serum sodium level below 130 mmol/L, low plasma osmolarity and simultaneous reduction in extracellular fluid volume. It can lead to weakness, apathy, irritability, dizziness, hypotension, nausea and vomiting in the clinic [20]. The development of severe hyponatremia (serum sodium level < 125 mmol/L), the presence of signs of HE worsening, muscle cramps, and acute kidney damage necessitate discontinuation of the drug. Loop diuretics can cause hypokalemia (serum potassium level less than 3 mmol/L), aldosterone antagonists can cause hyperkalemia (more than 6 mmol/L). In this case, diuretics should be discontinued.

Large volume paracentesis (LVP) is the preferred method in patients with third degree ascites. Removal of more than 5–6 L of acid fluid with LVP (albumin infusion 8 g/L acites removed), diuretic agents and a low sodium diet are recommended. Paracentesis with plasma support should be performed under sterile conditions using disposable material to prevent effective blood volume reduction after paracentesis circulatory impairment (PPCD). The procedure may cause very low local complications, especially bleeding. Clinical symptoms of PPCD are renal failure, dilutional hyponatremia, HE and decreased survival. Artificial plasma expanders such as dextran-70 (8 g/L ascites removed) or polygeline (150 ml/L), saline solution (170 ml/L) to prevent these complications (if less than 5 L ascites are discharged) only 20% albumin-like effect. Polygeline prions are not used in many countries due to the potential risk of contamination. Dextran carries the risk of severe allergic reactions and kidney failure.

According to recent studies, a reduction in short-term mortality has been reported in patients who underwent LVP. According to a meta-analysis, PPCD due to large volume paracentesis has been shown to be associated with acid recurrence, dilutional hyponatremia, development of hepatorenal syndrome, and high mortality [21]. The diagnosis of PPCD is made 5 days after LVP when the plasma renin concentration is 50% higher or 4 ng/ml compared to the basal value. Albumin infusion can prevent this complication with its increased oncotic pressure, anti-inflammatory and antioxidant properties. Alternative concentrated ascites reinfussion therapy (CART) is in the form of intravenous and reinfusion of proteins collected by concentrating and filtering acid fluid to maintain serum albumin level [22].

Since nonsteroidal anti-inflammatory drug (NSAIDs) inhibit prostaglandin synthesis and cause sodium retention, hyponatremia and acute kidney damage, they should not be used in acidic patients. Angiotensin converting enzyme inhibitors, angiotensin 2 antagonists or alpha 1 adrenergic receptor blockers are not used in patients with ascites due to an increased risk of renal failure [13].

2.1.2.2 Refractory ascites

The definition of refractory ascites is in the form of refractory ascites that cannot be mobilized with medical treatment or early recurrence (after LVP) according to the criteria of the IAC. Refractory ascites is associated with a poor prognosis. Average survival is about 6 months. These patients should be referred to transplant centers for transplantation. Diuretic resistant ascites: an acid that does not respond to sodium restriction and diuretic therapy or whose early recurrence cannot be prevented. Diuretic intractable ascites: Ascites that prevent the use of diuretics at effective doses and cannot be mobilized or early recurrence cannot be prevented due to the development of diuretic-related complications.

The duration of treatment should be salt restricted diet (less than 90 mmol/d) and at least one week of intensive diuretic therapy spirinolactone 400 mg/d, furosemide 160 mg/d. Lack of responce weight loss of less than 0.8 kg in 4 days and urine sodium should be less than the sodium intake.

Early acid development: Reappearance of Grade 2 or 3 acid within 4 weeks is the development of drug-induced HE in the absence of other predisposing factors, diuretic-induced renal failure, in patients with ascites serum creatinine level increases above 2 mg/dl. Diuretic-induced encephalopathy: The development of hepatic encephalopathy in the absence of any other precipitating factors.

Diuretic induced renal failure: an increase in serum creatinine level to >2 mg/dl (177 lmol/L) in patients with ascites. It is defined as a serum sodium level falling below 125 mmol/L. Diuretic-induced hypo or hyperkalemia is defined as serum potassium <3 mmol/L or > 6 mmol/L [23, 24].

First-line therapy combined with albumin infusion (8 g/L ascites removed) should be repeated every 2–3 weeks for LVP, and diuretics are only recommended when sodium concentration in urine is >30 mmol/d. Clonidine (alpha 2 presynaptic receptor agonist) may be considered to increase the effectiveness of the diuretic response and reduce the need for diuretics. Midodrine (alpha 1 receptor agonist) increases sodium excretion by decreasing plasma renin activity in patients with refractory ascites without azotemia. According to the meta-analysis results, it was shown that midodrine is effective therapeutically but does not have a statistically significant effect on survival [25]. The addition of clonidine or midodrine to diuretic therapy in resistant acids is not recommended according to current guidelines [13]. Despite controversial data on the use of non-selective beta-blockers (NSBBs) refractory ascites, high doses of NSBBs should be avoided in refractory ascites or circulatory dysfunction. (systolic blood pressure < 90 mmol Hg, serum sodium <130 mEq/L, sepsis, bleeding, AKI, SBP) (such as; propranolol >80 mg/d). Followed by an attempt at re-introduction of beta-blocker therapy after recovery. According to EASL, carvedilol is not recommended in this case. Terlipressin stimulates specific V1 receptors in arterial muscle cells, causing the arteries to contract. Reduced splanchnic vasodilation decreases the portal pressure and increases the effective blood volume and renal

No.	Factors
1.	MELD score > 25 and portasystemic pressure gradient <8 mm Hg
2.	INR value >2
3.	Ttotal serum bilirubin value >3 mg/dl and platelet count <75.000
4.	Serum creatinine >1.9 mg/dl
5.	GFR <90 ml/min and platelet count <125.000
6.	Recurrent HE (stage 2 and above)
7.	Diastolic diysfunction (E/A ratio ≤ 1)

MELD Model for End-Stage Liver disease, INR international normalized ratio, GFR glomerular filtration rate, HE hepatic encephelopathy, E/A: Echocardiographic E wave velocity, A wave velocity.

Table 2.
Factors negatively affecting the result in transjugular intrahepatic portosystemic shunt (TIPS).

perfusion pressure with a positive effect on hyperdynamic circulation, decreases plasma renin activity and noradrenaline level, and increases renal glomerular filtration rate and sodium excretion.

It has been shown that resistant acids can be successfully treated with transjugular intrahepatic portosystemic shunt (TIPS) [26]. TIPS improves cardiovascular function by causing a decrease in portal pressure, increased renal blood flow and glomerular filtration rate. According to current guidelines, cases where LVP is contraindicated (uncooperative patient, skin infection at the puncture site, pregnancy, severe abdominal distension, severe coagulopathy) and TIPS is recommended only when LVP is not effective. Diuretic and salt restriction after TIPS, close clinical monitoring is recommended until the acid regresses. The reason for this is the high mortality in decompensated cirrhotic patients and the development of HE associated with TIPS [27]. Patients undergoing TIPS should be selected carefully. TIPS is not recommended for patients with CTP C [23, 28] (**Table 2**).

The use of polytetrafluoroethylene (PTFE) stents is recommended for patients with TIPS dysfunction and high risk of HE. If the patient has contraindications for TIPS, implantation of a permanent peritoneal catheter may be an alternative. In addition, although the automatic low flow pump (alfa pump system) can reduce the need for paracentesis in patients with cirrhosis and refractory ascites, it remains unclear whether it has a significant advantage over LVP in improving survival. It is currently not considered a standard of medical care, but theoretically TIPS can serve as a bridge for liver transplantation in patients with contraindications [29].

2.2 Gastrointestinal bleeding

Gastrointestinal varices develop as a result of the dilation of abnormally enlarged submucosal veins in the digestive system as a result of PHT. The most important complication of PHT causing morbidity and mortality is gastrointestinal variceal bleeding. The most common gastrointestinal variceal type is esophageal varices 42.7% in CTP A, 70.7% in CTP B, and 75.5% in CTP C [30]. The prevalence of variceal veins increases with the severity of liver disease. Variceal veins can be in the form of esophagus, stomach or ectopic variceal (**Table 3**). Esophageal variceal incidence in cirrhosis patients is 5% in the first year and 28% in the third year. Small esophageal varices can progress to large varices at a rate of 10–12% annually. The risk of variceal bleeding is 5% annually in small variceal and 15% in large variceal veins (**Table 4**). Early mortality (6 weeks) rate after esophageal variceal bleeding is approximately 20%.

Esophageal varices		Stomach varices	
Grade	**Class of modified paquet**	**No**	**By anatomical location**
1	Lying on top of the mucosa	1	GOV-1 (most common type)
2	Covering 1/3 of a lumen	2	GOV-2
3	Covering 50% of the lumen	3	İsolated gastric varise- type 1
		4	Isolated gastric varise-type 2

GOV: gastroesophageal varices.

Table 3.
Esophageal varices according to the modified Paquet classification and gastric varices according to anatomical classification.

No of risk	Factors of risk
1	Hepatic venous pressure gradient>12 mm Hg
2	Medium and Large varices (varices veins>5 mm)
3	Increased varices wall tension and enlarged capillaries in the varices wall (red wale sign)
4	Small varices veins in patients with CTP C
5	Other factors (Coagulopathy, infection, presence of DS)

CTP: child turcotte pugh, DS: decompansated cirrhosis.

Table 4.
Risk factors for varices bleeding.

Endoscopy is the gold standard in the diagnosis of gastrointestinal variceal veins. Endoscopic ultrasonography (EUS) can be used to detect gastric varices, to evaluate the anatomical structure, and to evaluate the response to treatment with endoscopic variceal ligation [31]. Temporary elastography to predict PHT clinically, platelet count, spleen size, MR elastography, splenic stiffness are the most commonly used non-invasive parameters in cirrhotic patients. If the liver stiffness measured by transient elastography is <20 kPa and the thrombocyte count is>150.000 uL, the probability of high risk variceal is less than 5% [32]. Esophageal varices are the most common gastrointestinal varices. Endoscopy is recommended for all newly diagnosed cirrhosis patients. Endoscopy is recommended every 3 years in compensated cirrhotic patients without variceal veins, but if the patient has other predisposing factors such as HCV, alcohol use, obesity, endoscopic screening should be repeated every 2 years.

2.2.1 Non-bleeding variceal treatment

NSBBs (propranolol, nodolol), carvedilol, or endoscopic band ligation are recommended for patients with moderate or large variceal veins for primary prophylaxis. Primary prophylaxis should be initiated after the detection of small variceal veins with red sign, medium and large variceal veins, small variceal veins in patients with CTP C. NSBBs are recommended for patients with small variceal or CTP C with red wale marks. Patients with moderate to large variceal veins should be treated with NSBBs or endoscopic band ligations. Although there is no contraindication for ascites NSBBs, caution should be exercised in severe or refractory ascites cases and high dose NSBBs should be avoided. The EASL guideline does not recommend the use of carvedilol. NSBBs should be discontinued in patients with progressive hypotension (systolic blood pressure < 90 mm Hg), bleeding, sepsis, SBP and acute kidney injury. Endoscopic band ligation is recommended if the patient has NSBBs intolerance or contraindications. The NSBBs + EBL combination is recommended as it reduces the risk of bleeding compared to monotherapy [23, 32]. Primary prophylaxis of gastric varices NSBBs can be used in primary prophylaxis in the prevention of cardiofundal varices.

2.2.2 Treatment in acute variceal bleeding

Endoscopy should be performed within 12 hours after admission and when the patient is hemodynamically stable. Initially, the patient should be evaluated hemodynamically. Early TIPS should be considered in cases of resuscitation, vasoactive drugs, antibiotic therapy, early endoscopic evaluation, and endoscopic treatment (such as endoscopic band ligation) insufficiency.

Hemoglobin target should be kept between 7–9 g/dl. Antibiotic therapy (ceftriaxone 1 g/24 h, max. 7 days) has been associated with decreased mortality, reduced re-bleeding, and reduced hospital stay. Vasoactive drugs reduce portal blood flow. The use of agents such as octreotide, somatostatin and terlipressin is recommended in all main guidelines. When variceal bleeding is suspected, it should be started early and should be continued for 2–5 days. NSBBs should be initiated after stopping vasoactive drugs. Octireotide (somatostatin analogue) initially 50 microgram IV bolus, then 50 micrograms/hr. infusion 2–5 days. Somatostatin initially 250 microgram IV bolus, then 250 microgram/hr. 2–5 days.

Terlipressin (an analogue of vasopressin) initially 2 mg IV every 4 fours untill control of bleeding, maintenance therapy 1 mg IV every hours to prevent re-bleeding 2–5 days. Among the vasoactive agents, terlipressin was only associated with reduced mortality [33]. Endoscopic intervention (such as, endoscopic band ligation) constitutes the basis of treatment in variceal bleeding. Endoscopy should be performed within 24 hours after resuscitation.

Combination of NSBBs and endoscopic band ligation is first choice for preventing re-bleeding. In patients with high failure of endoscopic treatment or risk of re-bleeding (CTP C or endoscopic active bleeding CTP B, if bleeding recurs despite vasoactive drugs), an early TIPS within 72 hours may be beneficial in selected patients. TIPS is the recommended salvage therapy for recurrent bleeding despite NSBB and endoscopic band ligation treatment. Propranolol 20-40 mg orally, 2 times/day, the treatment goal should not be below the resting heart rate 55–60/min and systolic blood pressure < 90 mm Hg. Nadolol 20–40 mg/day oral, once/day. Endoscopic band ligation should be done at intervals of 1–4 weeks until variceal veins are eradicated. Endoscopy is recommended every 6 to 12 months after eradication [31].

Treatment of gastric varices endoscopic band ligation, cyanoacrylate injection, endoscopic ultrasound guided coil placement, TIPS and BRTO treatments require a multi-disciplinary approach. Patients with acute gastric variceal bleeding are initially performed similarly to esophageal varices (a restrictive transfusion policy, vasoactive drug infusion, and antibiotic prophylaxis). NSBBs can be used in primary prophylaxis to prevent cardio fundal varices. In the endoscopic treatment of gastric varices, mainly cyanoacrylate adhesives, fibrin and thrombin therapy, use of sclerosing agents such as endoscopic band ligation and alcohol are among the treatment options [34].

Endoscopic band ligation or cyanoacrylate glue injection are recommended treatments for bleeding GOV2 varices. In the secondary prophylaxis of GOV1 variceal bleeding, the combination of NSBBs and endoscopic variceal treatment (endoscopic band ligation or cyanoacrylate injection) is the first-line treatment to prevent re-bleeding. High dose NSBBs (propranolol>160 mg/d, nadolol>80 mg/d) should be avoided in patients with refractory ascites SBP. With refractory ascites and systolic blood pressure < 90 mm Hg, serum sodium level < 130 meq/L or hepatorenal syndrome (HRS) dose should be reduced [35].

It is an adhesive hemostatic powder. It forms a mechanical barrier that covers the bleeding area by contacting with blood or tissue. Its effect lasts about 24 hours [36]. There are case reports of the use of hemospray as a salvage therapy in the failure of cyanoacrylate injection [37]. There is little evidence to support its current use in active varices bleeding.

Balloon tamponade is a short-term measure. Sengstaken Blakemore (SB) tube, Minnesota tube, Linton-Nachlas tube. Because of the high risk of re-bleeding when the balloon is lowered and its complications, it should be considered as a temporary measure until definitive control of bleeding is achieved [38]. While the success rate with the use of balloon tamponade in gastric varices is 88%, the complication rate has been reported as 10% [39]. Complications include esophageal ulcers, necrosis, esophageal rupture, and aspiration pneumonia. Consequently, it is recommended that its use be limited to temporary control until a more precise method is applied [34].

TIPS is a shunt created by placing a stent between the portal vein and hepatic vein to reduce portal pressure. If variceal bleeding of the patient cannot be controlled due to medical and endoscopic treatment, early TIPS (24 hours) should be considered [31, 40]. Complications caused by TIPS include HE, heart failure and stent stenosis. Heart failure, severe pulmonary hypertension, severe tricuspid valve insufficiency, sepsis, unresolved bile duct obstruction are among the absolute contraindications for TIPS. Relative contraindications are portal vein thrombosis, hepatoma, uncorrected coagulopathy, and severe thrombocytopenia (<20,000 uL). Cardio fundal is increasingly used as a first-line treatment for the control of bleeding from varices (GOV2, IGV1) [41].

Balloon occluded retrograde transvenous obliteration (BRTO): It is an interventional radiology technique performed by accessing gastric varices through a gastrorenal shunt and injecting the variceal sclerosing agent. The current recommendation for BRTO can be applied as a salvage therapy in cases where TIPS such as advanced liver failure or HE is contraindicated. The main side effect of BRTO can be stated as causing vascular damage due to sclerosing substance and progression of esophageal varices in case of accidental displacement of the balloon. TIPS or BRTO is not recommended for primary prophylaxis in fundal varices without bleeding. However, fundal variceal veins are the first step treatments to prevent re-bleeding. Cyanoacrylate injection is recommended instead of TIPS in patients at high risk of advanced liver dysfunction and HE [42].

2.3 Hepatic encephalopathy

HE is a complication of liver failure characterized by reversible neuropsychiatric symptoms and signs ranging from disorientation to coma. High portosystemic shunting is an important cause of morbidity in acute and chronic liver diseases. It is the second most common complication of decompensated cirrhosis after acid. In addition, HE is the most common cause of hospitalization in decompensated cirrhosis patients. The incidence of symptomatic HE ranges from 30–40% and minimal encephalopathy from 20–80% [43, 44]. Although the pathogenesis of HE is not fully understood, ammonia toxicity is an important factor in its development, but inflammation (proinflammatory cytokines, TNF alpha, ınterleukin 1, ınterleukin 6) oxidative stress, changes in intestinal microbiota play a role [45, 46]. Intestinal flora changes play an important role in the development of HE. Ammonia, which is a product of intestinal metabolism in liver cirrhosis, cannot be effectively converted into urea in the liver. Serum ammonia level rises due to the passage of portal blood to the systemic circulation and the blood passes to the brain barrier. Astrocytes are neuroglial cells responsible for protecting the blood brain barrier and detoxifying it by converting ammonia to glutamine. Glutamine increase leads to astrocyte swelling, morphological changes and cell dysfunction [47]. Increased production of ammonia during HE triggers in the clinic (GIS bleeding, hypovolemia, hypokalemia, acidosis, diabetes, excessive diuresis, excessive protein intake), impaired ammonia excretion (constipation, renal failure, sarcopenia, portosystemic shunt, zinc deficiency, branched chain amino acid deficiency) and Increased neurotoxicity (infection, drug/substance abuse, hyponatremia, hyperglycemia).

Studies have shown a decrease in bile acid production in advanced stage liver disease, an increase in more pathogenic bacteria such as enterobacteia, and a decrease in protective bacteria such as lachnospiraceae [48]. Regarding the importance of gut-liver-brain axis in HE, it has been shown that patients with HE have more systemic inflammation, dysbiosis, hyperammonemia and neuronal/astrocytic dysfunction compared to controls and patients with cirrhosis without HE [49]. According to a recent meta-analysis, it has been reported that a decrease in serum ammonia and endotoxin levels can improve and prevent HE [50]. It has been shown that HE patients who underwent fecal microbiota transplantation (FMT) had fewer HE attacks and hospitalizations. In addition, albumin infusion can reduce the frequency and severity of HE in liver cirrhosis [51].

Current guidelines for the clinical management of HE suggest lactulosis and rifaximine as first-line therapy [44]. In HE patients, care needs to be initiated for a change in consciousness, which includes securing the airway, hemodynamic stabilization, and ensuring patient safety to prevent physical injury. Intubation is recommended in patients with HE 3 or above, Glasgow score (GCS) < 8, but this is not possible in many hospitals. Protection of the airway and close monitoring is recommended. CT scan is recommended to evaluate the causes of mental changes. Infection bleeding, constipation, dehydration, sedative drugs, alcohol intoxication, or electrolyte disturbances should be identified and corrected. The goal of many treatments is to reduce ammonia levels.

In the treatment of hepatic encephalopathy, lactulose, branched chain amino acids, rifaximine, and L-ornithine L-aspartate can be used. The current treatment in HE as the first step is lactulose 20 g/30 ml-30 g/45 ml orally 3–4 times a day, if not oral, similar dose nasogastric or 300 ml enema can be given 3–4 times a day. As a side effect, diarrhea is seen as abdominal swelling and taste disturbance. In the second step treatment, rifaximine 400–500 mg can be taken orally twice a day. An important side effect is the road. It is reported that percutaneous endoscopic gastrostomy, which has not yet been approved by food and drug administration (FDA), can be used in the third step.

Lactulose and rifaximine are recommended as primary care in the prevention of recurrent HE (**Figure 1**). Probiotics and fecal microbiota transplantation are included. There is no evidence yet for the use of probiotics in acute HE [52]. L ornithine L-Aspartate (LOLA) is a substrate for the urea cycle. It can be used in HE and other hyperammonemia conditions. According to a recent meta-analysis, it is reported that HE LOLA has a positive effect on decompensation and mortality.

The american association for the study of liver diseases (AASLD) and EASL guidelines suggest that LOLA oral therapy is not effective. The potential beneficial effect of LOLA remains unclear [53]. Osmotic laxatives, non-absorbable disaccharides lactulose and lactitol are recommended as first-line therapy. Lactulose is likely to increase intestinal transit, acidifying the intestinal environment, reducing ammonia production in the intestine, increasing fecal excretion and decreasing ammonia absorption. As an antimicrobial agent, Rifaximine is a semi-synthetic non-aminoglycoside substance effective against gram-positive, negative aerobic,

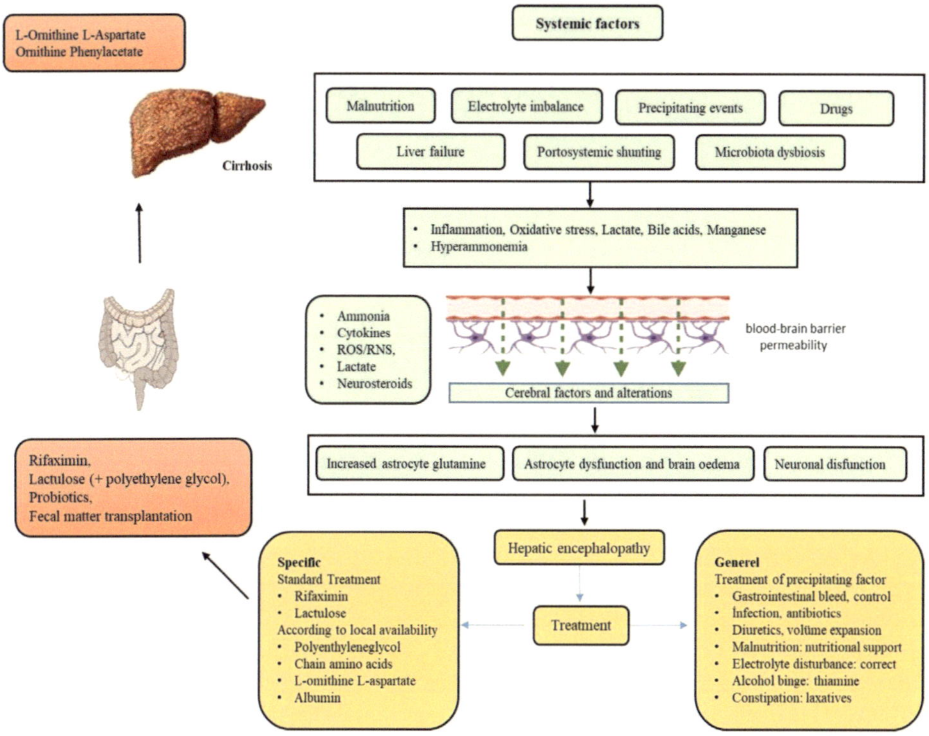

Figure 1.
Hepatic encephalopathy (HE) pathogenesis and treatment approaches.

anerobic enteric bacteria. It inhibits bacterial RNA synthesis. Rifaximine + lactulose has been shown to increase recovery in HE and decrease mortality.

In patients with recurrent HE, an improvement in FMT coordination has been shown to result in an improvement in the fecal microbiome profile with a decrease in the incidence of HE [54]. Other new treatments are changed to brain gamma-aminobutyric acid (GABA) receptors. Therapies focusing on *E. coli* are some of the new methods that are actively researched in HE but not currently close to clinical use.

2.4 Hepatorenal syndrome

Hepatorenal syndrome (HRS) is one of the most important complications in cirrhosis patients. In patients with cirrhotic portal hypertension in the pathophysiology of HRS, systemic and splanchnic vasodilation, bacterial translocation, inflammation, nitric oxide, increased prostacyclin, decrease in effective arterial blood volume (GIS bleeding, diuretics, lactulose, non-steroids, radiocontrast agent, oral intake failure) may cause hypovolemia. It causes vasoconstriction in renal artery tracts with RAAS and activation of sympathetic nervous system to decrease renal blood flow and HRS develops. It is evaluated in two groups in cirrhotic patients. (HRS AKI and non-HRS AKI) (**Table 5**). HRS AKI, decompensated cirrhosis is characterized by prerenal azotemia in patients with severe portal hypertension, nephrotoxicity, and worsening of renal functions in the absence of intrinsic renal disease. Non-HRS AKI may result from prerenal hypoperfusion bile acid nephropathy, nephrotoxicity, or acute parenchymal injury [55]. Although the best treatment option for HRS is liver transplantation, the basis of medical therapy is vasoconstrictor agents, such as terlipressin noradrenaline and dopamine in combination with albumin [56].

HRS subtypes according to the new classification	Criteria
HRS AKI	sCr ≥ 0.3 mg/dl increase up to 48 hours and/or
	Urine amount ≤ 0.5 ml/kg B.W. ≥6 h or
	sCr ≥ 50% according to basal value, increase within 3 months
HRS NAKI	eGFR <60 ml/min 1.73 m^2 in the absence of other structural causes
	<50% increase in sCr basal value within 3 months in outpatients

HRS AKI Hepatorenal sendrom acute kidney injury, NRS NAKI hepatorenal sendrom non acute kidney injury sCr, serum creatinine, eGFR estimated glomerular filtration rate.

Table 5.
Classification of Hepatorenal syndrome subtypes in cirrhosis.

In patients followed up with HRS in the intensive care unit, initial treatment is recommended as a combination of norepinephrine and albumin. (norepinephrine intravenously continuous infusion 0.5–3 mg/hr, albumin intravenous bolus 1 g/kg per day for at least two days). Terlipressin albumin combination is recommended as the initial therapy in HRS patients outside the intensive care unit. Terlipressin 1–2 mg is recommended as an intravenous bolus every 4 to 6 hours. Albumin is given for 2 days as intravenous bolus (1 gr/kg per day). During follow-up, terlipressin treatment is recommended as 25–50 g/day until discontinuation. TIPS therapy until liver transplantation can sometimes be successful in specially selected patients who are unresponsive to medical therapy [57–59].

2.5 Hepatopulmonary syndrome

Hepatopulmonary syndrome (HPS) is the most common cause of respiratory failure in patients with chronic liver disease. It is characterized by a gas exchange abnormality caused by intrapulmonary vascular dilatations (IPVD) in liver patients. Its incidence ranges from 4–47%. The pathogenesis of HPS includes a complex pathogenetic mechanism such as increased nitric oxide production, angiogenesis, intrapulmonary shunt and ventilation perfusion mismatch. Clinical consequences of hypoxemia can be seen together with progressive dyspnea, cyanosis, clubbing, platypnea and orthodoxy, and chronic pulmonary comorbidity (COPD, asthma bronchiale, idiopathic pulmonary fibrosis, restrictive lung disease).

Hepatopulmonary syndrome diagnostic criteria are partial oxygen pressure < 80 mmHg or alveolar-arterial oxygen gradient ≥15 mmHg (PO2 gradient) (or > 20 mmHg over 65 years of age). Detection of intrapulmonary vascular dilatation (Contrasted ECO cardıography or lung perfusion scan with radioactive albumin). Liver transplantation is the only successful treatment that alters the natural history of HPS and improves arterial hypoxemia. There is no effective treatment support for HPS other than long-term oxygen support [60–62].

2.6 Acute on chronic liver failure

Acute on chronic liver failure (ACLF) is a clinical sudden hepatic decompensation syndrome associated with one or more extra hepatic organ failure, increased mortality, observed in patients with pre-existing chronic liver disease. Hepatic causes include alcohol-related liver damage, drug-induced hepatic damage, viral hepatitis (A, B, C, D, and E), hypoxic damage or liver surgeries, including TIPS, in the etiology of pre-existing liver disease precipitating events. Extrahepatic causes are

DOI: http://dx.doi.org/10.5772/intechopen.96155

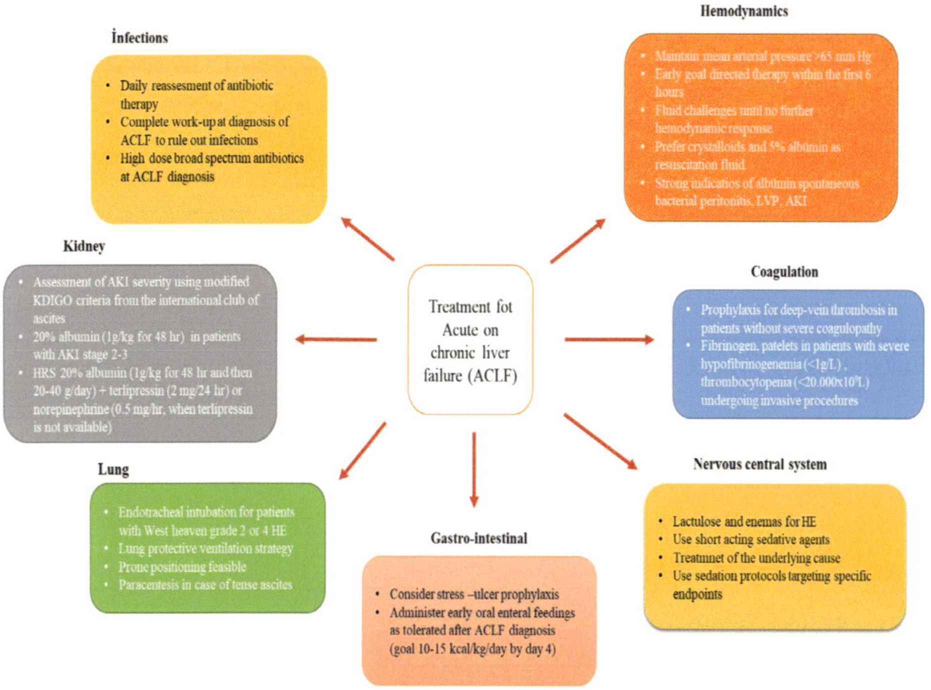

Figure 2.
Treatment approaches in organ failure due to acute on chronic liver failure (ACLF), AKI: Acute kidney ınjury, KDIGO: kidney disease improving globai outcomes, HE: Hepatic encephalopathy, HRS: Hepatorenal syndrome, LVP: large volume paracentesis.

bacterial infection and major surgical interventions. In patients with chronic liver disease, acute triggering agents trigger inflammatory cytokine cascade by causing hepatocyte damage, leading to further liver damage decompensation, multi-organ failure and death in the presence of insufficient hepatocyte regeneration [63, 64].

It consists of prevention of triggering factors that lead to acute decompensation, supportive therapy, early initiation of specific therapy and management of complications (**Figure 2**). All patients should be followed, preferably in a center with liver transplant facilities.

The essence of ACLF treatment is based on supportive treatment of organ failure in intensive care conditions. Liver transplantation is a good long-term effective treatment for selected patients. Potential treatment alternatives that will improve patient survival are highly awaited. There is currently no specific effective treatment for their patients. Therefore, treatment is based on organ support and treatment of associated complications.

2.7 Gut microbiota relationship in decompensated cirrhosis

Cirrhosis is associated with an altered immune response in the stool, potentially due to dysbiosis in the intestinal mucosa. Patients with cirrhosis have an altered gut-liver axis associated with changes in gut microbiota composition and function, associated with liver disease severity, intestinal barrier disorder, and changes in intestinal and systemic inflammation. Microbiota is one of the organs most exposed to intestinal toxins through the liver portal system. The gut microbiota is the first line of defense against toxic bacterial products in protecting the host's mucosal barrier integrity. Firmicutes, bacteroidetes, actinobacteria, proteobacteria, verrucomicrobia and fusobacteria are the main intestinal bacteria in the gastrointestinal flora. Firmicutes and bacteroidetes make up 90% of all bacteria [65]. Gastrointestinal system microbiota plays an important role in providing intestinal epithelial permeability and barrier function in NAFLD/NASH. Toxic bacterial products such as lipopolysaccharides bind to the CD14 receptor with Toll-like receptors (TLR), and stress-activated protein kinase, JNK, P38, interferon regulatory factor 3, nuclear factor JB play a role in the NASH process by initiating inflammatory cascade [66, 67]. In animal models, it has been shown that feeding mice with impaired intestinal barrier function with a diet containing high saturated fat, fructose and cholesterol leads to more severe steatohepatitis development compared to the control group [68]. Nutrition with a high fat diet; Atrophy in epithelial cell microvilli, disruption in the tight junction between cells, bacterial overgrowth in the small intestine (SIBO) is more severe in NASH than in NAFLD. Change in intestinal barrier function; Lipopolysaccharide and toxic bacterial products (other organic compounds such as ethanol, acetone, butanoic acid) cause the liver to be exposed to higher levels of inflammatory bacterial metabolites [69].

2.8 Artificial liver support systems

Artificial liver support systems (ALSS) are used to provide recovery in patients with acute liver failure (ALF) and acute-chronic liver failure and to act as a bridge until transplantation. There are two main types of devices, artificial and bioartificial. Artificial liver devices are detoxification of blood or plasma, removal of physical and chemical gradients, removal of toxic and metabolic wastes by means of albumin. There are artificial liver support systems used today, such as Molecular adsorbent recirculating system (MARS), single - pass albumin dialysis (SPAD), Prometheus, selective plasma filtration therapy and hemodiafiltration. There was no difference between Prometheus and standard medical treatment in terms of survival. The role of TPE2 in patients with ALF plasmapheresis ACLF is not known. Prospective studies are needed on this issue. Its effectiveness in hemodialysis patients with ALF and ACLF remains unclear. The effect of MARS therapy on ACLF and ALF survival has not been demonstrated [70, 71].

3. Conclusions

Portal hypertension has an important place in complications and deaths related to cirrhosis. Non-selective beta blockers occupy an important place in the medical treatment of portal hypertension, but their potential side effects limit their use. New agents that suppress fibrosis, tissue damage and angiogenesis are needed in cirrhosis. Statins and PPARα/y agonists may be an alternative in this regard. Intestinal microbiota (systemic inflammation, dysbiosis, increased intestinal permeability, endotoxemia, impaired intestinal motility, bacterial overgrowth, increased production of short-chain fatty acids and changes in metabolism) play an important role in the pathogenesis of liver diseases. Dysbiosis plays a key role in the development of cirrhosis-related complications. Moreover, modulation of the microbiome with current and future therapeutic strategies is thought to be the cornerstone of cirrhosis management. It is predicted that the microbiota will play an important role in developing new prognostic and therapeutic strategies in cirrhotic patients.

Conflict of interest

The authors declare no conflict of interest.

Author details

Anıl Delik* and Yakup Ülger
Department of Gastroenterology, Faculty of Medicine, Çukurova University, Adana, Turkey

*Address all correspondence to: anildelik@gmail.com

References

[1] Long, Brit, and Alex Koyfman. "The emergency medicine evaluation and management of the patient with cirrhosis." The American Journal of Emergency Medicine 2018:36.4: 689-698.

[2] P. Ichai, D. Samuel Epidemiology of liver failure Clin Res Hepatol Gastroenterol.2011:35(1), pp. 610-617. DOI: 10.1016/j.clinre.2011.03.010

[3] Wong MCS, Huang JLW, George J, et al. The changing epidemiology of liver diseases in the Asia-Pacific region. Nat Rev Gastroenterol Hepatol 2019;16:57-73. DOI: 10.1038/s41575-018-0055-0

[4] Asrani SK, Devarbhavi H, Eaton J, et al. Burden of liver diseases in the world. J Hepatol 2019;70:151-171. DOI: 10.1016/j.jhep.2018.09.014

[5] Hofmeister MG, Rosenthal EM, Barker LK, et al. Estimating prevalence of hepatitis C virus infection in the United States,2013-2016. Hepatology 2019;69:1020-1031. DOI: 10.1002/hep.30297

[6] D'Amico G, Garcia-Tsao G, Pagliaro L. Natural history and prognostic indicators of survival in cirrhosis: a systematic review of 118 studies. J Hepatol. 2006;44:217-231. DOI: 10.1016/j.jhep.2005.10.013

[7] Bernardi M, Moreau R, Angeli P, Schnabl B, Arroyo V. Mechanisms of decompensation and organ failure in cirrhosis: From peripheral arterial vasodilation to systemic inflammation hypothesis. J Hepatol 2015;63:1272-1284. DOI: 10.1016/j.jhep.2015.07.004

[8] Hotchkiss, RS. et al. Sepsis and septic shock. Nat. Rev. Dis. Primers. 2016:2, 16045. DOI: 10.1038/nrdp.2016.45

[9] Trautwein C, Friedman SL, Schuppan D, Pinzani M. Hepatic fibrosis: Concept to treatment. J Hepatol 2015;62:S15–S24. DOI: 10.1016/j.jhep.2015.02.039

[10] Schrier RW, Arroyo V, Bernardi M, Epstein M, Henriksen JH, Rodes J. Peripheral arterial vasodilation hypothesis: a proposal for the initiation of renal sodium and water retention in cirrhosis. Hepatology 1988;8:1151-1157. DOI: 10.1002/hep.1840080532

[11] Arroyo V, Fernandez J. Relationship Between Systemic Hemodynamics, Renal Dysfunction, and Fluid Retention in Cirrhosis. Clin Liver Dis 2013; 2: 120-122 [DOI: 10.1002/cld.185]

[12] Arroyo V, Terra C, Ginès P. Advances in the pathogenesis and treatment of type-1 and type-2 hepatorenal syndrome. J Hepatol 2007; 46: 935-946 [PMID: 17391801 DOI: 10.1016/j.jhep.2007.02.001]

[13] Garbuzenko, Dmitry Victorovich, and Nikolay Olegovich Arefyev. "Current approaches to the management of patients with cirrhotic ascites." World Journal of Gastroenterology 25.28 2019: 3738. DOI: 10.3748/wjg.v25.i28.3738

[14] Arroyo V, Ginès P, Gerbes AL, Dudley FJ, Gentilini P, Laffi G, Reynolds TB, Ring-Larsen H, Schölmerich J. Definition and diagnostic criteria of refractory ascites and hepatorenal syndrome in cirrhosis. International Ascites Club. Hepatology 1996; 23: 164-176 [PMID: 8550036 DOI: 10.1002/hep.510230122]

[15] Haberl J, Zollner G, Fickert P, Stadlbauer V. To salt or not to salt?-That is the question in cirrhosis. Liver Int 2018; 38: 1148-1159 [PMID: 29608812 DOI: 10.1111/liv.13750]

[16] Lenz K, Buder R, Kapun L, Voglmayr M. Treatment and management of ascites and

hepatorenal syndrome: an update. Therap Adv Gastroenterol 2015; 8: 83-100 [PMID: 25729433 DOI: 10.1177/1756283X14564673]

[17] Angeli P, Fasolato S, Mazza E, Okolicsanyi L, Maresio G, Velo E, etal. Combined versus sequential diuretic treatment of ascites in non-azotaemic patients with cirrhosis: results of an open randomised clinical trial. Gut 2010; 59: 98-104 [PMID: 19570764 DOI: 10.1136/gut.2008.176495]

[18] Piano S, Tonon M, Angeli P. Management of ascites and hepatorenal syndrome. Hepatol Int 2018; 12: 122-134 [PMID: 28836115 DOI: 10.1007/s12072-017-9815-0]

[19] Biecker E. Diagnosis and therapy of ascites in liver cirrhosis. World J Gastroenterol 2011; 17: 1237-1248 [PMID: 21455322 DOI: 10.3748/wjg.v17.i10.1237]

[20] Sahay M, Sahay R. Hyponatremia: A practical approach. Indian J Endocrinol Metab 2014; 18: 760-771 [PMID: 25364669 DOI: 10.4103/2230-8210.141320]

[21] Bernardi M, Caraceni P, Navickis RJ, Wilkes MM. Albumin infusion in patients undergoing largevolume paracentesis: a meta-analysis of randomized trials. Hepatology 2012; 55: 1172-1181 [PMID: 22095893 DOI: 10.1002/hep.24786]

[22] Kozaki K, IInuma M, Takagi T, Fukuda T, Sanpei T, etal. Cell-Free and Concentrated Ascites Reinfusion Therapy for Decompensated Liver Cirrhosis. Ther Apher Dial 2016; 20: 376-382 [PMID: 27523078 DOI: 10.1111/1744-9987.12469]

[23] European Association for the Study of the Liver. "EASL Clinical Practice Guidelines for the management of patients with decompensated cirrhosis." Journal of hepatology 69.2 2018: 406-460. DOI: 10.1016/j.jhep.2018.03.024.

[24] Runyon, Bruce A. "Introduction to the revised American Association for the Study of Liver Diseases Practice Guideline management of adult patients with ascites due to cirrhosis 2012." Hepatology 57.4 2013: 1651-1653. DOI: 10.1002/hep.26359

[25] Guo TT, Yang Y, Song Y, Ren Y, Liu ZX, Cheng G. Effects of midodrine in patients with ascites due to cirrhosis: Systematic review and meta-analysis. J Dig Dis 2016; 17: 11-19 [PMID: 26630543 DOI: 10.1111/1751-2980.12304]

[26] Bai M, Qi XS, Yang ZP, Yang M, Fan DM, Han GH. TIPS improves liver transplantation-free survival in cirrhotic patients with refractory ascites: an updated meta-analysis. World J Gastroenterol 2014; 20: 2704-2714 [PMID: 24627607 DOI: 10.3748/wjg.v20.i10.2704]

[27] Allegretti AS, Ortiz G, Cui J, Wenger J, etal. Changes in Kidney Function After Transjugular Intrahepatic Portosystemic Shunts Versus Large-Volume Paracentesis in Cirrhosis: A Matched Cohort Analysis. Am J Kidney Dis 2016; 68: 381-391 [PMID: 26994685 DOI: 10.1053/j.ajkd.2016.02.041]

[28] Hamel B, Guillaud O, Roman S, Vallin M, Pilleul F, Valette PJ, etal Prognostic factors in patients with refractory ascites treated by transjugular intrahepatic porto-systemic shunt: From the liver to the kidney. Dig Liver Dis 2014; 46: 1001-1007 [PMID: 25096966 DOI: 10.1016/j.dld.2014.06.013]

[29] Solà E, Sanchez-Cabús S, Rodriguez E, Elia C, Cela R, Moreira R, etal. Effects of alfapump™ system on kidney and circulatory function in patients with cirrhosis and refractory ascites. Liver Transpl 2017; 23: 583-593 [PMID: 28318147 DOI: 10.1002/lt.24763]

[30] Kovalak M, Lake J, Mattek N, Eisen G, Lieberman D, Zaman A. Endoscopic screening for varices in cirrhotic patients: data from a national endoscopic database. Gastrointest Endosc. 2007;65:82-88. DOI: 10.1016/j.gie.2006.08.023

[31] Lesmana, CRA, Raharjo, M, Gani, RA. Managing liver cirrhotic complications: Overview of esophageal and gastric varices. Clinical and molecular hepatology. 2020;26(4): 444. DOI:https://doi.org/10.3350/cmh.2020.0022

[32] Garcia-Tsao, Guadalupe, et al. "Portal hypertensive bleeding in cirrhosis: Risk stratification, diagnosis, and management: 2016 practice guidance by the American Association for the study of liver diseases." Hepatology 65.1 :2017: 310-335. DOI: 10.1002/hep.28906

[33] Zhou X, Tripathi D, Song T, Shao L, Han B, Zhu J, Han D, Liu F, Qi X. Terlipressin for the treatment of acute variceal bleeding: A systematic review and meta-analysis of randomized controlled trials. Medicine (Baltimore) 2018; 97: e13437 [PMID: 30508958 DOI: 10.1097/MD.0000000000013437]

[34] Tripathi D, Stanley AJ, Hayes PC, Patch D, Millson C, Mehrzad H, etal Clinical Services and Standards Committee of the British Society of Gastroenterology. U.K. guidelines on the management of variceal haemorrhage in cirrhotic patients. Gut 2015; 64: 1680-1704 [PMID: 25887380 DOI: 10.1136/gutjnl-2015-309262]

[35] McAvoy NC, Plevris JN, Hayes PC. Human thrombin for the treatment of gastric and ectopic varices. World J Gastroenterol 2012; 18: 5912-5917 [PMID: 23139607 DOI: 10.3748/wjg.v18.i41.5912]

[36] Ibrahim M, El-Mikkawy A, Abdel Hamid M, Abdalla H, Lemmers A, Mostafa I, Devière J. Early application of haemostatic powder added to standard management for oesophagogastric variceal bleeding: a randomised trial. Gut 2018 [PMID: 29730601 DOI: 10.1136/gutjnl-2017-314653]

[37] Holster IL, Poley JW, Kuipers EJ, Tjwa ET. Controlling gastric variceal bleeding with endoscopically applied hemostatic powder (Hemospray™). J Hepatol 2012; 57: 1397-1398 [PMID: 22864337 DOI: 10.1016/j.jhep.2012.07.024]

[38] Carbonell N, Pauwels A, Serfaty L, Fourdan O, Lévy VG, Poupon R. Improved survival after variceal bleeding in patients with cirrhosis over the past two decades. Hepatology 2004; 40: 652-659 [PMID: 15349904 DOI: 10.1002/hep.20339]

[39] Panés J, Terés J, Bosch J, Rodés J. Efficacy of balloon tamponade in treatment of bleeding gastric and esophageal varices. Results in 151 consecutive episodes. Dig Dis Sci 1988; 33: 454-459 [PMID: 3280273] DOI: 10.1097/MD.0000000000013437

[40] de Franchis R; Baveno VI Faculty. Expanding consensus in portal hypertension: Report of the Baveno VI Consensus Workshop: Stratifying risk and individualizing care for portal hypertension. J Hepatol. 2015;63:743-752. DOI: 10.1016/j.jhep.2015.05.022

[41] Vine, Louisa J., Mohsan Subhani, and Juan G. Acevedo. "Update on management of gastric varices." World Journal of Hepatology 11.3 :2019: 250. DOI: 10.4254/wjh.v11.i3.250

[42] Kim SK, Lee KA, Sauk S, Korenblat K. Comparison of Transjugular Intrahepatic Portosystemic Shunt with Covered Stent and Balloon-Occluded Retrograde Transvenous Obliteration in Managing Isolated Gastric Varices. Korean J Radiol 2017; 18: 345-354 [PMID: 28246514 DOI: 10.3348/kjr.2017.18.2.345].

[43] Dharel N, Bajaj JS. Definition and nomenclature of hepatic encephalopathy. J Clin Exp Hepatol. 2015;5:S37-S41. DOI: 10.1016/j.jceh.2014.10.001

[44] Vilstrup H., Amodio P., Bajaj J., Cordoba J., Ferenci P., Mullen K. D., Wong P. Hepatic encephalopathy in chronic liver disease: 2014 practice guideline by the American Association for the Study of Liver Diseases and the European Association for the Study of the Liver. Hepatology, 2014:60(2), 715-735. doi:10.1016/j.jhep.2014.05.042

[45] Tranah T., Paolino A., Shawcross D. Pathophysiologicalmechanismsofhepatic encephalopathy: Pathophysiological mechanisms. Clinical Liver Disease, 2015:5(3), 59-63. doi:10.1002/cld.445

[46] Butt Z., Jadoon N., Salaria O., Mushtaq K., Riaz I., Shahzad A., Sarwar S. Diabetes mellitus and decompensated cirrhosis: Risk of hepatic encephalopathy in different age groups. Journal of Diabetes, 2013:5(4), 449-455. doi:10.1111/1753-0407.12067

[47] Iwasa M., Takei Y. Pathophysiology and management of hepatic encephalopathy 2014 update: Ammonia toxicity and hyponatremia: Management of hepatic encephalopathy. Hepatology Research, 2015:45(12), 1155-1162. doi:10.1111/hepr.12495

[48] Liu Q, Duan ZP, Ha DK, et al. Synbiotic modulation of gut flora: effect on minimal hepatic encephalopathy in patients with cirrhosis. Hepatology 2004;39:1441-9. DOİ.org/10.1002/hep.20194

[49] Ahluwalia V, Betrapally NS, Hylemon PB. Impaired gut-liver-brain axis in patients with cirrhosis. Sci Rep 2016;6:26800. DOI: 10.1038/srep26800

[50] Cao Q, Yu CB, ang SG, et al. Effect of probiotic treatment on cirrhotic patients with minimal hepatic encephalopathy: a meta-analysis. HepatobiliaryPancreat Dis Int 2018;17(1):9-16. DOI: 10.1016/j.hbpd.2018.01.005

[51] Bai Z., Bernardi M., Yoshida EM., Li, H., Guo, X., Méndez-Sánchez, N. et al. Albumin infusion may decrease the incidence and severity of overt hepatic encephalopathy in liver cirrhosis. Aging (Albany NY), 2019:11(19), 8502. DOI: 10.18632/aging.102335.

[52] Dalal R, McGee RG, Riordan SM, et al. Probiotics for people with hepatic encephalopathy. Cochrane Database Syst Rev. 2017;2:CD008716. DOI: 10.1002/14651858.CD008716.pub3

[53] Rose CF, Amodio P, Bajaj JS, Dhiman RK, Montagnese S, taylor-Robinson SD, et al. Hepatic encephalopathy: Novel insights into classification, pathophysiology and therapy. Journal of Hepatology . 2020;73:1526-1547. DOI:https://doi.org/10.1016/j.jhep.2020.07.013

[54] Bajaj JS, Kassam Z, Fagan A, et al. Fecal microbiota transplant from a rational stool donor improves hepatic encephalopathy: a randomized clinical trial. Hepatology. 2017;66:1727-1738. DOI: 10.1002/hep.29306

[55] Amin AA, Alabsawy EI, Jalan R, davenport A. Epidemiology, Pathophysiology, and Management of Hepatorenal Syndrome. Seminars in Nephrology. 2019;39:1:17-30. DOI: 10.1016/j.semnephrol.2018.10.002.

[56] Zhang, J., Rössle, M., Zhou, X., Deng, J., Liu, L., Qi, X. Terlipressin for the treatment of hepatorenal syndrome: an overview of current evidence. Current medical research and opinion. 2019;35(5): 859-868. DOI: 10.1080/03007995.2018.1552575

[57] Rajesh, S., George, T., Philips, C. A., Ahamed, R., Kumbar, S., Mohan, N. et al. Transjugular intrahepatic

portosystemic shunt in cirrhosis: An exhaustive critical update. World Journal of Gastroenterology. 2020:26(37); 5561. DOİ: 10.3748/wjg.v26.i37.556.

[58] Bruce AR. Hepatorenal syndrome. UpToDate. 2020. www.uptodate.com/contents/hepatorenal-syndrome

[59] Angeli P, Garcia-Tsao G, Nadim MK, Parikh CR. News in pathophysiology, definition and classification of hepatorenal syndrome: A step beyond the ınternatıonal club of ascites (ıCA) consensus document. 2019;71:811-822. DOI: 10.1016/j.jhep.2019.07.002

[60] Krowka MJ, Fallon MB, Kawut SM, et al. International Liver Transplant Society Practice Guidelines: Diagnosis and Management of Hepatopulmonary Syndrome and Portopulmonary Hypertension. Transplantation 2016; 100:1440. DOI: 10.1097/TP.0000000000001229

[61] Nayyar D, Man HS, Granton J, et al. Proposed management algorithm for severe hypoxemia after liver transplantation in the hepatopulmonary syndrome. Am J Transplant 2015; 15:903. DOI: 10.1111/ajt.13177

[62] Zhao H, Liu F, Yue Z, et al. Clinical efficacy of transjugular intrahepatic portosystemic shunt in the treatment of hepatopulmonary syndrome. Medicine (Baltimore) 2017; 96:e9080. DOİ: 10.1097/MD.0000000000009080

[63] Arroyo V, Moreau R, Jalan R. Acute-on-Chronic Liver Failure. New England journal of Medicine. 2020;382:2137-2145. DOI: 10.1056/NEJMra1914900

[64] Zaccherini G, Weiss E, Moreau R. Acute-on-Chronic liver failure: Definitions pathophysiology and principles of treatment. JHEP Reports. 2020;100176. DOI: 10.1016/j.jhepr.2020.100176

[65] Zhou D, Fan JG. Gut microbiota and energy balance: role in obesity. Proc Nutr Soc. 2015;74:227-234. DOİ: 10.1017/S0029665114001700.

[66] Bajaj JS. Altered Microbiota in Cirrhosis and its relationship to the Development of infection. Clinical Liver Disease, 2019:14(3), 107. DOI: 10.1002/cld.827.

[67] Zheng, R., Wang, G., Pang, Z., Ran, N., Gu, Y., Guan, X. et al. Liver cirrhosis contributes to the disorder of gut microbiota in patients with hepatocellular carcinoma. Cancer Medicine. 2020. Jun;9(12):4232-4250. DOİ: 10.1002/cam4.3045.

[68] Rahman K, Desai C, Iyer SS, et al. Loss of junctional adhesion molecule A promotes severe steatohepatitis in mice on a diet high in saturated fat, fructose, and cholesterol. Gastroenterology. 2016;151:733-746 e712. DOİ: 10.1053/j.gastro.2016.06.022

[69] Mao JW, Tang HY, Zhao T, et al. Intestinal mucosal barrier dysfunction participates in the progress of nonalcoholic fatty liver disease. Int J Clin Exp Pathol. 2015;8:3648-3658. PMID: 26097546

[70] Larsen, FS. Artificial liver support in acute and acute-on-chronic liver failure. Current opinion in critical care, 2019;25(2):187-191. DOI: 10.1097/MCC.0000000000000584

[71] Tandon, R., and Froghi, S. Artificial liver support systems. Journal of Gastroenterology and Hepatology. 2020. DOİ: 10.1111/jgh.15255.

Chapter 14

Therapy that Targets Growth Factor Receptors: Novel Approach for Liver Cirrhosis Treatment

Halyna Kuznietsova and Olexandr Ogloblya

Abstract

The background of liver fibrous degeneration is excessive cell proliferation including hepatic stellate cells, inflammatory cells, fibroblasts and myofibroblasts. Often it is the consequence of increased growth factors and/or their receptors expression. Key contributors to the liver cell proliferation are EGFR, FGFR, PDGFR, VEGFR, TGFβR, the increased expression of which is indicated on *in vitro* and *in vivo* models of liver fibrosis and in patients who experienced fibrosis-accompanied liver diseases. Elimination of growth factors/suppression of their receptors is associated with the weakening/elimination of certain processes responsible for fibrogenesis. This chapter represents the evidences of the efficacy of growth factor receptors signaling downregulation for the suppression of liver fibrosis and cirrhosis and their individual manifestations. The data on established and experimental therapeutics – specific and multikinase growth factor receptor inhibitors which demonstrated antifibrotic and anticirrhotic activity under *in vitro* and *in vivo* models, are also presented.

Keywords: EGFR, VEGFR, PDGFR, FGFR, TGFβR, tyrosine kinase inhibitors

1. Introduction

If organs with high regenerative capacity undergo chronic injury and inflammation, their healing often occurs abnormally - due to replacement of the damaged elements with connective tissue. The most striking example of such distorted regeneration is the development of liver fibrosis and cirrhosis on the background of its chronic damage. Fibrosis is an "exceeding" healing accompanied with the formation of an excessive amount of connective tissue incorporated into liver parenchyma due to extracellular matrix (ECM) overproduction and/or its incomplete degradation.

The main etiological factors of liver fibrosis and cirrhosis are alcohol, storage diseases, hepatitis viruses, hepatotoxic drugs, cholestasis, and autoimmune reactions. The trigger of fibrogenesis is chronic injury accompanied by an inflammatory component, which causes the activation and expansion of mesenchymal cells (including fibroblasts, myofibroblasts, smooth muscle cells) and increased synthesis of ECM molecules, predominantly collagen. Cells involved into the inflammation actively produce soluble factors like pro-inflammatory cytokines, endothelins, growth factors, reactive oxygen and nitrogen species, which also promote fibrogenesis [1, 2]. The final stage of organ's fibrosis is cirrhosis - the irreversible replacement of a significant part of that by connective tissue, which leads to the organ's failure. The main cells which "trigger" liver fibrosis are hepatic stellate cells (HSC). Under liver injury and if being stimulated with cytokines produced by inflammatory cells, Kupffer cells and hepatocytes, HSCs are activated and transformed into myofibroblasts. The latters are able to migrate to the damaged area and produce a reduced number of matrix metalloproteinases (MMPs) and an increased number of their tissue inhibitors (TIMPs) and ECM proteins, causing the growth of connective tissue in liver and accumulation of fibrillar matrix into Disse spaces. Thick bundles of newly synthesized collagen fibers in the Disse spaces between hepatocytes are surrounded by fibroblasts, macrophages, HSCs, lymphocytes, polymorphonuclear leukocytes, eosinophils and plasmatic cells. These cells produce ROS, inflammatory mediators and growth factors, thus maintaining liver inflammation and promoting substantial disorders followed by cirrhosis development [3].

Cirrhosis is the endpoint of many liver diseases and causes the development of serious complications with possible fatal outcome. Those include: liver failure, gastrointestinal bleeding, portal hypertension, i.e. increased pressure in the portal vein, and hepatic coma. Thus, mortality from liver cirrhosis within 1 year after diagnosis varies from 1 to 57%, depending on the stage [4] and reaches more than 1.2 million deaths annually [5].

2. The role of growth factors and their receptors in fibrogenesis

Growth factor receptors are tightly involved in the pathogenesis of chronic inflammation due to their signaling close relationship with the major proinflammatory pathways. Those include, in particular, nuclear factor kappa B (NFκB), p38 mitogen-activated protein kinase (MAPK), phosphatidylinositol 3-kinase/Protein kinase B (PI3K/Akt), Janus kinase/signal transducer and activator of transcription (Jak/STAT) signaling pathways, which are activated not only by proinflammatory cytokines, but also by individual growth factors, such as transforming growth factor beta (TGFβ), TGFα, hepatocytes growth factor (HGF), epidermal growth factor (EGF), insulin-like growth factor (IGF) [6–9], associated with the "start" of regenerative processes.

The main proinflammatory pathways are also profibrogenic ones. Thus, NF-κB signaling provides not only survival and inflammatory reaction of Kupffer cells, but also survival, inflammatory response and activation of HSCs. Constitutive activity of this pathway in HSCs and/or hepatic myofibroblasts stimulates fibrous degeneration of the liver due to direct profibrogenic and antiapoptotic effects and by stimulating the secretion of cytokines - macrophage attractants [10]. Another proinflammatory pathway, STAT3, is involved in the control of MMPs and TIMPs transcription, TGF-β1 and ECM molecules synthesis and secretion, myofibroblasts proliferation and resistance to apoptosis, thus enhancing tissue regeneration. Activation of this pathway is observed in many tissues due to their fibrosis [11]. The PI3K/Akt pathway, in addition to its significant role in apoptosis inhibition and cell proliferation and survival, may promote epithelial-mesenchymal transition, thus contributing to fibrogenesis [12] (**Figure 1**). Furthermore, this pathway could be activated by EGF receptor (EGFR), the ligands of which are ones of the main profibrogenic growth factors [13]. P38 MAPK pathway is the one, the effects of the main profibrogenic cytokine TGF-β1 are realized through [14].

Macrophages and neutrophils, the first responders on damage and inducers of acute inflammation, also produce cytokines and chemokines, which serve as mitogens and chemoattractants for endothelial, epithelial and mesenchymal cells

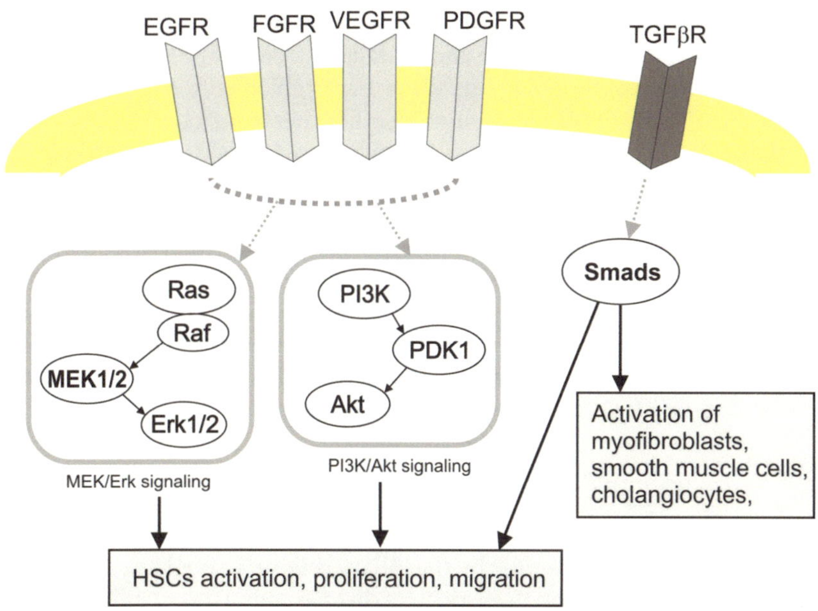

Figure 1.
The role of growth factor receptors in liver fibrogenesis.

(myofibroblasts, HSCs) migrating to the cites of injury. With the chronicity of the inflammatory process, these cells are activated and secrete profibrogenic cytokines and growth factors such as TGF-β1, interleukin 13 (IL-13) and platelet-derived growth factor (PDGF), which further activate macrophages and fibroblasts and promote proliferation of those in addition to epithelial cells. Wound/injury healing also includes ECM synthesis and remodeling. Under chronic inflammation, this process is violated: the synthesis of ECM molecules prevails on their cleavage, leading to accumulation of those, which called fibrosis [15].

Impaired activity of protein kinases, in particular growth factor receptors such as EGFR, vaso-endothelial growth factor receptor (VEGFR), PDGF receptor (PDGFR), fibroblast growth factor receptor (FGFR), play a significant role in development of numerous non-malignant liver diseases, including diseases associated with its fibrous degeneration [16]. Thus, PDGF is the most important cytokine responsible for the proliferation of HSCs; PDGF, VEGF and FGF2 induce their migration, TGF-β causes HSCs transformation to myofibroblasts, stimulates synthesis of ECM by those and inhibits its degradation. Inhibition of these growth factors receptors downregulates mentioned processes [17]. Furthermore, an excessive proliferation of cholangiocytes which express numerous cytokines, chemokines and growth factors is one of the main mechanisms of fibrogenesis. The proliferating cholangiocytes also involve myofibroblasts, fibroblasts and immune cells in this process [18, 19]. Therefore, activation of biliary proliferation (called ductular reaction) contributes a lot in the initiation and progression of liver fibrosis.

3. Growth factor receptors as the targets of antifibrotic therapy

There is no specific remedy for the liver fibrosis to date. Some compounds having therapeutic activity against liver fibrosis are undergoing preclinical and I-II phases of clinical trials. They include: (1) the monoclonal antibodies and low molecule inhibitors of key signaling pathways involved in the regulation of inflammation, HSCs life cycle and collagen metabolism [20]; (2) the broad-spectrum agents exhibiting antioxidant, anti-inflammatory, hepatoprotective, antilipotoxic activities such as ursolic, ursodeoxycholic and 24-norursodeoxycholic acids, resveratrol, silymarin [3]. However, the last agents are rather supplements, the positive effect of which is observed only in combination with other therapeutics.

Cytostatics like methotrexate and azathioprine are actively used for the treatment of diseases accompanied by fibrosis. However, due to the nonspecificity of action, they cause the development of numerous side effects. Therefore, the idea of using selective inhibitors of excessive cell proliferation can be fruitful. Impaired activity of tyrosine kinases, in particular growth factor receptors EGFR, VEGFR, PDGFR, TGFβR, and FGFR, contributes significantly to liver diseases associated with its fibrous degeneration [16]. Therefore, these receptors may be potential targets for antifibrotic therapy [21]. Among approved and experimental therapeutics tyrosine kinase inhibitors (TKIs) possess the leading position.

3.1 VEGFR

VEGF is a key regulator of liver cells proliferation. An increased expression of this growth factor and its receptors by the biliary cells was noted under liver biliary pathologies, in particular polycystic liver disease and primary biliary cirrhosis (PBC) [22]. PBC patients also demonstrated over-expression of the angiogenic factors Ang-1, Ang-2 and tyrosine kinase with immunoglobulin-like and EGF-like domains 2 (TIE2) their effects are realized by, in the epitheliocytes and periportal hepatocytes [23], suggesting, therefore, their contribution in fibrosis development. VEGF has been shown to stimulate also proliferation of sinusoidal endothelial cells and activated HSCs *in vitro*, indicating that VEGF-VEGFR interaction in HSCs plays an important role in liver fibrogenesis [24]. VEGFR inhibitor sunitinib significantly reduced the inflammatory infiltrate and collagen expression under liver cirrhosis [25]. Another small molecule tyrosine kinase inhibitor vatalanib, which is effective against all VEGF receptors, inhibited CCl_4-induced mice liver fibrosis, as evidenced by decrease of fibrous tissue accumulation and hepatic sinusoidal capillarization, and downregulation of α-smooth muscle actin (α-SMA), collagen I and TGF-β1 expression as well [26] (**Table 1**). Similar results were demonstrated for pan-VEGFR tyrosine kinase inhibitor PTK787/ZK222584 [27].

3.2 EGFR

The EGFR signaling plays an important role in proliferation of liver progenitor cells and their differentiation into hepatocytes or cholangiocytes during the hepatic regeneration. In liver samples of primary sclerosing cholangitic (PSC) patients, the upregulation of EGFR compared to that of healthy individuals was revealed. EGFR is also required for the induction of active pro-inflammatory response by the cholangiocytes [28]. Indeed, the panitumumab, anti-EGFR antibody, inhibited an excessive proliferation of the bile duct mucosa and accumulation of collagen fibers in chronic proliferative cholangitis [29]. In addition, anti-EGFR antibodies applied at bile duct ligation (BDL) model inhibited biliary epithelium hyperplasia and fibrosis. EGFR inhibitor erlotinib inhibited proliferation of the cholangiocytes and hepatocytes, and prevented activation of HSCs, which was demonstrated on different (CCl_4-, diethylnitrosamine (DEN)- and BDL-induced) rat models [30]. EGFR inhibition also significantly reduced viability and ECM production in activated HSCs, inhibited their proliferation and α-SMA production, but did not affect parenchymal cells [31, 32]. Moreover, inhibition of EGFR signaling by erlotinib and other specific inhibitors effectively prevented the progression of cirrhosis and regressed fibrosis in some animals [33, 34] (**Table 1**).

Drug	Target(s)	Cellular effects	Model/Patients	References
Panitumumab	EGFR	Inhibition of bile duct mucosa excessive proliferation and accumulation of collagen fibers	chronic proliferative cholangitis	Liu et al. 2019 [35]
Erlotinib	EGFR	Reduce the number of activated HSCs	DEN-, BDL-induced rats, CCl_4-induced mice	Fuchs et al. 2014 [36]
Vatalanib	VEGFR	Inhibition of α-SMA, collagen I and TGF-β1 expression	CCl_4-induced mice	Kong et al. 2017 [26]
Imatinib	PDGFR	Induce of HSC apoptosis, decrease HSC migration	CCl_4-, TAA-induced mice	Kim et al. 2012 [37]
Sunitinib	VEGFR, PDGFR, c-Kit	Decrease of vascular density, inflammatory infiltrate, α-SMA and collagen expression	CCl_4-induced rats	Tugues et al. 2007 [25]
Sorafenib	Raf, VEGFR2/3, PDGFR-β	Stimulation of HSCs autophagy and apoptosis, inhibition of HSCs proliferation and collagen deposition	High fat diet-, BDL-, DEN-induced mice	Wang et al. 2010 [38]
Pazopanib	VEGFR1, PDGFR-β, FGFR	Induce of HSCs apoptosis, inhibition of HSCs activation, α-SMA, MMP-2, TIMP-1 expression	CCl_4-induced mice	Elshal et al. 2015 [39]
Nilotinib	BCR-ABL, PDGFR, TGFβRII	Depression of HSCs activation, proliferation, migration, α-SMA formation, induce of HSCs apoptosis, reduce collagen deposition in activated HSCs and in liver tissues	CCl_4- and BDL-induced rats	Liu et al. 2011 [40]
Nintedanib	PDGFR, VEGFR, FGFR	Depression of HSCs activation, contractility, migration, collagen deposition, inhibition of macrophage migration	CCl_4-induced mice	Acora et al. 2017 [41]
Regorafenib	VEGFR1–3, PDGFR-β and FGFR, TIE2	Reduce portal hypertension, NO effects on HSCs activation and fibrosis progression or regression	BDL-, CCl_4-induced mice	Uschner et al. 2018 [42]
Brivanib	VEGFR, FGFR	Decrease of HSCs proliferation	BDL-, CCl_4-, TAA-induced mice	Nakamura et al. 2014 [17]

Table 1.
TKIs which demonstrated antifibrotic effects, their molecular targets and cellular effects.

3.3 FGFR

FGF family includes 7 subfamilies of growth factors (1, 4, 8, 9, 10, 11, 19) and four isoforms of their receptors (FGFR1, FGFR2, FGFR3, FGFR4), and all of them are involved in liver injury and regeneration. There is coordinated regulation of

FGFR activation and FGFs secretion during liver injury and subsequent healing: hepatocyte-derived FGFs activate FGFRs on HSCs, and FGFs produced by HSCs activate FGFRs on hepatocytes [38]. FGF signaling during liver damage enhances liver regeneration, however, its chronic production can also lead to the abnormal regeneration with subsequent fibrosis development.

FGF2, a main FGFR1 binding partner, is a mitogen for HSCs. FGFR1 overexpression has been reported in human liver myofibroblasts and activated HSCs compared to the non-activated ones [37]. Then, FGF2 also induces chemotaxis and chemoinvasion by HSCs and may participate in the recruitment and activation of HSCs in acute liver injury. Thus, Yu et al. demonstrated, that chronic hepatic fibrosis is markedly reduced in FGF1/FGF2-deficient mice. However, the absence of FGF1 and FGF2 did not impair the total number of HSCs and their migration into the areas of injury, but overproduction of matrix components, especially collagen α1(I), by those, and therefore excessive fibrous tissue accumulation. The probable explanation is that FGF1 and FGF2 are not essential activating ligands for proliferation and migration of activated HSCs *in vivo*, but the important ones for fibrosis progression [43].

Furthermore, blockade of FGFR1 by small molecule inhibitors prevents HSCs activation (as evidenced by diminishing of α-SMA expression by those), inhibits their proliferation and release of the inflammatory cytokines by those both *in vitro* and *in vivo*. *In vivo* experiments also demonstrated that such inhibition significantly ameliorates CCl_4-induced hepatic fibrosis in a rat model [44, 45].

The ability of FGFs to regulate HSCs proliferation, migration, and transdifferentiation makes FGFR signaling an attractive target for the treatment of hepatic fibrosis. Therapeutic agents which are developing now aim to inhibit FGFRs, to modulate FGF expression, are recombinant FGF proteins, therefore achieving to inhibit EGFR signaling in all levels [37].

3.4 PDGFR

PDGF is the most prominent cytokine that regulates HSCs activation, proliferation and migration. Primary producers of PDGF are platelets, vascular endothelial cells, pericytes and Kupffer cells. PDGFR, tyrosine kinase receptor, is primarily located in vascular endothelial cells, fibroblasts and Kupffer cells. Under the liver injury macrophages, injured endothelial cells and activated HSCs synthesize and secrete PDGF which stimulates proliferation of fibroblasts and vascular endothelial cells via autocrine and paracrine mechanisms. Additionally, PDGF promotes HSCs transformation into myofibroblasts and collagen production by those. Marked upregulation of PDGFR expression on the membranes of activated HSCs have been shown under various chronic liver diseases associated with its fibrosis. Hence, PDGFR overexpression contributes to HSCs activation by synthesized PDGF via the autocrine mechanism and enhances cellular chemotaxis [46]. Additionally, clinical studies demonstrated an excessive activation of PDGF and its downstream molecules, and association of those with the extent of fibrosis in patients with hepatic damage.

There are four PDGF subunits (A, B, C and D) and 2 types of PDGFRs (α and β), and all of them are involved in different stages of hepatic fibrogenesis. Thus, PDGF-B is elevated during the early stage of the disease and is the most potent factor associated with HSCs activation, whereas PDGF-C and -D levels continuously rise during the whole process of HSCs transformation into myofibroblasts and demonstrate relatively high level at the late stage of hepatic fibrosis. Then, quiescent HSCs express PDGFR-α only, and activated ones – predominantly PDGFR-β.

The latter is substantially upregulated, and together with PDGF-B and -D serves important role in hepatic fibrosis [46].

Activated PDGFR induces many signaling pathways, which regulate cell proliferation, migration and survival. In particular, activated Ras system through MAPK signaling cascade regulates the expression of collagen type I, MMPs, TIMPs genes responsible for ECM synthesis and degradation; phospholipase Cγ (PLCγ) signaling contributes to HSCs mitosis; PDGFR-activated PI3K/Akt and JAK/STAT pathways promote cell migration, mediate metabolic regulation, stimulate cell growth and inhibit cellular apoptosis.

Blocking of PDGF signaling has been suggested to inhibit HSCs proliferation and to ameliorate liver fibrogenesis, so the strategies aimed to regulate that have been explored in preclinical and clinical investigations. Application of PDGF isoform antagonists, blocking of PDGFR activation and its downstream pathway regulation are considered as those ones. Thus, sorafenib (a first-line oral chemotherapy drug towards advanced hepatocellular carcinoma (HCC)) is a multikinase inhibitor that targets Raf, VEGFR2/3, and PDGFR-β and has been demonstrated to be a potent antifibrotic agent. The mechanisms of its antifibrotic action were revealed on mice models (high fat diet-, BDL- and DEN- induced ones) and include HSCs autophagy and apoptosis induction (through activation of Akt/mTOR and MAPK signaling pathways), suppression of neovascularization and oxidative stress (through PDGF, STAT3 and mitochondrial respiration downregulation), and inhibition of collagen deposition [47]. Imatinib, another selective TKI, which specifically targets PDGFR, attenuates liver fibrosis and additionally inhibits PDGFR-β expression and decreases the levels of proinflammatory cytokines. The ability of imatinib to induce HSCs apoptosis and substantially decrease their migration could contribute a lot to antifibrotic activity of that and was proven *in vitro* and on CCl_4- and thioacetamide (TAA)-induced mice models [35] (**Table 1**). Strong antifibrotic activity under cholestatic liver diseases has been demonstrated for small molecule roseotoxin B, and investigation of its possible mechanisms revealed its ability to block the PDGF-B/PDGFR-β pathway in HSCs directly [48].

The great potency of PDGFR inhibitors was demonstrated on numerous animal and *in vitro* models. However, it is difficult and often impossible to distinguish the antifibrotic activity from anticancer one due to analysis of clinical trials outcomes. The first reason is that these agents are tested as anti-HCC therapeutics, and outcomes important for anticancer assessment only (like overall survival, disease-free survival etc.) are considered. The second possible reason is strong stratification of HCC patients involved in clinical trial according to their cirrhotic stage, and, despite "anticancer-important" outcomes are monitored thoroughly, the level of cirrhosis is not reassessed. So anticancer activity of the chemicals might be accompanied with antifibrotic one, however, it should be checked additionally. Furthermore, due to high similarity of the homologous domains of PDGFR and VEGFR, applied TKIs like sorafenib, sunitinib and pazopanib could not only inhibit PDGFR activation but also downregulate VEGFR (**Table 1**). It could indicate the complex and therefore more powerful action of these drugs on liver fibrogenesis, but, on the other hand, could also lead to non-target cells impairment and additional toxicity [49].

3.5 TGFβR

TGF-β is a cytokine which plays a prominent role in transformation of HSCs to myofibroblasts. Indeed, many of TGF-β pathological effects could be related with its ability to regulate cell plasticity – change of cell phenotype and function due to genetic and epigenetic changes and cytoskeleton remodeling. One of the most striking events of cell plasticity is epithelial-mesenchymal transition (EMT). Activation of HSCs and their transformation to myofibroblasts is an example of that one. Moreover, another example of cell transformation caused by TGF-β is EMT in hepatocytes accompanied with loss of cell–cell contacts and polarity [50]. Actually, TGF-β stimulates almost of all liver cell populations (portal and resident fibroblasts, bone marrow-derived fibrocytes, endothelial cells, vascular smooth muscle cells, pericytes and cholangiocytes additionally to hepatocytes and HSCs) to change into a more fibroblastic phenotype [40] and to release profibrogenic transcriptional program manifested by upregulation of collagen expression [41] and disturbances in ECM turnover through imbalance between MMPs and TIMPs. TGF-β receptors (TGFβRI and TGFβRII) are Ser/Tre protein kinases expressed on the membranes of various cells including all above mentioned ones. TGF-β is secreted by these cells and regulates their activity by autocrine and paracrine mechanisms. Moreover, both monocyte-derived macrophages and Kupffer cells (liver resident macrophages) produce this cytokine and some other profibrogenic factors like PDGF and connective tissue growth factor (CTGF), contributing, therefore, to HSCs activation and transdifferentiation, and promoting fibrosis [39]. Thus, TGF-β plays a master role in the activation of HSCs to myofibroblasts. In fact, some of the previous factors stimulate the expression, production and activation of TGF-β, which is responsible finally for the activation of HSCs, and the higher the level of TGF-β the more expressed fibrotic changes in the tissue.

The main mediators of the TGF-β-induced fibrogenic transcriptional program are SMADs (*Caenorhabditis elegans* Sma genes and the *Drosophila* Mad, Mothers against decapentaplegic) [41] (**Figure 1**). Moreover, proteins enriched in TGFR signaling involve Src, cAMP response element-binding protein (CREBP) and others, and some of them belong to EGFR signaling, indicating the crosstalk between these pathways [51]. Additionally, TGF-β1 also mediates the role of FGF1 and FGF2 in the deposition of ECM, or FGF1 and FGF2 mediate the TGF-β activity, or both factors play independent roles through convergent signaling pathways *in vivo* [43].

4. Multikinase inhibitors

Some TKIs have been shown to release antifibrotic activity do not demonstrate exact specificity against their targets and could inhibit more than one receptor. So, it is difficult to explain the mechanism of their action precisely. Nevertheless, these agents attract the attention and reveal the antifibrotic potency even more than specific inhibitors because of multiplicity of mechanisms and downregulated signaling pathways, and therefore, ability to avoid drug resistance through the compensatory mechanisms and signaling crosstalk.

For example, multikinase TKI nilotinib, which is a breakpoint cluster region protein (Bcr)-tyrosine-protein kinase ABL (Abl) inhibitor, also significantly inhibited PDGFR and TGFβRII, which contributes to depression of HSCs activation, proliferation, migration, and α-SMA formation, induction of their apoptosis, reduce collagen deposition in activated HSCs and in liver tissues of CCl_4- and BDL-induced rats experienced liver fibrosis [52]. Moreover, the effects of nilotinib also include diminished expression of VEGF and VEGFR, which, however, is expected due to high similarity of PDGFR and VEGFR kinase domains. These results indicated that nilotinib may represent a putative antifibrotic treatment due to its combined inhibition of non-receptor tyrosine kinases (nonRTK) (Abl) and RTK (PDGFR-β, TGFβRII and VEGFR) (**Table 1**).

Treatment of CCl_4-induced fibrotic mice with nintedanib that blocks PDGFR, VEGFR and FGFR, in addition to depression of HSCs activation, contractility, migration, and collagen deposition, inhibited macrophage migration, intrahepatic inflammation and angiogenesis as well [36]. Another oral multitargeted TKI pazopanib (approved for renal cell sarcoma treatment) directly inhibits PDGFRs, FGFRs, mast/stem cell growth factor receptor (KIT) and selectively suppresses VEGFR-mediated angiogenesis. The drug can halt liver fibrosis progression through modulating inflammatory cytokines, suppressing HSCs activation, inducing their apoptosis, and regulating angiogenesis [53]. Regorafenib could affect similar targets (VEGFR1–3, PDGFR-β and FGFR) and also potently inhibits another angiogenic RTK TIE2. This drug has recently been approved as a second-line therapy for HCC and demonstrated depression of cirrhotic-associated systemic changes and portal hypertension in HCC patients. Moreover, regorafenib might also be beneficial towards fibrosis and portal hypertension even in absence of HCC [42]. Despite regorafenib treatment had no direct observable effect on HSCs activation and fibrosis progression or regression (as evidenced by liver histopathology, α-SMA and hydroxyproline deposition), however, even its acute administration improved cirrhotic portal hypertension (BDL and CCl_4 models of liver fibrosis) and also hemodynamic circulation in an animal model mimicking portal vein thrombosis [54] (**Table 1**). These findings might explain the anticirrhotic effects of the drug in HCC patients by normalization of liver blood circulation in fibrotic liver and therefore exhausting the inflammatory microenvironment which leads to fibrosis progression.

Brivanib is a selective inhibitor of VEGFR and FGFR and also affects liver fibrosis through multiple signaling pathways. Nakamura et al. demonstrated that brivanib decreased HSCs proliferation induced by PDGF, VEGF and FGF treatment, and also abrogated the phosphorylation of PDGFRβ, which was confirmed *in vitro* and on BDL-, CCl_4- and TAA-induced mice models and supported by histopathological evidences of liver fibrosis alleviation [17] (**Table 1**).

Our team developed the set of multikinase inhibitors, and one of them (1-(4-Cl-benzyl)-3-chloro-4-(CF3-phenylamino)-1H-pyrrole-2,5-dione, called MI1) demonstrated high inhibitory activity against EGFR, VEGFR1,2,3 (the most prominent results), FGF-R1, IGF1-R, spleen associated tyrosine kinase (Syk), 3-phosphoinositide-dependent protein kinase-1 (PDK1), and Src [55]. Besides anticancer and anti-inflammatory activity having been revealed in our previous investigations [56, 57], we showed that MI1 could inhibit liver fibrosis development on rat acute (3 days) and chronic (28 days) cholangitis models, as evidenced by substantially depleted connective tissue deposits in liver and improved liver general state (according to plasma biochemical tests). Moreover, antifibrotic effects of MI1 preserved through at least 28 days since the interventions were terminated (unpublished data, under consideration).

Thus, multikinase inhibitors might be more potent antifibrotic treatments through their impact on several signaling pathways. However, this task should be explored in more detail because of high probability of adverse effects due to multiplicity of these drugs' targets.

5. Small molecule inhibitors of RTK signaling – "noncanonical" approach

Inhibitors of RTK signaling include not only molecules designed to block ATP-binding sites of the kinase, but also small therapeutic molecules with different activities, which, however, could additionally inhibit RTK. For example, natural antioxidant of polyphenol origin resveratrol despite of different therapeutic activities (anti-inflammatory, antitumor, antiaging, protective etc.) demonstrated also strong antifibrotic effect against liver cirrhosis (CCl_4- model) [58]. The mechanisms of its action are different and include predominantly antioxidant capability, but also impact on gene expression and ability to modulate different signaling pathways through interaction with their key molecules. Among others, resveratrol could downregulate EGFR/Akt/ERK1/2 signaling pathway particularly by decrease of EGFR activation [59]. Furthermore, this polyphenol could scavenge VEGF, altering, therefore, its binding with VEGFR and activation of the latter [60]. Of course, this action could not be interpreted as direct impact on VEGFR. However, it deserves to be considered as an approach for modulation of this signaling activity on its initial stages.

Another plant-derived polyphenol curcumin among various types of biological activities (anticancer, antiviral, antioxidant, anti-inflammatory ones) had beneficial effects in animal models of liver injury and cirrhosis [61]. While studying the possible mechanisms of its action, substantial reduce of TGFβRII levels and its downstream molecules Smad2/3 phosphorylation in response to added TGF-β was found [62]. Furthermore, curcumin revealed anti-EGFR activity: firstly, it was able to inhibit directly the enzymatic activity of the EGFR intracellular domain, and, secondly, it could influence the cell membrane environment of the receptor [63, 64].

Ability to affect the membrane environment of the receptor and thus alter its binding with ligand and subsequent activation has been shown for biologically active indolic related compounds including melatonin, 3-indoleacetic acid, 5-hydroxytryptophol, and serotonin. These chemicals are proven to significantly inhibit VEGF-induced VEGFR2 activation in human umbilical vein endothelial cells through interacting with the cell surface components in a way that prevents VEGF from activating the receptor [65]. This property could contribute to the hepatoprotective and antifibrotic efficacy of melatonin realizing by inhibition of inflammation, HSCs proliferation and hepatocyte apoptosis [66]. The similar mechanism of RTK inhibition has been considered for natural cyclopeptide destruxin A5, that effectively downregulate PDGF-B-induced PDGFR-β signaling. Destruxin A5 does not bind to the ATP-binding pocket of PDGFR-β, so the inhibitory mechanism of that is distinct from the mechanism of "canonical" TKIs. It looks like this chemical selectively targets PDGF-β/PDGFR-β interaction interface and blocks this signaling [67].

However, some non-specific small molecules are able to inhibit RTK by "classical" mechanism – through binding to receptor and preventing its activation by ligand. A naturally occurring flavone 4′,5,7-trihydroxy-3′,5′-dimethoxyflavone (tricin) is one of them. Tricin affected HSCs *in vitro* exploring its potential as antifibrotic therapeutic, as evidenced by inhibiting of human HSC line LI90 and culture-activated HSCs proliferation and migration by that. This flavone reduced the phosphorylation of PDGFRβ and downstream signaling molecules ERK1/2 and Akt, which might be due to its TKI properties rather than inhibition of the direct binding between PDGF-B and its receptor [68]. Flavonoid quercetin was reported to exhibit a wide range of pharmacological properties, including its ability to attenuate liver fibrosis by multiple mechanisms involving several signaling pathways [69]. In particular, quercetin was found to suppress the phosphorylation of EGFR by direct binding with its ATP-binding site [70]. A powerful free radical scavenger carbon-based nanoparticle C60 fullerene could be considered as another unusual RTK inhibitor. It explores wide range of biological activities including antifibrotic and anticirrhotic ones [71–75] probably realized by its antioxidant capacity. However, we also demonstrated its ability to bind to ATP-binding pockets of EGFR and FGFR and to avoid interaction of those with ATP [75], which could be an alternative mechanism of this nanoparticle's antifibrotic action.

6. Conclusions

Growth factor receptors, in particular EGFR, VEGFR, PDGFR, FGFR, and TGFβR are proven to be key regulators of various liver cell populations behavior under hepatic injury and reparation, and subsequent fibrosis development if "something has been going wrong". Upregulation of related signaling pathways has been shown in numerous *in vitro* and *in vivo* models, and for patients who experienced liver diseases accompanied by its fibrosis as well. Inhibiting of those by specific and non-specific compounds followed by fibrosis depression. Above mentioned suggests the potency of RTK inhibition as an antifibrotic treatment. However, all the clinical evidences dedicated to that are rather "concomitant" to TKIs anticancer activity because of predominant focus of these studies on the therapy of liver malignancies developed on cirrhotic background. However, we should remember that liver fibrosis and subsequent cirrhosis are severe high-morbidity diseases themselves. And our knowledge about mechanisms of liver fibrosis development and essential RTKs involvement in that, as well as our achievements in the field of liver fibrosis therapy by TKIs should not be neglected.

Conflict of interest

The authors declare that they have no conflict of interest.

Author details

Halyna Kuznietsova* and Olexandr Ogloblya
Taras Shevchenko National University of Kyiv, Kyiv, Ukraine

*Address all correspondence to: biophyz@gmail.com

References

[1] Qiao J. Occurrence, diagnosis and management of hepatic fibrosis and cirrhosis: An updated literature review. Arch Hepat Res.2019;5(1):022-026. DOI: 10.17352/ahr.000023.

[2] Rieder F, Fiocchi C, Rogler G. Mechanisms, Management, and Treatment of Fibrosis in Patients With Inflammatory Bowel Diseases. Gastroenterology. 2017;152(2):340-350. e6. doi:10.1053/j.gastro.2016.09.047

[3] Zhang CY, Yuan WG, He P, Lei JH, Wang CX. Liver fibrosis and hepatic stellate cells: Etiology, pathological hallmarks and therapeutic targets. World J. Gastroenterol. 2016;22:1051210522. doi: 10.3748/wjg. v22.i48.10512

[4] Li J., Zhao YR, Tian Z. Roles of hepatic stellate cells in acute liver failure: From the perspective of inflammation and fibrosis. World J Hepatol. 2019;11(5):412-420. doi: 10.4254/wjh. v11.i5.412

[5] Mattiuzzi C, Lippi G. Current Cancer Epidemiology. J Epidemiol Glob Health. 2019;9(4):217-222. doi: 10.2991/ jegh.k.191008.001

[6] Kostenko S, Dumitriu G, Lægreid KJ, Moens U. Physiological roles of mitogen-activated-proteinkinase-activated p38-regulated/ activated protein kinase. World J Biol Chem. 2011;2(5):73-89. doi: 10.4331/ wjbc. v2.i5.73

[7] Hers I, Vincent EE, Tavaré JM. Akt signalling in health and disease. Cell Signal. 2011;23(10):1515-1527. doi: 10.1016/j.cellsig.2011.05.004.

[8] Neurath MF, Finotto S. IL-6 signaling in autoimmunity, chronic inflammation and inflammation-associated cancer. Cytokine Growth Factor Rev. 2011;22(2):83-89. doi: 10.1016/j. cytogfr.2011.02.003

[9] Hayden MS, Ghosh S. Shared principles in NF-kappaB signaling. Cell. 2008;132(3):344-362. doi: 10.1016/j. cell.2008.01.020

[10] Luedde T, Schwabe RF. NF-κB in the liver--linking injury, fibrosis and hepatocellular carcinoma. Nat Rev Gastroenterol Hepatol. 2011;8(2):10818. doi: 10.1038/nrgastro.2010.213

[11] Kasembeli MM, Bharadwaj U, Robinson P, Tweardy DJ. Contribution of STAT3 to Inflammatory and Fibrotic Diseases and Prospects for its Targeting for Treatment. Int J Mol Sci. 2018;19(8):2299. doi: 10.3390/ ijms19082299

[12] Zhang XL, Xing RG, Chen L, Liu CR, Miao ZG. PI3K/Akt signaling is involved in the pathogenesis of bleomycin-induced pulmonary fibrosis via regulation of epithelialmesenchymal transition. Mol Med Rep. 2016;14(6): 5699-5706. doi: 10.3892/mmr.2016.5960

[13] Le Cras TD, Korfhagen TR, Davidson C, Schmidt S, Fenchel M, Ikegami M, Whitsett JA, Hardie WD. Inhibition of PI3K by PX-866 prevents transforming growth factor-alphainduced pulmonary fibrosis. Am J Pathol. 2010;176(2):679-686. doi: 10.2353/ajpath.2010.090123

[14] Choi ME, Ding Y, Kim SI. TGF-β signaling via TAK1 pathway: role in kidney fibrosis. Semin Nephrol. 2012;32(3):244-252. doi:10.1016/j. semnephrol.2012.04.003

[15] Wynn TA. Cellular and molecular mechanisms of fibrosis. J Pathol. 2008;214(2):199-210. doi:10.1002/ path.2277

[16] Friedman SL. Mechanisms of hepatic fibrogenesis. Gastroenterology. 2008;134(6):1655-1669. doi:10.1053/j. gastro.2008.03.003

[17] Nakamura I, Zakharia K, Banini BA, Mikhail DS, Kim TH, Yang JD, Moser CD, Shaleh HM, Thornburgh SR, Walters I, Roberts LR. Brivanib attenuates hepatic fibrosis in vivo and stellate cell activation in vitro by inhibition of FGF, VEGF and PDGF signaling. PLoS One. 2014;9(4):e92273. doi: 10.1371/journal.pone.0092273

[18] Karlsen TH, Folseraas T, Thorburn D, Vesterhus M. Primary sclerosing cholangitis - a comprehensive review. J Hepatol. 2017;67(6):1298-1323. doi: 10.1016/j.jhep.2017.07.022

[19] Hall C, Sato K, Wu N, Zhou T, Kyritsi K, Meng F, Glaser S, Alpini G. Regulators of Cholangiocyte Proliferation. Gene Expr. 2017;17(2):155-171. doi: 10.3727/105221616X692568

[20] Koyama Y, Xu J, Liu X, Brenner DA. New Developments on the Treatment of Liver Fibrosis. Dig Dis. 2016;34(5):58996. doi: 10.1159/000445269

[21] Qu K, Huang Z, Lin T, Liu S, Chang H, Yan Z, Zhang H, Liu C. New Insight into the Anti-liver Fibrosis Effect of Multitargeted Tyrosine Kinase Inhibitors: From Molecular Target to Clinical Trials. Front Pharmacol. 2016;6:300. doi: 10.3389/ fphar.2015.00300.

[22] Glaser SS, Gaudio E, Miller T, Alvaro D, Alpini G. Cholangiocyte proliferation and liver fibrosis. Expert Rev Mol Med. 2009;11:e7. doi: 10.1017/S1462399409000994

[23] Fabris L, Cadamuro M, Fiorotto R, Roskams T, Spirlì C, Melero S, Sonzogni A, Joplin RE, Okolicsanyi L, Strazzabosco M. Effects of angiogenic factor overexpression by human and rodent cholangiocytes in polycystic liver diseases. Hepatology. 2006 May;43(5):1001-1012. doi: 10.1002/hep.21143

[24] Yoshiji H, Kuriyama S, Yoshii J, Ikenaka Y, Noguchi R, Hicklin DJ, Wu Y, Yanase K, Namisaki T, Yamazaki M, Tsujinoue H, Imazu H, Masaki T, Fukui H. Vascular endothelial growth factor and receptor interaction is a prerequisite for murine hepatic fibrogenesis. Gut. 2003;52(9):1347-1354. doi: 10.1136/gut.52.9.1347

[25] Tugues S, Fernandez-Varo G, Muñoz-Luque J, Ros J, Arroyo V, Rodés J, Friedman SL, Carmeliet P, Jiménez W, Morales-Ruiz M. Antiangiogenic treatment with sunitinib ameliorates inflammatory infiltrate, fibrosis, and portal pressure in cirrhotic rats. Hepatology. 2007;46(6):1919-1926. doi: 10.1002/hep.21921

[26] Kong LJ, Li H, Du YJ, Pei FH, Hu Y, Zhao LL, Chen J. Vatalanib, a tyrosine kinase inhibitor, decreases hepatic fibrosis and sinusoidal capillarization in CCl4-induced fibrotic mice. Mol Med Rep. 2017;15(5):2604-2610. doi: 10.3892/mmr.2017.6325

[27] Ornitz DM, Itoh N. The Fibroblast Growth Factor signaling pathway. Wiley Interdiscip Rev Dev Biol. 2015;4(3):21566. doi: 10.1002/wdev.176.

[28] Schumacher JD, Guo GL. Regulation of Hepatic Stellate Cells and Fibrogenesis by Fibroblast Growth Factors. Biomed Res Int. 2016;2016:8323747. doi: 10.1155/2016/8323747

[29] Liu Y, Lui EL, Friedman SL, Li L, Ye T, Chen Y, Poon RT, Wo J, Kok TW, Fan ST. PTK787/ZK22258 attenuates stellate cell activation and hepatic fibrosis in vivo by inhibiting VEGF signaling. Lab Invest. 2009;89(2):20921. doi: 10.1038/labinvest.2008.127

[30] Yu C, Wang F, Jin C, Huang X, Miller DL, Basilico C, McKeehan WL. Role of fibroblast growth factor type 1 and 2 in carbon tetrachloride-induced hepatic injury and fibrogenesis. Am J Pathol. 2003 Oct;163(4):1653-1662. doi: 10.1016/S0002-9440(10)63522-5

[31] Lin N, Chen S, Pan W, Xu L, Hu K, Xu R. NP603, a novel and potent inhibitor of FGFR1 tyrosine kinase, inhibits hepatic stellate cell proliferation and ameliorates hepatic fibrosis in rats. Am J Physiol Cell Physiol. 2011;301(2):C469-C477. doi: 10.1152/ ajpcell.00452.2010;

[32] Lou D, Han J, Zhou L, Ma H, Xv J, Shou J, Xu Z, Jiang L, Qian Y. Fibroblast growth factor receptor 1 antagonism attenuates lipopolysaccharide-induced activation of hepatic stellate cells via suppressing inflammation. Exp Ther Med. 2018 Oct;16(4):2909-2916. doi: 10.3892/etm.2018.6586

[33] Trussoni CE, Tabibian JH, Splinter PL, O'Hara SP. Lipopolysaccharide (LPS)-induced biliary epithelial cell NRas activation requires epidermal growth factor receptor (EGFR). PLoS One. 2015;10(4):e0125793. doi: 10.1371/ journal.pone.0125793

[34] Breitkopf K, Roeyen Cv, Sawitza I, Wickert L, Floege J, Gressner AM. Expression patterns of PDGF-A, -B, -C and -D and the PDGFreceptors alpha and beta in activated rat hepatic stellate cells (HSC) Cytokine. 2005;31:349-357. doi: 10.1016/j. cyto.2005.06.005

[35] Liu SH, Chen XF, Xie ZB, Zhou J. EGFR monoclonal antibody panitumumab inhibits chronic proliferative cholangitis by downregulating EGFR. Int J Mol Med. 2019;44(1):79-88. Doi: 10.3892/ ijmm.2019.4190

[36] Fuchs BC, Hoshida Y, Fujii T, Wei L, Yamada S, Lauwers GY, McGinn CM, DePeralta DK, Chen X, Kuroda T, Lanuti M, Schmitt AD, Gupta S, Crenshaw A, Onofrio R, Taylor B, Winckler W, Bardeesy N, Caravan P, Golub TR, Tanabe KK. Epidermal growth factor receptor inhibition attenuates liver fibrosis and development of hepatocellular carcinoma. Hepatology. 2014;59(4):1577-1590. doi: 10.1002/ hep.26898.

[37] Kim Y, Fiel MI, Albanis E, Chou HI, Zhang W, Khitrov G, Friedman SL. Anti-fibrotic activity and enhanced interleukin-6 production by hepatic stellate cells in response to imatinib mesylate. Liver Int. 2012;32:1008-1017. doi: 10.1111/j.1478-3231.2012.02806.x

[38] Wang Y, Gao J, Zhang D, Zhang J, Ma J, Jiang H. New insights into the antifibrotic effects of sorafenib on hepatic stellate cells and liver fibrosis. J Hepatol. 2010;53:132-144. doi: 10.1016/j. jhep.2010.02.027

[39] Elshal M, Abu-Elsaad N, El-Karef A, Ibrahim TM. The multi-kinase inhibitor pazopanib targets hepatic stellate cell activation and apoptosis alleviating progression of liver fibrosis. Naunyn Schmiedebergs Arch Pharmacol. 2015;388(12):1293-1304. doi: 10.1007/ s00210-015-1157-7

[40] Liu Y, Wang Z, Kwong SQ, Lui ELH, Friedman SL, Li FR, Lam RWC, Zhang GC, Zhang H, Ye T. Inhibition of PDGF, TGF-β, and Abl signaling and reduction of liver fibrosis by the small molecule Bcr-Abl tyrosine kinase antagonist Nilotinib. J Hepatol. 2011;55(3):612-625. doi: 10.1016/j. jhep.2010.11.035

[41] Akcora BO, Storm G, Prakash J, Bansal R. Tyrosine kinase inhibitor BIBF1120 ameliorates inflammation, angiogenesis and fibrosis in CCl4-induced liver fibrogenesis mouse model. Sci Rep. 2017;7:44545.

[42] Uschner FE, Schueller F, Nikolova I, Klein S, Schierwagen R, Magdaleno F, Gröschl S, Loosen S, Ritz T, Roderburg C, Vucur M, Kristiansen G, Lammers T, Luedde T, Trebicka J. The multikinase inhibitor regorafenib decreases angiogenesis and improves portal hypertension. Oncotarget. 2018;9(90):36220-36237. doi: 10.18632/oncotarget.26333

[43] Wang X, Gao Y, Li Y, Huang Y, Zhu Y, Lv W, Wang R, Gou L, Cheng C, Feng Z, Xie J, Tian J, Yao R. Roseotoxin B alleviates cholestatic liver fibrosis through inhibiting PDGF-B/PDGFR-β pathway in hepatic stellate cells. Cell Death Dis. 2020;11(6):458. doi: 10.1038/s41419-020-2575-0

[44] Ying HZ, Chen Q, Zhang WY, Zhang HH, Ma Y, Zhang SZ, Fang J, Yu CH. PDGF signaling pathway in hepatic fibrosis pathogenesis and therapeutics (Review). Mol Med Rep. 2017;16(6):7879-7889. doi: 10.3892/mmr.2017.7641

[45] Wells RG. Cellular sources of extracellular matrix in hepatic fibrosis. Clin Liver Dis. 2008;12:759-768. Doi: 10.1016/j.cld.2008.07.008

[46] Lazaridis KN, Strazzabosco M, Larusso NF. The cholangiopathies: disorders of biliary epithelia. Gastroenterology. 2004;127:1565-1577. Doi: 10.1053/j.gastro.2004.08.006

[47] Pellat A, Vaquero J, Fouassier L. Role of ErbB/HER family of receptor tyrosine kinases in cholangiocyte biology. Hepatology. 2018;67(2):762773. doi: 10.1002/hep.29350

[48] Fabregat I, Caballero-Díaz D. Transforming Growth Factor-βInduced Cell Plasticity in Liver Fibrosis and Hepatocarcinogenesis. Front Oncol. 2018;8:357. Doi: 10.3389/fonc.2018.00357

[49] Wynn TA, Barron L. Macrophages: master regulators of inflammation and fibrosis. Semin Liver Dis. 2010;30:24557. Doi: 10.1055/s-0030-1255354

[50] Hassan S, Zil-E-Rubab, Shah H, Shawana S. Dysregulated epidermal growth factor and tumor growth factorbeta receptor signaling through GFAPACTA2 protein interaction in liver fibrosis. Pak J Med Sci. 2020;36(4):782787. doi: 10.12669/pjms.36.4.1845

[51] Wilhelm SM, Dumas J, Adnane L, Lynch M, Carter CA, Schütz G, Thierauch KH, Zopf D. Regorafenib (BAY 73-4506): a new oral multikinase inhibitor of angiogenic, stromal and oncogenic receptor tyrosine kinases with potent preclinical antitumor activity. Int J Cancer. 2011;129(1):245-255. doi: 10.1002/ ijc.25864

[52] Xu H, Liu L, Cong M, Liu T, Sun S, Ma H, You H, Jia J, Wang P. EGF neutralization antibodies attenuate liver fibrosis by inhibiting myofibroblast proliferation in bile duct ligation mice. Histochem Cell Biol. 2020;154(1):107116. doi: 10.1007/s00418-020-01867-9.

[53] Arabpour M., Poelstra K., Helfrich W., Bremer E., Haisma H.J. Targeted elimination of activated hepatic stellate cells by an antiepidermal growth factor-receptor single chain fragment variable antibody-tumor necrosis factor-related apoptosisinducing ligand (scFv425-sTRAIL) J Gene Med. 2014;16:281-290. doi: 10.1002/jgm.2776

[54] Liang D, Chen H, Zhao L, Zhang W, Hu J, Liu Z, Zhong P, Wang W, Wang J, Liang G. Inhibition of EGFR attenuates fibrosis and stellate cell activation in diet-induced model of nonalcoholic fatty liver disease. Biochim Biophys Acta Mol Basis Dis. 2018;1864(1):133-142. doi: 10.1016/j.bbadis.2017.10.016

[55] Kuznietsova H, Dziubenko N, Byelinska I, Hurmach V, Bychko A, Lynchak O, Milokhov D, Khilya O, Rybalchenko V. Pyrrole derivatives as potential anti-cancer therapeutics: synthesis, mechanisms of action, safety. J Drug Target. 2020;28(5):547-563. doi: 10.1080/1061186X.2019.1703189

[56] Kuznietsova HM, Yena MS, Kotlyar IP, Ogloblya OV, Rybalchenko VK. Anti-Inflammatory Effects of Protein Kinase Inhibitor Pyrrol Derivate. ScientificWorldJournal.

2016;2016:2145753. doi: 10.1155/2016/2145753

[57] Kuznietsova HM, Lynchak OV, Danylov MO, Kotliar IP, Rybal'chenko VK. [Effect of dihydropyrrol and maleimide derivatives on the state of the liver and colon in normal rats and those with colorectal carcinogenesis induced by dimethylhydrazine]. Ukr Biokhim Zh (1999). 2013;85(3):74-84. Ukrainian. PMID: 23937051.

[58] ChávezE, Reyes-GordilloK, SegoviaJ, Shibayama M, Tsutsumi V, Vergara P, Moreno MG, Muriel P. Resveratrol prevents fibrosis, NF-kappaB activation and TGF-beta increases induced by chronic CCl4 treatment in rats. J Appl Toxicol. 2008;28(1):35-43. doi: 10.1002/jat.1249

[59] Li W, Ma X, Li N, Liu H, Dong Q, Zhang J, Yang C, Liu Y, Liang Q, Zhang S, Xu C, Song W, Tan S, Rong P, Wang W. Resveratrol inhibits Hexokinases II mediated glycolysis in non-small cell lung cancer via targeting Akt signaling pathway. Exp Cell Res. 2016;349(2):320-327. doi: 10.1016/j.yexcr.2016.11.002

[60] Hu WH, Duan R, Xia YT, Xiong QP, Wang HY, Chan GK, Liu SY, Dong TT, Qin QW, Tsim KW. Binding of Resveratrol to Vascular Endothelial Growth Factor Suppresses Angiogenesis by Inhibiting the Receptor Signaling. J Agric Food Chem. 2019;67(4):1127-1137. doi: 10.1021/acs. jafc.8b05977

[61] Vera-Ramirez L, Pérez-Lopez P, Varela-Lopez A, Ramirez-Tortosa M, Battino M, Quiles JL. Curcumin and liver disease. Biofactors. 2013;39(1):88100. doi: 10.1002/biof.1057

[62] Yao QY, Xu BL, Wang JY, Liu HC, Zhang SC, Tu CT. Inhibition by curcumin of multiple sites of the transforming growth factor-beta1 signalling pathway ameliorates the progression of liver fibrosis induced by carbon tetrachloride in rats. BMC Complement Altern Med. 2012;12:156. doi: 10.1186/1472-6882-12-156

[63] Starok M, Preira P, Vayssade M, Haupt K, Salomé L, Rossi C. EGFR Inhibition by Curcumin in Cancer Cells: A Dual Mode of Action. Biomacromolecules. 2015;16(5):163442. doi: 10.1021/acs.biomac.5b00229

[64] Tang Y. Curcumin targets multiple pathways to halt hepatic stellate cell activation: updated mechanisms in vitro and in vivo. Dig Dis Sci. 2015;60(6):1554-1564. doi: 10.1007/s10620-014-3487-6

[65] Cerezo AB, Hornedo-Ortega R, Álvarez-Fernández MA, Troncoso AM, García-Parrilla MC. Inhibition of VEGFInduced VEGFR-2 Activation and HUVEC Migration by Melatonin and Other Bioactive Indolic Compounds. Nutrients. 2017;9(3):249. doi: 10.3390/nu9030249

[66] Hu C, Zhao L, Tao J, Li L. Protective role of melatonin in early-stage and end-stage liver cirrhosis. J Cell Mol Med. 2019;23(11):7151-7162. doi: 10.1111/jcmm.14634

[67] Wang X, Wu X, Zhang A, Wang S, Hu C, Chen W, Shen Y, Tan R, Sun Y, Xu Q. Targeting the PDGF-B/PDGFR-β Interface with Destruxin A5 to Selectively Block PDGF-BB/PDGFR-ββ Signaling and Attenuate Liver Fibrosis. EBioMedicine. 2016;7:146-156. doi: 10.1016/j.ebiom.2016.03.042

[68] Seki N, Toh U, Kawaguchi K, Ninomiya M, Koketsu M, Watanabe K, Aoki M, Fujii T, Nakamura A, Akagi Y, Kusukawa J, Kage M, Shirouzu K, Yamana H. Tricin inhibits proliferation of human hepatic stellate cells in vitro by blocking tyrosine phosphorylation of PDGF receptor and its signaling pathways. J Cell Biochem. 2012;113(7):2346-2355. doi: 10.1002/jcb.24107

[69] Wang R, Zhang H, Wang Y, Song F, Yuan Y. Inhibitory effects of quercetin on the progression of liver fibrosis through the regulation of NF-κB/IκBα, p38 MAPK, and Bcl-2/Bax signaling. Int Immunopharmacol. 2017;47:126-133. doi: 10.1016/j.intimp.2017.03.029

[70] Fridrich D, Teller N, Esselen M, Pahlke G, Marko D. Comparison of delphinidin, quercetin and (−)-epigallocatechin-3-gallate as inhibitors of the EGFR and the ErbB2 receptor phosphorylation. Mol Nutr Food Res. 2008;52(7):815-822. doi: 10.1002/mnfr.200800026

[71] Kuznietsova HM, Lynchak OV, Dziubenko NV, Osetskyi VL, Ogloblya OV, Prylutskyy YuI, Rybalchenko VK, Ritter U, Scharff P. Water-soluble C60 fullerenes reduce manifestations of acute cholangitis in rats. Appl Nanosci. 2019;9:601-608. Doi: 10.1007/s13204-018-0700-5

[72] Kuznietsova H, Lynchak O, Dziubenko N, Herheliuk T, Prylutskyy Y, Rybalchenko V, Ritter U. Water-soluble pristine C60 fullerene attenuates acetaminophen-induced liver injury. Bioimpacts. 2019;9(4):227-237. doi: 10.15171/bi.2019.28

[73] Kuznietsova HM, Dziubenko NV, Lynchak OV, Herheliuk TS, Zavalny DK, Remeniak OV, Prylutskyy YI, Ritter U. Effects of Pristine C60 Fullerenes on Liver and Pancreas in α-Naphthylisothiocyanatelnduced Cholangitis. Dig Dis Sci. 2020;65(1):215-224. doi: 10.1007/ s10620-019-05730-3

[74] Kuznietsova H, Dziubenko N, Herheliuk T, Prylutskyy Y, Tauscher E, Ritter U, Scharff P. WaterSoluble Pristine C60 Fullerene Inhibits Liver Alterations Associated with Hepatocellular Carcinoma in Rat. Pharmaceutics. 2020;12(9):794. doi: 10.3390/pharmaceutics12090794

[75] Kuznietsova H, Dziubenko N, Hurmach V, Chereschuk I, Motuziuk O, Ogloblya O, Prylutskyy Y. Water-Soluble Pristine C60 Fullerenes Inhibit Liver Fibrotic Alteration and Prevent Liver Cirrhosis in Rats. Oxid Med Cell Longev. 2020;2020:8061246. doi: 10.1155/2020/8061246